Insurance Handbook
for the Medical Office

STUDENT WORKBOOK

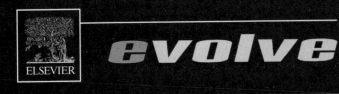

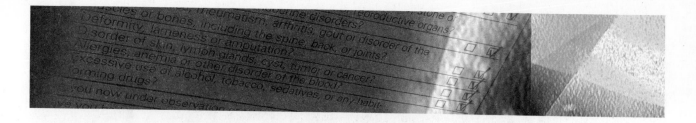

Insurance Handbook for the Medical Office

STUDENT WORKBOOK

TENTH EDITION

Marilyn Takahashi Fordney, CMA-AC

Formerly Instructor of Medical Insurance, Medical Terminology,
Medical Machine Transcription, and Medical Office Procedures
Ventura College
Ventura, California

TECHNICAL COLLABORATOR:

Karen Levein, CPC
Instructor
Monrovia Adult School
Monrovia, California

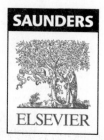

SAUNDERS

ELSEVIER

SAUNDERS
ELSEVIER

11830 Westline Industrial Drive
St. Louis, Missouri 63146

Notice

Neither the Publisher nor the Author assumes any responsibility for any loss or injury and/or damage
to persons or property arising out of or related to any use of the material contained in this book. It is
the responsibility of the treating practitioner, relying on independent expertise and knowledge of the
patient, to determine the best treatment and method of application for the patient.

The Publisher

ISBN 13: 978-1-4160-3663-0

Publishing Director: Andrew Allen
Executive Editor: Susan Cole
Associate Developmental Editor: Jennifer Presley
Publishing Services Manager: Patricia Tannian
Senior Project Manager: Anne Altepeter
Designer: Amy Buxton

Printed in the United States of America

Last digit is the print number: 9 8 7 6 5 4 3 2 1

Working together to grow
libraries in developing countries

www.elsevier.com | www.bookaid.org | www.sabre.org

ELSEVIER   BOOK AID International   Sabre Foundation

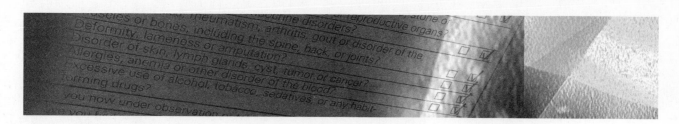

Acknowledgments

This edition of the *Workbook* for *Insurance Handbook for the Medical Office* has had considerable input from many medical professionals. Expert consultation has been necessary because of the complexities of the managed care environment, intricacies of procedural and diagnostic coding, impact of technology on insurance claims processing, and the more sophisticated role the insurance billing specialist has in today's work force.

I owe an immense debt of gratitude to Karen Levein, instructor at Monrovia Adult School, who helped me update the coding data and developed assignments for the practice management software. Also a debt of gratitude is extended to Linda French, CMA-C, NCICS, CPC, and Karen Hawkins, RN, who acted as technical collaborators and helped me update the clinical and coding information of the patient records in the *Workbook* exercises and tests for a previous edition.

Thank you to my assistant, Barbara Evans, who enthusiastically and competently did the typing, filing, mailing, and many other tasks necessary to meet the target dates.

Most important, I express overwhelming gratitude to the professional consultants who provided vital information to make this *Workbook* better than previous editions. They are:

Deborah Emmons, CMA
President
S.T.A.T. Transcription Service
Port Hueneme, California

Sandy Gutt
Instructor
Southern California Regional Occupational Center
Torrance, California

Ronna Jurow, MD
Active Staff and Attending Physician in Obstetrics, Gynecology, and Infertility
Community Memorial Hospital
Ventura, California

Lucille M. Loignon, MD, FACS
Diplomate, American Board of Ophthalmology
Oxnard, California

Maria Reyes
Ventura Anesthesia Medical Group
Ventura, California

Walter A. Shaff
President
CPR
Lake Oswego, Oregon

Lita Starr
Office Manager
Oxnard, California

Paul Wertlake, MD
Medical Director and Chief Pathologist
Unilab Corporation
Tarzana, California

Shirley Wertlake, CLS
Technical Specialist
Clinical Laboratories
University of California—Los Angeles Medical Center
Los Angeles, California

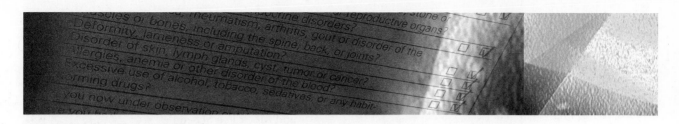

Contents

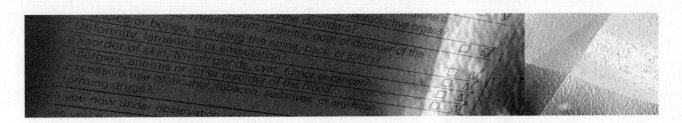

Instruction Guide to the Workbook

LEARNING OBJECTIVES

The student will be able to:

- Define and spell key terms and key abbreviations for each chapter.
- Answer review questions for each chapter of the *Handbook.*
- Complete assignments to enhance and develop better critical thinking skills.
- Define abbreviations as they appear on a patient record.
- Abstract subjective and objective data from patient records.
- Review documentation on patient records.
- Prepare legally correct medicolegal forms and letters.
- Code professional services properly, using the *Current Procedural Terminology* (CPT) Code Book or appendices A and B.
- Select diagnostic code numbers, using the *International Classification of Diseases, Ninth Revision, Clinical Modification* (ICD-9-CM).
- Locate errors on insurance claims before submission to insurance companies.

- Locate errors on returned insurance claims.
- Complete an insurance claim tracer form.
- Carry out collection procedures on delinquent accounts.
- Execute financial management procedures for tracing managed care plans.
- Abstract information necessary to complete insurance claim forms from patient records and billing statement/ledger cards.
- Complete and electronically transmit insurance claim forms commonly used in medical offices.
- Post payments, adjustments, and balances to patients' statement/ledger cards when submitting insurance claims.
- Compute mathematical calculations for Medicare and TRICARE cases.
- Analyze insurance claims in both hospital inpatient and outpatient settings.
- Prepare a cover letter, resume, job application, and follow-up letter when searching for employment.
- Access the Internet and visit websites to research and/or obtain data.

Instructions to the Student

The tenth edition of *Workbook for Insurance Handbook for the Medical Office* has been prepared for those who use the textbook, *Insurance Handbook for the Medical Office* (hereafter referred to as the *Handbook*). It is designed to assist the learner in a practical approach to doing insurance billing and coding. It will also develop a better understanding of the differences among the insurance programs when completing and electronically transmitting the 837 P (Professional) or paper claim the CMS-1500 (08-05).

The key terms and key abbreviations are repeated for quick reference when studying. Each chapter's outline serves as a lecture guide to use for note taking. The review questions in the form of short answer, true/false, multiple choice, and matching are presented to reinforce learning of key concepts for each topic.

Some assignments give students hands-on experience in typing claim forms for optical character recognition (OCR) scanning equipment, which is used in many states for insurance claims processing and payment. Insurance claim forms and other sample documents that are easily removable are included for typing practice.

Current procedural and diagnostic code exercises are used throughout to facilitate and enhance coding skills for submitting a claim or making up an itemized billing statement.

Icons appearing throughout the *Workbook* are used to indicate assignment types. An illustration of each icon, along with its description, is outlined below.

Self-study assignments encompass important points from each chapter and allow you to study at your own pace.

Critical thinking assignments require skills that help prepare you for real-world scenarios encountered in insurance billing.

The **Practice Management and Billing Software CD-ROM** found at the back of the *Workbook* is required for completing selected assignments for many chapters.

Internet assignments point you to the World Wide Web for resources.

Key Terms and Key Abbreviations

Key terms and key abbreviations are presented for each chapter, and definitions may be located in the glossary at the end of the *Handbook*. It is suggested that you make up 3- by 5-inch index cards for each term or abbreviation and write in the definitions as you encounter them while reading each chapter in the *Handbook*. Doing this will reinforce your knowledge and help you learn the words and abbreviations. Your instructor may wish to select certain words to study for "pop" quizzes.

Note Taking

Taking notes is an important key to success in studying and learning. Note taking helps an individual pay attention during class and retain information. Each chapter has a study outline for organizational purposes, and the outline may be used as a guide for writing down key points during lectures or when studying or reviewing from the *Handbook* for tests. Use file cards, notepads, or a notebook for taking notes. Underline or highlight important words or phrases. To improve the usefulness of notes, try the following format:

1. On a notepad sheet or file card, draw a margin 3 inches from the left.
2. Use the left side for topic headings and the right side for notes.
3. Skip a few lines when the topic changes.
4. Write numbers or letters to indicate sub-ideas under a heading.
5. Be brief; do not write down every word except when emphasizing a quotation, rule, or law. Write notes in your own words, since that is what you will understand.
6. Use abbreviations that you know how to translate.
7. Listen carefully to the lecture.
8. After the lecture, reread your notes. Highlight the word(s) on the left side of the page to identify the topic of the notes on the right.
9. For study purposes, cover the right side and see if you can explain to yourself or someone else the topic or word.
10. Remember—learning is by doing, and doing is up to you. So take notes for better understanding.

Review Question Assignments

Review questions have been designed to encompass important points for each chapter to assist you in studying insurance billing and coding theory. Additional quizzes are available at the Evolve website.

Simulation Assignments

Assume that you have been hired as an insurance billing specialist and that you are working in a clinic setting for an incorporated group of medical doctors, other allied health specialists, and a podiatrist. You will be asked to complete various assignments. These doctors will be on the staff of a nearby hospital. Appendix A details this clinic's policies and procedures, which you must read completely before beginning the competency-based assignments. Within each chapter, the simulation assignments progress from easy to more complex. Some assignments are given with critical thinking problems, which the instructor may use for class discussion.

Always read the assignment entirely before beginning it. There are *Workbook* assignments. Table I.1 is a reference guide that lists chapter numbers and titles, along with the corresponding assignment numbers.

Medical Terminology and Abbreviations

A list of abbreviations is provided in Appendix A to help you learn how to abstract and read physicians' notes. Decode any abbreviations that you do not understand or that are unfamiliar to you. To reinforce learning these abbreviations, write their meanings on the assignment pages. If you do not have a background in medical terminology, it may be wise to use a good medical dictionary as a reference or, better yet, enroll in a terminology course to master that skill.

Patient Records

Patient records, financial accounting records (ledgers), and encounter forms are presented as they might appear in a physician's office, so the learner may have the tools needed to extract information to complete claim forms. Patient records have been abbreviated because of space and page constraints. The records contain pertinent data for each type of case, but it was necessary to omit a lengthy physical examination. Because detailed documentation is encouraged in medical practices, the records all appear typewritten rather than in handwritten notes. The physician's signature appears after each dated entry on the record.

All the materials included in the assignments have been altered to prevent identification of the cases or parties involved. The names and addresses are fictitious, and no reference to any person living or dead is intended. No evaluation of medical practice or medical advice is to be inferred from the patient records, nor is any recommendation made toward alternative treatment methods or prescribed medications.

Financial Records

Financial accounting record (ledger) assignments provide you with experience in posting, totaling the fees, and properly recording appropriate information on the ledger when the insurance claim is submitted. Financial accounting record statement/ledger cards are

TABLE I-1

Workbook Assignments

Handbook Chapter	Corresponding Workbook Chapter	Assignments
1	Role of an Insurance Billing Specialist	1–1 through 1–3
2	HIPAA Compliance and Privacy in Insurance Billing	2–1 through 2–5
3	Basics of Health Insurance	3–1 through 3–9
4	Medical Documentation	4–1 through 4–8
5	Diagnostic Coding	5–1 through 5–13
6	Procedural Coding	6–1 through 6–11
7	The Health Insurance Claim Form	7–1 through 7–9
8	Electronic Data Interchange (EDI)	8–1 through 8–13
9	Receiving Payments and Insurance Problem Solving	9–1 through 9–11
10	Office and Insurance Collection Strategies	10–1 through 10–9
11	The Blue Plans, Private Insurance, and Managed Care Plans	11–1 through 11–7
12	Medicare	12–1 through 12–14
13	Medicaid and Other State Programs	13–1 through 13–5
14	TRICARE and CHAMPVA	14–1 through 14–6
15	Workers' Compensation	15–1 through 15–6
16	Disability Income Insurance and Disability Benefit Program	16–1 through 16–6
17	Hospital Billing	17–1 through 17–9
18	Seeking a Job and Attaining Professional Advancement	18–1 through 18–8

also included for typing practice. Refer to Appendix A to obtain information about the Mock Fee Schedule and the physicians' fees for posting to the statements.

CMS-1500 (08-05) Claim Form

If you have access to a computer, use the practice management software that accompanies the *Workbook* to complete each assignment and print it out for evaluation. To complete the CMS-1500 (08-05) claim form properly for each type of program, refer to the section in Chapter 7 of the *Handbook* that describes in detail the correct information to be put in each block. Also view the templates found at the end of Chapter 7 for each insurance type.

Complete all insurance forms in OCR style, since this is the format in which insurance carriers process claims most expediently. Chapter 7 gives instructions on OCR do's and don'ts. If you do not have access to a computer, type or neatly write in the information on the insurance form as you abstract it from the patient record.

Performance Evaluation Checklist

The tenth edition features a competency-based format for each assignment indicating performance objectives to let you know what is to be accomplished. The task (job assignment), conditions (elements needed to perform and complete the task), and standards (time management), as well as directions for the specific task, are included. Use of a checklist with points projected and points earned is available at the Evolve website; the checklist assists in scoring the assignments and helps you develop the skill of speed in completing tasks.

A two-part performance evaluation checklist used when completing a CMS-1500 (08-05) claim form is depicted in Figures I-1 and I-2. Reproduce these sheets only for the assignments that involve completing the CMS-1500 (08-05) claim form. Your instructor will give you the number of points to be assigned for each step.

Appendices

Refer to Table I.2, which shows what is included in each of the appendices.

Student Reference Notebook

A student reference notebook is recommended so that you can access information quickly to help you complete the *Workbook* assignments. Before beginning the assignments, tear out Appendix A and place it in a three-ring binder with chapter indexes. Appendix A includes the clinic policies and guidelines, data about the clinic staff, medical and laboratory abbreviations, and mock fee schedule used while working as an insurance billing specialist for the College Clinic.

Besides these suggestions, you may wish either to tear out or make photocopies of other sections of the *Handbook* for your personal use. In addition, your instructor may give you handouts from time to time, pertaining to regional insurance program policies and procedures, to place in your notebook.

Content Suggestions from Workbook

✓ Appendix A: College Clinic policies, data about staff physicians, medical and laboratory abbreviations, and mock fee schedule
✓ Appendix B: HCPCS codes
✓ CMS-1500 (08-05) claim form (photocopy if extra copies are needed for making rough drafts or retyping an assignment)

TABLE I-2	
Appendix	**Contents**
A	College Clinic Staff (Provider) Information
	College Clinic Information
	Medical Abbreviations and Symbols
	Laboratory Abbreviations
	College Clinic Mock Fee Schedule
B	Medicare Level II Healthcare Common Procedure Code System (HCPCS) Codes
C	Instructions and Guide to Using AltaPoint Practice Management Software

PERFORMANCE EVALUATION CHECKLIST

Assignment No. _____

Name: _____ Date: _____

Performance Objective

Task: Given access to all necessary equipment and information, the student will complete a CMS-1500 health insurance claim form.

Standards: Claim Productivity Management
Time _____ minutes
Note: Time element may be given by instructor.

Directions: See assignment.

NOTE TIME BEGAN_____ **NOTE TIME COMPLETED**_____

PROCEDURE STEPS	ASSIGNED POINTS	STEP PERFORMED SATISFACTORY	COMMENTS
1. Assembled CMS-1500 claim form, patient record, E/M code slip, ledger card, typewriter or computer, pen or pencil, and code books.	_____	_____	_____
2. Posed ledger card correctly.	_____	_____	_____
3. Proofread form for spelling and typographical errors while form remained in typewriter or on computer screen.	_____	_____	_____
4. Points earned for correct completion of CMS-1500 block-by-block data.	_____	_____	_____

Figure I–1

Content Suggestions from Handbook

✓ Evaluation and Management CPT codes: Tables 6–3 and 6–4
✓ Insurance form templates from Chapter 7: Figures 7–5 through 7–14
✓ Medical terminology (lay and medical terms): Table 4–1
✓ Terminology used in coding procedures: CMS-1500 (08-05) block-by-block claim form instructions from Chapter 7
✓ Glossary (key terms and key abbreviations)

PERFORMANCE EVALUATION CHECKLIST

BLOCK	INCORRECT	MISSING	NOT NEEDED	REMARKS	BLOCK	INCORRECT	MISSING	NOT NEEDED	REMARKS
					18				
1A					19				
2					20				
3					21				
4									
5					22				
6					23				
7					24A				
8					24B				
					24C				
9					24D				
9A									
9B									
9C					24E				
9D									
					24F				
10A					24G				
10B					24H, 24I				
10C					24J				
10D					24K				
11					25, 26				
11A					27				
11B					28				
11C					29				
11D									
12					30				
13									
14					31				
15									
16					32				
17									
17A					33				
					Reference Initials				

TOTAL POINTS EARNED: _____   TOTAL POINTS POSSIBLE: _____

Evaluator's signature _____   NEED TO REPEAT: _____

Figure I–2

Tests

Tests are provided at the end of the *Workbook* to provide a complete, competency-based educational program.

Reference Material

To do the assignments in this *Workbook* and gain expertise in coding and insurance claims completion, an individual must have access to the books listed here. Addresses for obtaining these materials are given in parentheses. Additional books and booklets on these topics, as well as Medicaid, Medicare, TRICARE, and more, are listed in the appendix in the *Handbook*.

Dictionary

Dorland's Illustrated Medical Dictionary, 31st edition, Elsevier, 2007 (6277 Sea Harbor Drive, Orlando, FL 32821-9989; 1-800-545-2522).

Code Books

Current Procedural Terminology, American Medical Association, published annually (515 North State Street, Chicago, IL 60610; 1-800-621-8335).

International Classification of Diseases, Ninth Revision, Clinical Modification (An inexpensive soft-cover generic physician version of volumes 1 through 3 is available from Channel Publishing Limited, 4750 Longley Lane, Suite 100, Reno, NV 89502; 1-800-248-2882.)

Word Book

Medical Abbreviations and Eponyms by Sheila Sloane, Elsevier, 1997 (6277 Sea Harbor Drive, Orlando, FL 32821-9989; 1-800-545-2522).

Pharmaceutical Book

Optional publications for drug names and descriptions might be either drug books used by nurses (e.g., *Mosby's Gen RX*, Elsevier, published annually [11830 Westline Industrial Drive, St. Louis, MO 63146; 1-800-325-4177; www.elsevier.com]) or ones used by physicians (e.g., *Physician's Desk Reference* [PDR], Medical Economics Company, published annually [5 Paragon Drive, Montvale, NJ, 07645; 1-800-432-4570]).

Employee Insurance Procedural Manual

If you currently work in a medical office, you may custom design an insurance manual for your physician's practice as you complete insurance claims in this *Workbook*. Obtain a three-ring binder with indexes and label them "Group Plans," "Private Plans," "Medicaid," "Medicare," "Managed Care Plans," "State Disability," "TRICARE," and "Workers' Compensation." If many of your patients have group plans, complete an insurance data or fact sheet for each plan and organize them alphabetically by group plan. For managed care plans, type a form as shown in Figure 11-5 of the *Handbook*.

An insurance manual with fact sheets listing benefits can keep you up to date on policy changes and ensure maximum reimbursement. Fact sheets can be prepared from information obtained when patients bring in their benefit booklets. Obtain and insert a list of the procedures that must be performed as an outpatient and those that must have second opinions for each of the insurance plans.

As you complete the assignments in this *Workbook*, place them in the insurance manual as examples of completed claims for each particular program.

PRACTICE MANAGEMENT AND BILLING SOFTWARE

Because more and more medical practices use computer technology to perform financial operations, Elsevier has teamed up with the software company AltaPoint to provide students with a real-life practice management and billing software experience. The software program is located on the CD-ROM that accompanies the *Workbook*, and corresponds with special exercises located in Chapters 3 through 12. By following the instructions located in Appendix C of the *Workbook*, you can install the practice management software on your computer to complete the corresponding exercises.

INSURANCE DATA

1. Employer's name _____

2. Address _____ Telephone Number _____

3. Insurance Company Contact Person _____

4. Insurance Carrier _____

5. Address _____ Telephone Number to Call for Benefits _____

6. Group Policy Number_____

7. Group Account Manager_____ Telephone Number _____

8. **Insurance Coverage:**

   Annual Deductible_____ Patient Copayment Percentage _____

   Noncovered Procedures _____

   Maximum Benefits _____

9. **Diagnostic Coverage:**

   Limited Benefits _____

   Maximum Benefits _____

   Noncovered Procedures _____

10. **Major Medical:**

    Annual Deductible_____ Patient Copayment Percentage _____

    Limited Benefits _____

    Maximum Benefits _____

    Noncovered Procedures _____

Mandatory Outpatient Surgeries _____

Second Surgical Opinions _____

Preadmission Certification   Yes _____ No _____   Authorized Labs_____

Payment Plan:

UCR _____ Schedule of Benefits _____ CPT _____RVS _____

Send claims to: _____

_____

Date Entered _____ Date Updated _____

Figure I–3

SPECIAL FEATURES

AltaPoint Practice Management Software

AltaPoint Data Systems, LLC, is a private software company that has developed practice management systems for professionals in fields such as medical, dental, legal, optometric/ophthalmologic, chiropractic, and veterinary. Through a special partnership, Elsevier has customized AltaPoint's innovative practice management system into the CD-ROM that accompanies the *Workbook*. More information regarding AltaPoint can be found at www.altapoint.com.

Source Documents

Authentic source documents such as encounter forms (p. 268), medical records with progress notes, and more are provided to give students the opportunity to enter pertinent information into the software as they would in an actual practice environment.

Fee Schedule/Billing Codes

Based on the College Clinic fee schedule printed in the back of this and past *Workbooks*, fees automatically appear when the CPT and diagnostic codes are entered.

Claims Transmission

Using the software and specialized assignments in the *Workbook*, students can transmit an insurance claim electronically or on hard copy to individual insurance companies.

Patient Database

To provide an authentic practice management setting, Elsevier has customized the practice management software program to include a database of patients, including names, telephone numbers, birthdates, addresses, photographs, and outstanding balances.

Detailed Instructions

Detailed instructions are provided in Appendix C to explain simple procedures or more complex functions of the software. For each set of instructions, screen shots are provided. Examples of the screen shots are depicted here.

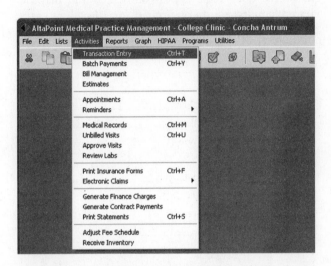

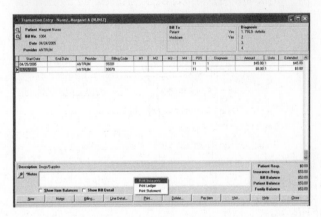

Software installation instructions begin on p. 587 in Appendix C of the *Workbook*.

STUDENT SOFTWARE CHALLENGE

The Student Software Challenge is another user-friendly software program located on the CD-ROM that accompanies the *Workbook*. The software simulates a realistic experience by having students gather necessary documents and extract specific information to complete the CMS-1500 (08-05) insurance claim form. All source documents appear on screen and may be viewed simultaneously or printed for 10 patient cases that escalate in difficulty.

Student Software Challenge exercises are located in Chapters 7, 12, and 14.

An added feature on the CD are blank forms that students can print for additional practice or for use in the classroom. Documents avaible for printing include letterheads, authorization request forms, financial acounting statements (ledgers), and the CMS-1500 (08-05) form.

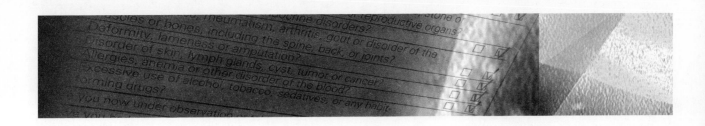

Insurance Handbook
for the Medical Office

STUDENT WORKBOOK

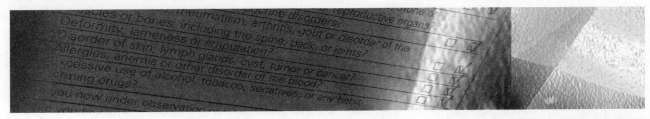

Role of an Insurance Billing Specialist

KEY TERMS

Your instructor may wish to select some specific words pertinent to this chapter for a test. For definitions of the terms, further study, and/or reference, the words, phrases, and abbreviations may be found in the glossary at the end of the Handbook. *Key terms for this chapter follow.*

American Health Information Management
  Association (AHIMA)

American Medical Association (AMA)

cash flow

claims assistance professional (CAP)

ethics

etiquette

insurance billing specialist

list service (listserv)

medical billing representative

multiskilled health practitioner (MSHP)

reimbursement specialist

respondeat superior

senior billing representative

KEY ABBREVIATIONS

See how many abbreviations and acronyms you can translate and then use this as a handy reference list. Definitions for the key abbreviations are located near the back of the Handbook *in the glossary.*

AAMA _____

ACA _____

AHIMA _____

AMA _____

ASHD _____

CAP _____

CCS _____

CPC _____

e-mail _____

GED _____

HIPAA _____

listserv _____

MSHP _____

MSO _____

NPP _____

PERFORMANCE OBJECTIVES

The student will be able to:

■ Define and spell the key terms and key abbreviations for this chapter, given the information from the *Handbook* glossary, within a reasonable time period and with enough accuracy to obtain a satisfactory evaluation.

■ Answer the fill-in-the-blank, multiple choice, and true/false review questions after reading the chapter, with enough accuracy to obtain a satisfactory evaluation.

■ Use critical thinking to write one or two grammatically correct paragraphs with sufficient information to obtain a satisfactory evaluation.

■ Visit websites and site-search information via the Evolve website, with sufficient information to obtain a satisfactory evaluation.

STUDY OUTLINE

Background of Insurance Claims, Coding, and Billing

Role of the Insurance Billing Specialist
    Job Responsibilities
    Educational and Training Requirements
    Career Advantages
    Qualifications

Medical Etiquette
Medical Ethics
Employer Liability
Employee Liability
Scope of Practice
Future Challenges

 ASSIGNMENT 1–1 ▸ REVIEW QUESTIONS

Part I Fill in the Blank

    Review the objectives, key terms, and chapter information before completing the following review questions.

1. Read the job descriptions in Chapter 1 in the *Handbook*. Ability to input data and transmit insurance claims accurately, either directly or through a clearinghouse as well as update and maintain software applications to requirements of third-party payers are technical skills required in the job of a/an _____.

2. Name some of the facilities where facility billing is used.

    a. _____

    b. _____

    c. _____

    d. _____

    e. _____

3. Name examples of nonphysician practitioners (NPPs).

a. _____

b. _____

c. _____

d. _____

e. _____

f. _____

g. _____

h. _____

4. Identify three career opportunities (job titles) available after training in diagnostic and procedural coding and insurance claims completion.

a. _____

b. _____

c. _____

5. List some of the responsibilities and duties an insurance billing specialist might perform generally as well as when acting as a collection manager.

a. _____

b. _____

c. _____

d. _____

e. _____

f. _____

g. _____

6. List the duties of a claims assistance professional.

a. _____

b. _____

c. _____

7. Insurance claims must be promptly submitted within _____ business days to ensure continuous cash flow.

8. Define cash flow.

   _____

9. Reasons for a medical practice's large accounts receivable are

   a. _____

   b. _____

   c. _____

   d. _____

10. Skills required for an insurance billing specialist are

   a. _____

   b. _____

   c. _____

   d. _____

   e. _____

   f. _____

   g. _____

   h. _____

   i. _____

   j. _____

11. Standards of conduct by which an insurance billing specialist determines the propriety

    of his or her behavior in a relationship are known as _____.

12. Complete these statements with either the word *illegal* or *unethical*.

    a. To report incorrect information to the Aetna Casualty Company is _____.

    b. To report incorrect information to a Medicare fiscal intermediary is _____.

    c. In certain circumstances, it may be _____ for two physicians to treat the same patient for the same condition.

13. When a physician is legally responsible for an employee's conduct performed during

    employment, this is known as _____.

14. A claims assistance professional neglects to submit an insurance claim to a Medicare supplemental insurance carrier within the proper time limit. What type of insurance is needed for protection against this loss for the client?

    _____

Part II Multiple Choice

Choose the best answer.

15. Two billing components are facility billing and professional billing. Professional billing is done for

    a. hospitals

    b. skilled nursing facilities

    c. ambulatory surgical centers

    d. physicians

16. *Physician extenders* are health care personnel trained to provide medical care under the direct or indirect supervision of a physician, such as

    a. multiskilled health practitioners (MSHPs)

    b. claims assistance professionals (CAPs)

    c. nonphysician practitioners (NPPs)

    d. insurance billing specialists

17. The individual responsible for documenting the patient's clinical notes and assigning a diagnosis code and a procedure code for medical services rendered is a/an

    a. physician

    b. insurance biller

    c. office manager

    d. financial accounting clerk

18. An individual cross-trained to function in more than one job is known as a/an

    a. administrative medical assistant

    b. receptionist

    c. claims assistance professional

    d. multiskilled health practitioner

19. Third-party payers that require the provider to submit insurance claims for the patient are

    a. federal and state programs

    b. private insurance plans

    c. managed care programs

    d. healthcare insurance plans

Part III True/False

Write "T" or "F" in the blank to indicate whether you think the statement is true or false.

_____ 20. Physicians are paid according to relative value units that are based on cost of delivering care, malpractice insurance, and the physician's work.

_____ 21. It is not necessary to use coding books to refer to because medical practices use a fee schedule.

_____ 22. It is the coder's responsibility to inform administration or his or her immediate supervisor if unethical or illegal coding practices are occurring.

_____ 23. When one code is available that includes all of the services, it is permissible to bill using separate codes for the services.

_____ 24. Depending on the circumstances of the case, an insurance billing specialist can be held personally responsible under the law for billing errors.

CRITICAL THINKING

To enhance your critical thinking skills, problems will be interspersed throughout the *Workbook*. Thinking is the goal of instruction and a student's responsibility. When trying to solve a problem by critical thinking, it is desirable to have more than one solution and to take time to think out answers. Remember that an answer may be changed when additional information is provided in a classroom setting.

ASSIGNMENT **1–2** ▸ **CRITICAL THINKING**

Performance Objective

Task: Describe why you are training to become an insurance billing specialist.

Conditions: Use one or two sheets of white typing paper and pen or pencil.

Standards: Time:_____ minutes

              Accuracy: _____

              (Note: The time element and accuracy criteria may be given by your
              instructor.)

Directions. Write one or two paragraphs describing why you are training to become an
insurance billing specialist. Or, if enrolled in a class that is part of a medical assisting
course, explain why you are motivated to seek a career as a medical assistant. Make sure
grammar, punctuation, and spelling are correct.

A S S I G N M E N T **1 – 3** ▸ **V I S I T W E B S I T E S**

Performance Objective

Task: Access the Internet and visit several websites of the World Wide Web.

Conditions: Use a computer with printer and/or pen or pencil to make notes.

Standards: Time: _____ minutes

                    Accuracy: _____

                    (Note: The time element and accuracy criteria may be given by your
                    instructor.)

Directions. For active web links to the following resources, visit the Evolve website online
at http://evolve.elsevier.com/Fordney/handbook and do the following three site searches:

1. Access an Internet server and find one of the web search engines (Yahoo, Excite, Google,
   Alta Vista). Begin a web search (e.g., key in "insurance billers") to search for information
   about insurance billers, or go to the career path website listed on Evolve. List three to
   five websites found. Go to one or more of those resources and list the benefits that those
   sites might have for a student in locating job opportunities or networking with others for
   professional growth and knowledge. Bring the website addresses to share with the class.

2. Site-search information on standards of ethical coding by visiting the website of the
   American Health Information Management Association. Download and print a hard
   copy of this code of ethics developed by AHIMA. Next, obtain information on eHealth
   code of ethics by visiting the website of the Internet Healthcare Coalition organization.
   Click on "eHealth Code of Ethics," download the file, print a hard copy, read the
   document, and respond to the following:

   A. Write a brief definition for each of the following terms: health information, health
      products, and health services.
   B. State the eight guiding principles of organizations and individuals who provide
      health information over the Internet.

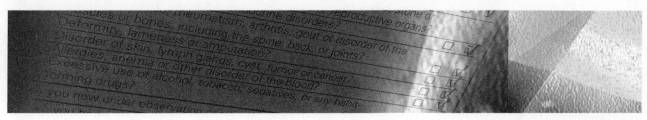

HIPAA Compliance and Privacy in Insurance Billing

KEY TERMS

Your instructor may wish to select some specific words pertinent to this chapter for a test. For definitions of the terms, further study, and/or reference, the words, phrases, and abbreviations may be found in the glossary at the end of the Handbook. *Key terms for this chapter follow.*

abuse

authorization

authorization form

breach of confidential communication

business associate

clearinghouse

code set

compliance

compliance plan

confidential communication

confidentiality

consent

consent form

covered entity

disclosure

e-health information management (eHIM)

electronic media

embezzlement

fraud

health care provider

individually identifiable health information (IIHI)

nonprivileged information

Notice of Privacy Practices (NPP)

phantom billing

privacy

privacy officer, privacy official (PO)

privileged information

protected health information (PHI)

security officer

Security Rule

standard

state preemption

transaction

use

KEY ABBREVIATIONS

See how many abbreviations and acronyms you can translate and then use this as a handy reference list. Definitions for the key abbreviations are located near the back of the Handbook *in the glossary.*

CCI _____

CD _____

CDT _____

CLIA _____

CMP _____

CMS _____

CPT _____

DHHS _____

DOJ _____

EDI _____

eHIM _____

EIN _____

ePHI _____

FBI _____

FCA _____

FDIC _____

FTP _____

HCFAP _____

HCPCS _____

HIPAA _____

HIV _____

HL7 _____

ICD-9-CM _____

IIHI _____

MCO _____

MIP _____

NCVHS _____

NDC _____

NHII _____

NPI _____

NPP _____

NSF _____

OCR _____

OIG _____

ORT _____

OSHA _____

P&P _____

PHI _____

PO _____

SNOMED _____

TCS _____

TPA _____

TPO _____

PERFORMANCE OBJECTIVES

The student will be able to:

- Define and spell the key terms and key abbreviations for this chapter, given the information from the *Handbook* glossary, within a reasonable time period and with enough accuracy to obtain a satisfactory evaluation.
- Answer the fill-in-the-blank, multiple choice, and true/false review questions after reading the chapter, with enough accuracy to obtain a satisfactory evaluation.
- Make decisions after reading scenarios whether the situations are considered fraud, abuse, or neither,

with sufficient information to obtain a satisfactory evaluation.
- Decide when a situation is an incidental disclosure, HIPAA violation, or neither, with sufficient information to obtain a satisfactory evaluation.
- Make a choice after reading scenarios whether to ask for consent or authorization, or perform other office procedures, with sufficient information to obtain a satisfactory evaluation.
- Visit websites and site-search information via the Evolve website, with sufficient information to obtain a satisfactory evaluation.

STUDY OUTLINE

Compliance Defined

Health Information Using Electronic Technologies
E-Health Information Management
National Health Information Infrastructure
Health Level Seven

Systemized Nomenclature of Human and Veterinary Medicine (SNOMED) International

Health Insurance Portability and Accountability Act (HIPAA)
Title I: Health Insurance Reform
Title II: Administrative Simplification
Defining Roles and Relationships: Key Terms
HIPAA in the Practice Setting

The Privacy Rule: Confidentiality and Protected Health Information
Confidential Information
Patients' Rights
Privacy Rules: Patient Rights Under HIPAA
Right to Notice of Privacy Practices
Right to Request Restrictions on Certain Uses and Disclosures of PHI
Right to Request Confidential Communications
Right to Access, Inspect, and Obtain PHI
Right to Request Amendment of PHI
Right to Receive an Accounting of Disclosures of PHI
Verification of Identity and Authority
Validating Patient Permission
Training
Safeguards: Ensuring that Confidential Information is Secure
Complaints to Health Care Practice and Workforce Sanctions
Mitigation
Refraining from Intimidating or Retaliatory Acts

Transaction and Code Set Regulations: Streamlining Electronic Data Interchange
Standard Unique Identifiers

The Security Rule: Administrative, Physical, and Technical Safeguards
Guidelines for HIPAA Privacy Compliance

Consequences of Noncompliance with HIPAA

Office of the Inspector General
Fraud and Abuse Laws
Federal False Claims Act
Qui Tam "Whistleblower"
Civil Monetary Penalties Law
Criminal False Claims Act
Stark I and II Laws
Anti-Kickback Statute
Safe Harbors
Additional Laws and Compliance
Operation Restore Trust
Medicare Integrity Program
Correct Coding Initiative
Increased Staffing and Expanded Penalties for Violations
Special Alerts, Bulletins, and Guidance Documents
Exclusion Program

Application to Practice Setting

Organization and Staff Responsibilities in Protecting Patient Rights

Compliance Program Guidance for Individual and Small Group Physician Practices
Increased Productivity and Decreased Penalties with Plan

Seven Basic Components of a Compliance Plan
Conducting Internal Monitoring and Auditing
Implementing Compliance and Practice Standards
Designating a Compliance Officer or Contact
Conducting Appropriate Training and Education
Responding Appropriately to Detected Offenses and Developing Corrective Action
Developing Open Lines of Communication
Enforcing Disciplinary Standards through Well-Publicized Guidelines

What to Expect from Your Health Care Practice

Compliance Lessons Learned

A S S I G N M E N T   **2 – 1** ▸ **R E V I E W   Q U E S T I O N S**

Part I Fill in the Blank

Review the objectives, key terms, and chapter information before completing the following review questions.

1. Compliance is the process of

_____

_____

2. Transactions in which health care information is accessed, processed, stored, and

    transferred using electronic technologies is known as _____ and

    its acronym is _____.

3. Baby Nelson was born on January 20, 2005, at 7:15 AM. When using the required
   Health Level 7 (HL7) format for transmission, how would this appear?

    _____

4. A code system used for managing patient electronic health records, informatics, indexing,

    and billing laboratory procedures is called _____

    and its acronym is _____.

5. What is the primary purpose of HIPAA Title I: Insurance Reform?

    _____

    _____

6. The focus on the health care practice setting and reduction of administrative costs and
   burdens are the goals of which part of HIPAA?

    _____

7. An independent organization that receives insurance claims from the physician's office,
   performs edits, and transmits claims to insurance carriers is known as a/an

    _____.

8. Under HIPAA guidelines, a health care coverage carrier, such as Blue Cross/Blue Shield
   that transmits health information in electronic form in connection with a transaction,

    is called a/an _____.

9. Dr. John Doe contracts with an outside billing company to manage claims and accounts receivable. Under HIPAA guidelines, the billing company is considered a/an

   _____ of the provider.

10. An individual designated to assist the provider by putting compliance policies and

    procedures in place and training office staff is known as a/an _____

    _____ under HIPAA guidelines.

11. If you give, release, or transfer information to another entity, this is known as

    _____.

12. Define protected health information (PHI).

    _____

    _____

    _____

    _____

13. Unauthorized release of a patient's health information is called

    _____.

14. A confidential communication related to the patient's treatment and progress that may be disclosed only with the patient's permission is known as

    _____.

15. Under HIPAA, exceptions to the right of privacy are those records involving

    a. _____

    b. _____

    c. _____

    d. _____

    e. _____

    f. _____

    g. _____

    h. _____

    i. _____

16. At a patient's first visit under HIPAA guidelines, the document that must be given so the patient acknowledges the provider's confidentiality of their protected health

    information is the _____.

17. Under HIPAA Privacy Regulation, state the types of information that patients do not have the right to access.

    a. _____

    b. _____

    c. _____

18. Name the three main sections of the HIPAA Security Rule for protecting electronic health information.

    a. _____

    b. _____

    c. _____

19. Indicate whether the situation is one of fraud or abuse in the following situations.

    a. Under the False Claims Act, billing a claim for services not medically necessary _____

    b. Changing a figure on an insurance claim form to get increased payment_____

    c. Dismissing the copayment owed by a Medicare patient _____

    d. Neglecting to refund an overpayment to the patient_____

    e. Billing for a complex fracture when the patient suffered a simple break_____

Part II Multiple Choice

Choose the best answer.

20. A standards developing organization whose mission is to provide standards for the exchange, management and integration of data that support clinical patient care and the management, delivery, and evaluation of health care services is called

    a. American Medical Association

    b. American Hospital Association

    c. Medicare Integrity Program

    d. Health Level Seven (HL7)

21. HIPAA transaction standards apply to the following, which are called covered entities. They are

    a. health care third-party payers

    b. health care providers

    c. health care clearinghouses

    d. all of the above

22. Enforcement of the privacy standards of HIPAA is the responsibility of

    a. Health Care Fraud and Abuse Control Program (HCFAP)

    b. National Committee on Vital and Health Statistics (NCVHS)

    c. Office for Civil Rights (OCR)

    d. Federal Bureau of Investigation (FBI)

23. Verbal or written agreement that gives approval to some action, situation, or statement is called

    a. authorization

    b. consent

    c. disclosure

    d. release

24. An individual's formal written permission to use or disclose his or her personally identifiable health information for purposes other than treatment, payment, or health care operations is called

    a. authorization

    b. disclosure

    c. release

    d. consent

Part III True/False

Write "T" or "F" in the blank to indicate whether you think the statement is true or false.

_____ 25. Individually identifiable health information (IIHI) is any part of a person's health data (e.g., demographic information, address, date of birth) obtained from the patient that is created or received by a covered entity.

_____ 26. HIPAA requirements protect disclosure of protected health information outside of the organization but not for internal use of health information.

_____ 27. Under HIPAA, patients may request confidential communications and may restrict certain disclosures of protected health information.

_____ 28. A national provider identifier (NPI) number is issued for 5 years and must be renewed.

_____ 29. To submit an insurance claim for medical services that were not medically necessary is a violation of the False Claims Act (FCA).

ASSIGNMENT **2–2** ▸ **CRITICAL THINKING: INCIDENTAL DISCLOSURE VERSUS HIPAA VIOLATION**

Performance Objective

Task: Make a decision using your best judgment after reading each case study, whether it should be considered an incidental disclosure, an HIPAA violation, or neither.

Conditions: Use pen or pencil.

Standards: Time: _____ minutes

Accuracy: _____

(Note: The time element and accuracy criteria may be given by your instructor.)

Directions. Read through each case study. Use your best judgment and circle whether you think it is an incidental disclosure issue (ID), an HIPAA violation (V), or neither (N).

Scenarios

1. Dr. Practon's office sign-in sheets ask patients to fill in their names, appointment times, and physicians' names.

   ID   V   N

2. It is Monday morning and you are inundated with work that needs to be done. You receive a telephone call and give patient information without confirming who is on the line.

   ID   V   N

3. You send a fax but accidentally you switch the last two digits of the fax number and the patient's billing information is received in the wrong location.

   ID   V   N

4. You are in a high-traffic area where patients might overhear protected health information and you are careful to keep your voice down.

   ID   V   N

5. It is 10:30 AM and you go on a coffee break leaving two patients' charts on the checkout counter.

   ID   V   N

6. In the reception room, a patient, Martha Havasi, overhears your telephone conversation even though you spoke quietly and shut the glass window.

   ID   V   N

7. You telephone a patient, Alex Massey, to remind him of tomorrow's appointment and leave a voice mail message on his answering machine.

   ID   V   N

8. Three patients near the reception area of the office overhear you telling another staff member that Daisy Dotson is scheduled for a Pap smear tomorrow at 4:00 PM.

   ID   V   N

9. You telephone a patient, Janet Hudson. She is not home so you leave a message on her answering machine that her breast cancer biopsy results came back negative.

   ID   V   N

10. You call out Fran O'Donnell's complete name in the waiting room where other patients are sitting.

    ID   V   N

11. You do not close the glass window to the reception room when talking on the telephone with your sister.

    ID   V   N

12. The office nurse tells a patient, Hugo Wells, his test results in front of his relatives.

    ID   V   N

13. You leave Katy Zontag's medical chart open at the receptionist's counter.

    ID   V   N

14. You telephone a patient, Jose Ramirez, and leave your name, the physician's name, and telephone number on his answering machine.

    ID   V   N

15. A patient, Kim Lee, is in the examination room and overhears a conversation concerning blood test results of another patient in an adjoining room.

    ID   V   N

16. While waiting in the reception room, a patient, Xavier Gomez, overhears a receptionist talking with another patient on the telephone about a colonoscopy appointment.

    ID   V   N

17. Betty Burton, a patient who is being weighed on the office scale by the medical assistant, overhears a conversation between an insurance billing specialist and an insurance company representative in which she is trying to obtain preauthorization for another patient's medical procedure.

    ID   V   N

18. In a restaurant, a waitress overhears an insurance biller talking to a friend and telling her about a famous actress who visited her physician's office yesterday.

    ID   V   N

A S S I G N M E N T   **2 – 3** ▶ **CRITICAL THINKING: FRAUD VERSUS ABUSE**

Performance Objective

Task: Make a decision after reading each case study, whether it is considered fraud, abuse, or neither.

Conditions: Use pen or pencil.

Standards: Time: _____ minutes

                   Accuracy: _____

                   (Note: the time element and accuracy criteria may be given by your instructor.)

Directions. Read through each scenario and circle whether it is a fraud (F) issue, practice of abuse (A), or neither (N). To distinguish the difference between fraud and abuse situations, remember that under the Medicare program, abuse relates to incidents or practices that are inconsistent with accepted sound business practices whereas fraud is intentional deception that an individual knows, or should know, to be false, and the individual knows the deception could result in some unauthorized benefit to himself or some other person(s).

Scenarios

1. Dr. Pedro Atrics has a friend and his child needs elective surgery. He agrees to perform the surgery and bill as an "insurance only" case.

   F   A   N

2. A patient, Carl Skinner, calls the office repeatedly about his prescriptions. When seen in the office the next time, Dr. Input bills a higher level of evaluation and management service to allow for the additional time.

   F   A   N

3. Dr. Skeleton sets a simple fracture and puts a cast on Mr. Davis. He bills for a complex fracture.

   F   A   N

4. A patient, Maria Gomez, asks a friendly staff member to change the dates on the insurance claim form. The medical assistant complies with the request.

   F   A   N

5. A patient, Roberto Loren, asks the physician to restate a diagnosis so the insurance company will pay because payment would be denied based on the present statement. The physician complies with the request.

   F   A   N

6. Dr. Rumsey sees a patient twice on the same day but bills as though the patient was seen on two different dates.

   F   A   N

7. A Medicare patient, Joan O'Connor, is seen by Dr. Practon, and the insurance claim shows a charge to the Medicare fiscal intermediary at a fee schedule rate higher than and different from that of non-Medicare patients.

   F   A   N

8. A patient, Hazel Plunkett, receives a service that is not medically necessary to the extent rendered and an insurance claim is submitted.

   F   A   N

9. A patient, Sun Cho, paid for services that were subsequently declared not medically necessary, and Dr. Cardi failed to refund the payment to the patient.

   F   A   N

10. Dr. Ulibarri tells the insurance biller not to collect the deductible and copayments from Mrs. Gerry Coleman.

    F   A   N

ASSIGNMENT **2-4 ▸ CRITICAL THINKING: CONSENT VERSUS AUTHORIZATION**

Performance Objective

Task: Make a decision using your best judgment after reading each scenario, and determine whether you should ask for consent or authorization, or do other procedures.

Conditions: Use pen or pencil.

Standards: Time: _____ minutes

               Accuracy: _____

               (Note: The time element and accuracy criteria may be given by your instructor. Class discussion may offer other possible ways of handling the given situations.)

Directions. Read through each case study and determine whether you should ask for consent or authorization, or perform other office procedures.

Scenarios

1. Dr. Practon's patient, Mary Ann Bailey, goes to the College Hospital's emergency department complaining of severe stomach cramps. Subsequently she is admitted to the hospital for pancreatitis. The floor nurse at the hospital telephones Dr. Practon's office asking for the patient's medical records to be brought over immediately. What should you do?

   Response _____

   _____

   _____

2. Robert Fellow, a patient, telephones the College Clinic and states that he has hired a lawyer and is filing a lawsuit against another driver for an automobile accident that happened about a month ago. The attorney for the other driver needs your patient's medical records to find out what injuries your patient suffered as a result of the accident. The attorney also wants to know if there are any preexisting injuries. Mr. Fellow requests that you send a copy of his medical records to the other attorney. What should you do?

   Response _____

   _____

   _____

3. Consuelo Lopez, the mother of a minor patient, Johnnie Lopez, telephones your office stating that Johnnie is having difficulty staying focused and loses his concentration during classroom activities at school. Mrs. Lopez has made an appointment for him to be seen by a psychologist and has requested that you send his medical records to the psychologist before the date of the appointment. What should you do?

Response _____

_____

_____

4. Eric Jacobs, a patient, receives psychiatric counseling as well as treatment for diabetes at the College Clinic. The patient requests a copy of his medical record. (A) Is it necessary to remove the documentation pertaining to the psychiatric counseling sessions before giving the patient a copy of his medical record? (B) Can you disclose to the patient his medical records? Explain.

Response (A) _____

_____

Response (B) _____

_____

_____

ASSIGNMENT **2–5** ▸ **VISIT WEBSITES**

Performance Objective

Task: Access the Internet and visit several websites of the World Wide Web.

Conditions: Use a computer with printer and/or pen or pencil to make notes.

Standards: Time: _____ minutes

                         Accuracy: _____

                         (Note: The time element and accuracy criteria may be given by your instructor.)

Directions. For active weblinks to the following resources, visit the Evolve website online at: http://evolve.elsevier.com/ Fordney/handbook and do the following three site searches.

1. Site-search information on patient confidentiality by visiting the website of the American Medical Association. Under "ethics, education, science, public health, quality, and accreditation," Click on "legal issues of physicians." Then click on "patient-physician relationship issues." Then click on "patient confidentiality." Make notes or print a hard copy of the pages while remaining online.

2. Site-search information on patient confidentiality by visiting the website of the American Health Information Management Association. Click on "site search" at that website. Key in "patient confidentiality." Then click on "search for matching documents." List a recent question asked about this topic and record the answer or print a hard copy of all the questions and answers while remaining online.

3. Site-search for information on fraud and abuse by visiting one or more of the federal websites. See what you can discover and either print out or take notes and bring back information to share with the class for discussion. Try one or more of the CMS websites listed on Evolve.

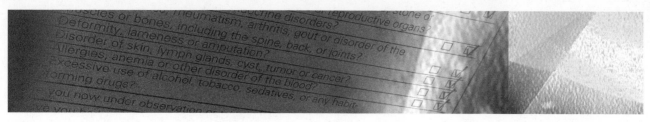

Basics of Health Insurance

KEY TERMS

Your instructor may wish to select some words pertinent to this chapter for a test. For definitions of the terms, further study, and/or reference, the words, phrases, and abbreviations may be found in the glossary at the end of the Handbook. *Key terms for this chapter follow.*

accounts receivable management

applicant

assignment

blanket contract

capitation

The Civilian Health and Medical Program of the Department of Veterans Affairs (CHAMPVA)

claim

coinsurance

competitive medical plan (CMP)

conditionally renewable

contract

coordination of benefits (COB)

daysheet

deductible

disability income insurance

electronic signature

eligibility

emancipated minor

encounter form

exclusions

exclusive provider organization (EPO)

expressed contract

extended

financial accounting record

foundation for medical care (FMC)

guaranteed renewable

guarantor

health insurance

health maintenance organization (HMO)

high risk

implied contract

indemnity

independent or individual practice association (IPA)

insured

major medical

Maternal and Child Health Program (MCHP)

Medicaid (MCD)

Medicare (M)

Medicare/Medicaid (Medi-Medi)

member

noncancelable policy

nonparticipating provider (nonpar)

optionally renewable

participating provider (par)

patient registration form

personal insurance

point-of-service (POS) plan

posted

preauthorization

precertification

predetermination

preexisting conditions

preferred provider organization (PPO)

premium

running balance

State Disability Insurance (SDI)

subscriber

TRICARE

Unemployment Compensation Disability (UCD)

Veterans Affairs (VA) outpatient clinic

workers' compensation (WC) insurance

KEY ABBREVIATIONS

See how many abbreviations and acronyms you can translate and then use this as a handy reference list. Definitions for the key abbreviations are located near the back of the Handbook *in the glossary.*

AAMB _____

AAPC _____

ADSM _____

AHIMA _____

A/R _____

CMP _____

CMS _____

COB _____

COBRA _____

copay _____

DDE _____

DoD _____

DOS _____

EFT _____

EOB _____

EPO _____

FMC _____

FSA _____

HBMA _____

HDHP _____

HFMA _____

HMO _____

HRA _____

HSA _____

HIPAA _____

IPA _____

M _____

MAB _____

MCD _____

MCHP _____

Medi-Medi _____

MGMA _____

MSA _____

nonpar _____

NPP _____

OIG _____

PAHCOM _____

par _____

PMS _____

POS _____

POS plan _____

PPO _____

RA _____

ROA _____

SOF _____

TPO _____

UCD _____

VA _____

WC _____

PERFORMANCE OBJECTIVES

The student will be able to:

- Define and spell the key terms and key abbreviations for this chapter, given the information from the *Handbook* glossary, within a reasonable time period and with enough accuracy to obtain a satisfactory evaluation.

- Answer the fill-in-the-blank, multiple choice, and true/false review questions after reading the chapter, with enough accuracy to obtain a satisfactory evaluation.

- Arrange 18 administrative processing steps of an insurance claim in proper sequence, given data from the textbook, within a reasonable time period and with enough accuracy to obtain a satisfactory evaluation.

- Use critical thinking to explain some of the differences in insurance key terms, given data from the textbook, within a reasonable time period and with enough accuracy to obtain a satisfactory evaluation.

- Prepare a financial accounting record, given data from the textbook, within a reasonable time period and with enough accuracy to obtain a satisfactory evaluation.

- Abstract data from some insurance identification cards, given data from the textbook, within a reasonable time period and with enough accuracy to obtain a satisfactory evaluation.

ALTAPOINT PRACTICE MANAGEMENT SOFTWARE OBJECTIVES

The student will be able to:

- Use a patient ledger to find information on a patient account.
- Locate information on an insurance company.

STUDY OUTLINE

History

Insurance in the United States

Legal Principles of Insurance
Insurance Contracts

Physician–Patient Contracts and Financial Obligation
Implied or Expressed Contracts

The Insurance Policy
Policy Application
Policy Renewal Provisions
Policy Terms
Coordination of Benefits
General Policy Limitations

Choice of Health Insurance
Group Contract
Individual Contract
Prepaid Health Plan

Types of Health Insurance Coverage
CHAMPVA
Competitive Medical Plan

Disability Income Insurance
Exclusive Provider Organization
Foundation for Medical Care
Health Maintenance Organization
Independent or Individual Practice Association
Maternal and Child Health Program
Medicaid
Medicare
Medicare/Medicaid
Point-of-Service Plan
Preferred Provider Organization
TRICARE
Unemployment Compensation Disability
Veterans Affairs Outpatient Clinic
Workers' Compensation Insurance

Examples of Insurance Billing

Keeping Up to Date

Procedure: Handling and Processing Insurance Claims

Procedure: Prepare and Post to a Patient's Financial Accounting Record

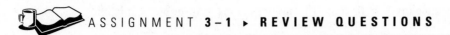

ASSIGNMENT 3-1 ▸ REVIEW QUESTIONS

Part I Fill in the Blank

Review the objectives, key terms, glossary definitions to key terms, chapter information, and figures before completing the following review questions.

1. A/an _____ is a legally enforceable agreement or contract.

2. An individual promising to pay for medical services rendered is known as a/an

_____.

3. List five health insurance policy renewal provisions.

   a. _____

   b. _____

   c. _____

   d. _____

   e. _____

4. Insurance reimbursement or payment is also called

_____.

5. Name two general health insurance policy limitations.

   a. _____

   b. _____

6. The act of determining whether treatment is covered under an individual's health

   insurance policy is called _____.

7. The procedure to obtain permission for a procedure before it is done, to determine whether the insurance program agrees it is medically necessary, is termed

_____.

8. Determining the maximum dollar amount the insurance company will pay for a

   procedure before it is done is known as _____.

9. Name three ways an individual may obtain health insurance.

   a. _____

   b. _____

   c. _____

10. List four methods a physician's practice may use to submit insurance claims to insurance companies.

    a. _____

    b. _____

    c. _____

    d. _____

11. A document signed by the insured directing the insurance company to pay benefits

    directly to the physician is known as a/an _____.

12. A patient service slip personalized to the practice of the physician and used as a communications/billing tool during routing of the patient is also known as a/an

    a. _____

    b. _____

    c. _____

    d. _____

13. Electronic access to computer data may consist of the following verification or access methods.

    a. _____   d. _____

    b. _____   e. _____

    c. _____   f. _____

14. Guidelines for avoiding unauthorized use and preventing problems when a medical practice uses a facsimile signature stamp are

    a. _____

    b. _____

    c. _____

    d. _____

Part II Mix and Match

15. Match the following insurance terms in the right column with their descriptions and fill in the blank with the appropriate letter.

_____ An insurance company takes into account benefits payable by another carrier in determining its own liability.

a. adjuster

_____ Benefits paid by an insurance company to an insured person.

b. assignment

_____ Transfer of one's right to collect an amount payable under an insurance contract.

c. carrier

_____ Time that must elapse before an indemnity is paid.

d. coordination of benefits

_____ Acts for insurance company or insured in settlement of claims.

e. deductible

_____ Periodic payment to keep insurance policy in force.

f. exclusions

_____ Amount insured person must pay before policy will pay.

g. indemnity

_____ Time period in which a claim must be filed.

h. premium

_____ Certain illnesses or injuries listed in a policy that the insurance company will not cover.

i. subscriber

_____ Insurance company that carries the insurance.

j. time limit

_____ One who belongs to an insurance plan.

k. waiting period

Part III Multiple Choice

Choose the best answer.

16. When a patient goes to a physician's office seeking medical services, the physician accepts the patient and agrees to render treatment, and both parties agree, this contract is known as a/an

    a. expressed contract

    b. agreed contract

    c. implied contract

    d. written contract

17. The process of checking and confirming that a patient is covered under an insurance plan is known as

    a. precertification

    b. eligibility verification

    c. coordinating benefits

    d. predetermination

18. A provision that allows the policyholder the right to refuse to renew the insurance policy on a premium due date is called

    a. conditionally renewable

    b. guaranteed renewable

    c. optionally renewable

    d. noncancelable

19. A provision in a health insurance policy in which two insurance carriers work together for payment so that there is no duplication of benefits paid between the primary insurance carrier and the secondary insurance carrier is called

    a. copayment

    b. coinsurance

    c. coordination of benefits

    d. cost-share rider

20. Type of tax-free savings account that allows individuals and their employers to set aside money to pay for health care expenses is known as

    a. health savings accounts

    b. medical savings account

    c. flexible spending account

    d. all of the above

21. Time limits for filing insurance claims may have a range of

    a. 10 days from the date medical service is received to 1 year

    b. 30 days from the date of service to 1½ years

    c. 60 days from the date of service

    d. there is no time limit

Part IV True/False

Write "T" or "F" in the blank to indicate whether you think the statement is true or false.

_____ 22. If a physician belongs to a preferred provider organization (PPO) and does not follow his or her contract with the PPO, the patient is liable for the bill.

_____ 23. The birthday law is a change in the order of determination of coordination of benefits regarding primary and secondary insurance carriers for dependent children.

_____ 24. The Consolidated Omnibus Budget Reconciliation Act of 1985 (COBRA) mandates that when an employee is laid off from a company, the group health insurance coverage must continue at group rates for up to 18 months.

_____ 25. Capitation is a system of payment used by managed care plans in which a member physician is paid different amounts monthly for each patient enrolled.

_____ 26. Provider's signatures on a CMS-1500 claim form is acceptable either handwritten, facsimile stamp, or electronic signature.

 ASSIGNMENT 3-2 ▸ CRITICAL THINKING: ADMINISTRATIVE SEQUENCE OF PROCESSING AN INSURANCE CLAIM

Performance Objective

Task: Number from 1 to 18 the proper sequence of processing an insurance claim.

Conditions: Use given data and pen or pencil.

Standards: Time: _____minutes

                    Accuracy: _____

                    (Note: The time element and accuracy criteria may be given by your instructor.)

Directions. Arrange the listed steps 1 through 18 in proper sequence by placing the correct number to the left of the statement.

_____ 16 Bank deposit made and unpaid claims followed up

_____ 7 Patient account established in practice management software

_____ 2 Insurance information obtained and verified

_____ 15 Claim processed by insurance payer and payment posted

_____ 928 Patient's financial data posted

_____ 1 Appointment made and patient preregistration obtained

_____ 11 CMS-1500 (08-05) paper claim forms submitted

_____ 3 4 Provider's signature requirements

_____ 12 Electronic (HIPAA X12 837) claims transmitted

_____ 10 Insurance claims generated

_____ 3 HIPAA Notice of Privacy Practices presented

_____ 17 Claim transaction completed and monthly statement sent to patient

_____ 14 Pending insurance claims tracked

_____ 5 Patient's signature obtained

_____ 6 Assignment of benefits obtained

_____ 8A Services performed and encounter form completed

_____ 4 Patients's insurance identification card photocopied

_____ 18 Financial records retained

ASSIGNMENT 3-3 ▸ CRITICAL THINKING: DIFFERENCES IN INSURANCE KEY TERMS

Performance Objective

Task: Describe and/or explain your response to five questions.

Conditions: Use one or two sheets of white typing paper and pen or pencil.

Standards: Time: _____ minutes

                   Accuracy: _____

                   (Note: The time element and accuracy criteria may be given by your instructor.)

Directions. Respond verbally or in writing to these questions or statements.

1. Explain the difference between the following:

   Blanket contract _____

   Individual contract _____

2. Explain the difference between a participating provider and a nonparticipating provider for the following:

   Commercial insurance company or managed care plan participating provider:

   _____

   Commercial insurance company or managed care plan nonparticipating provider:

   _____

   Medicare participating provider:

   _____

   Medicare nonparticipating provider:

   _____

3. State the difference between the following:

   Implied contract _____

   Expressed contract _____

4. Explain the birthday law (rule) and when it is used.

   _____

ASSIGNMENT 3-4 ▸ PREPARE A FINANCIAL ACCOUNTING RECORD

Performance Objective

Task: Prepare, insert descriptions, and post fees, payments, credit adjustments, and balances due to a patient's ledger card. If you have access to copy equipment, make a photocopy.

Conditions: Use one patient accounts or ledger form (Figure 3–1), pen or pencil, and calculator.

Standards: Time: _____ minutes

                      Accuracy: _____

                      (Note: The time element and accuracy criteria may be given by your instructor.)

Directions:

1. Locate a financial accounting record (ledger) (Figure 3–1) form. Refer to the step-by-step procedures at the end of Chapter 3 in the *Handbook*. In addition, see Figures 3–16 and 10–3 in the *Handbook* for graphic examples of financial accounting records (ledgers).

2. Insert the patient's name and address, including ZIP code in the box.

3. Enter the patient's personal data.

4. Ledger lines: Insert date of service (DOS), reference (CPT code number, check number, or dates of service for posting adjustments or when insurance was billed), description of the transaction, charge amounts, payments, adjustments, and running current balance. The posting date is the actual date the transaction is recorded. If the DOS differs from the posting date, list the DOS in the reference or description column.

Note: A good bookkeeping practice is to use a red pen to draw a line across the financial accounting record (ledger) from left to right to indicate the last entry billed to the insurance company.

Account No. ___3-3___

FINANCIAL STATEMENT
PRACTION MEDICAL GROUP, INC.
4567 Broad Avenue
Woodland Hills, XY 12345-0001
Tel. 555-486-9002
Fax No. 555-487-8976

Phone No. (H) _____ (W) _____   Birthdate _____

Primary Insurance Co. _____   Policy/Group No. _____

	REFERENCE	DESCRIPTION	CHARGES	CREDITS PYMNTS.	ADJ	BALANCE
			BALANCE FORWARD➤			

PLEASE PAY LAST AMOUNT IN BALANCE COLUMN ⬆

THIS IS A COPY OF YOUR FINANCIAL ACCOUNT AS IT APPEARS ON OUR RECORDS

Figure 3–1

Scenario: A new patient, Miss Carolyn Wachsman, of 4590 Ashton Street, Woodland Hills, XY 12345, was seen by Dr. Practon; her account number is 2-3. Her home telephone number is (555) 340-8876 and her work telephone number is (555) 509-7091. She was born on 5-8-75. She is insured by Blue Cross, and her subscriber number is 540-xx-3209.

Miss Wachsman was seen on March 24 of the current year for a level III evaluation and management office visit ($). She also received an ECG ($). Locate these fees in the Mock Fee Schedule in Appendix A of this *Workbook*.

An insurance claim form was sent to Blue Cross on March 25. On May 15, Blue Cross sent an explanation of benefits stating the patient had previously met her deductible. Check number 433 for $76 was attached to the EOB and $19 was indicated as the adjustment to be made by the provider. On May 25, the patient was billed for the balance.

After the instructor has returned your work to you, either make the necessary corrections and place it in a three-ring notebook for future reference, or, if you received a high score, place it in your portfolio for reference when applying for a job.

A S S I G N M E N T   3 - 5 ▸ A B S T R A C T   D A T A   F R O M   A N   I N S U R A N C E
I D E N T I F I C A T I O N   C A R D

Performance Objective

Task: Answer questions in reference to an insurance identification card for Case A.

Conditions: Use an insurance identification card (Figure 3–2), the questions presented, and pen or pencil.

Standards: Time: _____ minutes

                         Accuracy: _____

                         (Note: The time element and accuracy criteria may be given by your instructor.)

Directions. An identification card provides much of the information needed to establish a patient's insurance coverage. You have photocopied the front and back sides of three patients' cards and placed copies in their patient records, returning the originals to the patients. Answer the questions by abstracting or obtaining the data from the cards.

CASE A

1. Name of patient covered by the policy _____

2. Provide the insurance policy's effective date. _____

3. List the telephone number for preauthorization. _____

4. State name and address of insurance company. _____

5. List the telephone number to call for provider access. _____

6. Name the type of insurance plan. _____

7. List the insurance identification number (a.k.a. subscriber, certificate, or member numbers). _____

8. Furnish the group number. _____ Plan or coverage code. _____

9. State the copay requirements _____

10. Does the card indicate the patient has hospital coverage? _____

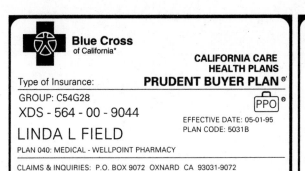

Figure 3–2

ASSIGNMENT **3-6** ▸ *ABSTRACT DATA FROM AN INSURANCE IDENTIFICATION CARD*

Performance Objective

Task: Answer questions in reference to the insurance identification card for Case B.

Conditions: Use an insurance identification card (Figure 3–3), the questions presented, and pen or pencil.

Standards: Time: _____ minutes

Accuracy: _____

(Note: The time element and accuracy criteria may be given by your instructor.)

CASE B

1. Patient's name covered by the policy. _____

2. Provide the insurance policy's effective date. _____

3. List the telephone number for preauthorization. _____

4. State name of insurance company. _____

5. List the telephone number to call for patient benefits and eligibility. _____

6. Name the type of insurance plan. _____

7. List the insurance identification number (a.k.a. subscriber, certificate, or member

   numbers). _____

8. Furnish the group number. _____ Plan or coverage code. _____

9. State the copay requirements, if any. _____

10. List the Blue Shield website. _____

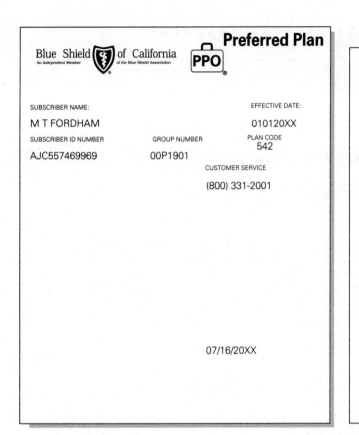

Blue Shield of California
An Independent Member / of the Blue Shield Association

PPO

Preferred Plan

SUBSCRIBER NAME:

M T FORDHAM

EFFECTIVE DATE:

010120XX

SUBSCRIBER ID NUMBER   GROUP NUMBER   PLAN CODE
                                                     542
AJC557469969   00P1901

CUSTOMER SERVICE

(800) 331-2001

07/16/20XX

Use Blue Shield of California Preferred Physicians and Hospitals to receive maximum benefits.

Carry the Blue Shield Identification Card with you at all times and present it whenever you or one of your covered dependents receives medical services. Read your employee booklet/Health Services Agreement which summarizes the benefits, provisions, limitations and exclusions of your plan. Your health plan may require prior notification of any hospitalization and notification, within one business day, of an emergency admission. Review of selected procedures may be required before some services are performed. To receive hospital pre-admission and pre-service reviews, call 1-800-343-1691. Your failure to call may result in a reduction of benefits.

For questions, including those related to benefits, and eligibility, call the customer service number listed on the front of this card.

The PPO logo on the front of this ID Card identifies you to preferred providers outside the state of California as a member of the Blue Card PPO Program.

When you are outside of California call 1-800-810-2583 to locate the nearest PPO Provider. Remember, any services you receive are subject to the policies and provisions of your group plan.

ID-23200-PPO REVERSE   www.blueshieldca.com

Figure 3–3

ASSIGNMENT 3-7 ▶ ABSTRACT DATA FROM AN INSURANCE IDENTIFICATION CARD

Performance Objective

Task: Answer questions in reference to the insurance identification card for Case C.

Conditions: Use an insurance identification card (Figure 3–4), the questions presented, and pen or pencil.

Standards: Time: _____ minutes

Accuracy: _____

(Note: The time element and accuracy criteria may be given by your instructor.)

CASE C

1. Patient's name covered by the policy. _____

2. Provide the insurance policy's effective date, if there is one. _____

3. List the number to call for out-of-network preauthorization. _____

4. State name and address of insurance company. _____

5. List the telephone number to call for member inquiries. _____

6. Name the type of insurance plan. _____

7. List the insurance identification number (a.k.a. subscriber, certificate, or member numbers).

   _____

8. Furnish the group number. _____

9. State the copay requirements, if any. _____

10. Who is the patient's primary care physician? _____

UNITEDhealthcare

LINDA L. FLORES
Member # 52170-5172 _____

CALMAT

Group # 176422
COPAY: Office Visit $10 ER $50
    Urgent $35

Electronic Claims Payor ID 87726 _____

Call 800-842-5751 for Member Inquiries

POS PCP Plan
WITH RX D - UHC
and MH/CD
PCP: G. LOMAN
805-643-9973

MTH

This identification card is not proof of membership nor does it guarantee coverage. Persons with coverage that remains in force are entitled to benefits under the terms and conditions of this group health benefit plan as detailed in your benefit description.

IMPORTANT MEMBER INFORMATION
In non-emergencies, call your Primary Care Physician to receive the highest level of benefits. If you have an emergency and are admitted to a hospital, you are required to call your Primary Care Physician within two working days.
For out of network services that require authorization, call the Member Inquiries 800 number on the front of this card.

Claim Address: P.O. Box 30990, Salt Lake City, UT 84130-0990

Figure 3–4

ALTAPOINT PRACTICE MANAGEMENT SOFTWARE ASSIGNMENTS

ASSIGNMENT 3-8 ▸ VIEW A PATIENT FINANCIAL ACCOUNT RECORD (LEDGER) AND FIND INFORMATION ON A PATIENT ACCOUNT

Performance Objective

Task: View a patient's financial account record (ledger) and find information

Conditions: Use Teri E. Simpson's financial account record (ledger), patient's electronic data, and computer.

Standards: Time: _____ minutes

                Accuracy: _____

                (Note: The time element and accuracy criteria may be given by your instructor.)

Directions: Before attempting the Practice Management software assignment, refer to Appendix C and follow the instructions provided to familiarize yourself with the software. Then refer to the Practice Management software on the CD that accompanies the *Workbook*. Follow the instructions for viewing a patient's financial account record (ledger) and open the financial account record (ledger) for Teri E. Simpson.

1. What is Teri E. Simpson's balance due amount? _____

2. What was the fee for her billing code 99070 on November 7, 2005? _____

ASSIGNMENT 3-9 ▸ **LOCATE INFORMATION ABOUT AN INSURANCE COMPANY**

Performance Objective

Task: Locate information about an insurance company

Conditions: Onscreen list of insurance companies and computer

Standards: Time: _____ minutes

                  Accuracy: _____

                  (Note: The time element and accuracy criteria may be given by your instructor.)

Directions: Before attempting the Practice Management software assignment, refer to Appendix C and follow the instructions provided to familiarize yourself with the software. Then refer to the Practice Management software on the CD that accompanies the *Workbook*. For this assignment, follow the instructions for viewing the list of insurance compaines and view the information on United Western Benefit Insurance.

1. What is the adddress for United Western Benefit Insurance company?

   _____

2. What is the Practice Group ID? _____

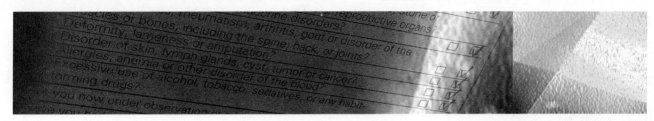

Medical Documentation

KEY TERMS

Your instructor may wish to select some words pertinent to this chapter for a test. For definitions of the terms, further study, and/or reference, the words, phrases, and abbreviations may be found in the glossary at the end of the Handbook. *Key terms for this chapter follow.*

acute

attending physician

chief complaint (CC)

chronic

comorbidity

comprehensive (C)

concurrent care

consultation

consulting physician

continuity of care

counseling

critical care

detailed (D)

documentation

electronic health record (EHR)

emergency care

eponym

established patient

expanded problem focused (EPF)

external audit

facsimile (fax)

family history (FH)

health record/medical record

high complexity (HC)

history of present illness (HPI)

internal review

low complexity (LC)

medical decision making (MDM)

medical necessity

medical report

moderate complexity (MC)

new patient (NP)

nonphysician practitioner (NPP)

ordering physician

past history (PH)

physical examination (PE or PX)

primary care physician (PCP)

problem focused (PF)

prospective review

referral

referring physician

resident physician

retrospective review

review of systems (ROS)

social history (SH)

straightforward (SF)

subpoena

subpoena duces tecum

teaching physician

treating or performing physician

KEY ABBREVIATIONS

See how many abbreviations and acronyms you can translate and then use this as a handy reference list. Definitions for the key abbreviations are located near the back of the Handbook *in the glossary.*

AHIMA _____

AMA _____

C _____

CC _____

CCU _____

CHEDDAR _____

CMS _____

CPT _____

D _____

DOS _____

dx, Dx _____

ED or ER _____

EHR _____

E/M service _____

EMR _____

EPF level of history or examination _____

fax _____

FH _____

HC medical decision making _____

HHS _____

HIM _____

HIPAA _____

HIV _____

HPI _____

ICU _____

imp _____

LC medical decision making _____

LLQ _____

LUQ _____

MC medical decision making _____

NLP _____

NPP _____

OIG _____

PCP _____

PDA _____

PE or PX _____

PF level of history or examination _____

PFSH _____

PH _____

PHI _____

PI _____

POR system _____

POS _____

RCU _____

RLQ _____

R/O _____

ROS _____

RUQ _____

SF medical decision making _____

SH _____

SOAP style _____

SOR system _____

TOS _____

WNL _____

PERFORMANCE OBJECTIVES

The student will be able to:

- Define and spell the key terms and key abbreviations for this chapter, given the information from the *Handbook* glossary, within a reasonable time period and with enough accuracy to obtain a satisfactory evaluation.
- Answer the fill-in-the-blank, mix and match, multiple choice, and true/false review questions after reading the chapter, with enough accuracy to obtain a satisfactory evaluation.
- Use critical thinking to solve an office problem about patients' medical records.
- Abstract subjective and objective data from patient records, within a reasonable time period and with enough accuracy to obtain a satisfactory evaluation.
- Review a patient record and obtain answers to questions about the documentation presented, within a reasonable time period and with enough accuracy to obtain a satisfactory evaluation.
- Select the correct medicolegal form, create a letter with appropriate content, prepare an envelope, and properly complete U.S. Postal Service documents for the physician's signature, given the patients' chart notes and ledger cards, within a reasonable time period and with enough accuracy to obtain a satisfactory evaluation.

ALTAPOINT PRACTICE MANAGEMENT SOFTWARE OBJECTIVES

The student will be able to:

- Enter a new patient into the practice management system.

STUDY OUTLINE

The Documentation Process
 Health Record
 Documenters
 Reasons for Documentation
General Principles of Health Record Documentation
 Medical Necessity
 External Audit Point System
 Legalities of Health Record Documentation
Documentation Guidelines for Evaluation and Management Services
Contents of a Medical Report
 Documentation of History
 Documentation of Examination
 Documentation of Medical Decision-Making Complexity

Documentation Terminology
 Terminology for Evaluation and Management Services
 Diagnostic Terminology and Abbreviations
 Directional Terms
 Surgical Terminology
Review and Audit of Health Records
 Internal Reviews
 External Audit
 Retention of Records
 Termination of a Case
 Prevention of Legal Problems
Procedure: Abstract Data from a Health Record
Procedure: Compose, Format, Key, Proofread, and Print a Letter

ASSIGNMENT **4-1** ▸ **REVIEW QUESTIONS**

Part I Fill in the Blank

Review the objectives, key terms, glossary definitions to key terms, chapter information, and figures before completing the following review questions.

1. Written or graphic information about patient care is termed a/an _____.

2. _____ is written or dictated to record chronologic facts and observations about a patient's health.

3. Performance of services or procedures consistent with the diagnosis, done with standards of good medical practice and a proper level of care given in the appropriate setting is

   known as _____.

4. If a medical practice is audited by Medicare officials and intentional miscoding is

   discovered, _____ may be levied and providers

   may be _____.

5. A list of all staff members' names, job titles, signatures, and their initials is known as a/an

   _____.

6. How should an insurance billing specialist correct an error on a patient's record?

   _____

   _____

7. Name the six documentation components of a patient's history.

   a. _____

   b. _____

   c. _____

   d. _____

   e. _____

   f. _____

8. An inventory of body systems by documenting responses to questions about symptoms

   that a patient has experienced is called a/an _____.

9. Define the following terms in relationship to billing.

   a. New patient _____

   _____

b. Established patient _____

_____

10. Explain the difference between a consultation and the referral of a patient.

a. Consultation _____

_____

b. Referral _____

11. If two physicians see the same patient on the same day, one for the patient's heart condition and the other for a diabetic situation, this medical care situation is called

_____.

12. Medical care for a patient who has received treatment for an illness and is referred to a second physician for treatment of the same condition is a situation called

_____.

13. A patient's protected health information may be disclosed for treatment, payment, or health care operations but for other situations and especially when faxing a patient's

medical records, a signed document for _____

_____ must be obtained from the patient.

14. If a fax is misdirected, either_____

or_____.

15. Indicate either indefinite retention or number of years for keeping records in the following situations:

a. Computerized payroll records _____

b. Insurance claim for Medicare patient _____

c. Medical record of a deceased patient _____

d. Active patient medical records _____

e. Telephone records _____

16. Is it proper for an insurance billing specialist to receive a subpoena for his or her physician?

_____

17. Can a physician terminate a contract with a patient?_____ If so, how?

_____

Part II Mix and Match

18. Match the following terms in the right column with their descriptions and fill in the blank with the appropriate letter.

___I___ Renders a service to a patient

___D___ Directs selection, preparation, and administration of tests, medication, or treatment

___A___ Legally responsible for the care and treatment given to a patient

___B___ Gives an opinion regarding a specific problem that is requested by another doctor

___F___ Sends the patient for tests or treatment or to another doctor for consultation

___e___ Oversees care of patients in managed care plans and refers patients to see specialists when needed

___H___ Responsible for training and supervising medical students

___C___ Clinical nurse specialist or licensed social worker who treats a patient for a specific medical problem and uses the results of a diagnostic test in managing a patient's medical problem

___g___ Performs one or more years of training in a specialty area while working at a hospital (medical center)

a. Attending physician

b. Consulting physician

c. Nonphysician practitioner

d. Ordering physician

e. Primary care physician

f. Referring physician

g. Resident physician

h. Teaching physician

i. Treating or performing physician

Part III Multiple Choice

Choose the best answer.

19. During the performance of an external audit to review a medical practice's health records, the system used to show deficiencies in documentation is called a/an

    a. CHEDDAR system

    b. electronic recording system

    c. information record system

    (d.) point system

20. The SOAP style of documentation that a physician uses to chart a patient's progress in the health record means

    a. signature, observations, assessment, and progress

    (b.) subjective, objective, assessment, and plan

    c. symptoms, objective findings, and professional services

    d. subjective, opinions, assistance, and present illness

21. A physical examination of a patient performed by a physician is

   a. descriptive

   b. comprehensive

   c. subjective

   (d.) objective

22. A health care management process after doing a history and physical examination on a patient that results in a plan of treatment is called

   a. selecting a treatment option

   (b.) medical decision making

   c. establishing a diagnosis

   d. choosing a management option

23. When there is an underlying disease or other conditions are present at the time of the patient's office visit, this is termed

   a. mortality

   b. continuity

   (c.) comorbidity

   d. complexity

Part IV True/False

Write "T" or "F" in the blank to indicate whether you think the statement is true or false.

___F___ 24. A patient's hospital discharge summary contains the discharge diagnosis but not the admitting diagnosis.

___F___ 25. An eponym should not be used when a comparable anatomic term can be used in its place.

___F___ 26. If the phrase "rule out" appears in a patient's health record in connection with a disease, then code the condition as if it existed.

___T___ 27. During a prospective review or prebilling audit, all procedures or services and diagnoses listed on the encounter form must match the data on the insurance claim form.

___T___ 28. Assigned insurance claims for Medicaid and Medicare cases must be kept for a period of 7 years.

ASSIGNMENT 4-2 ▸ REVIEW DIAGNOSTIC TERMINOLOGY AND
ABBREVIATIONS

In the *Handbook*, review Table 4–1 and anatomic figures, as well as Appendix A in the *Workbook*, which has a list of abbreviations and symbols.

1. Match the following terms in the right column with the descriptions and fill in the blank with the appropriate letter.

____D____ Pertaining to both sides   a. acute

____e____ Decubitus ulcer   b. chronic

____A____ Condition that runs a short but severe course   c. menopause

____C____ Change of life   d. bilateral

____f____ Tinnitus   e. bed sore

____B____ Condition persisting over a long period of time   f. ringing sensation in ears

2. Write in the meaning for these abbreviations and/or symbols commonly encountered in a patient's medical record.

RLQ   Right Lower Quadrant

DC   Doctor of chiropractic

WNL   w/in normal limits

R/O   Rule out

URI   upper respiratory infection

c̄   w/

⊕   positive

3. When documenting incisions, the unit of measure length should be listed in

Cm

Multiple Choice

Circle the letter that gives the best answer to each question.

4. If a physician called and asked for a patient's medical record STAT, what would he or she mean?

a. The physician wants a statistic from a patient's record.

b. The physician wants the record delivered on Tuesday.

c. The physician wants the record delivered immediately.

5. If a physician asks you to locate the results of the last UA, what would you be searching for?

   a. a urinalysis report

   b. an x-ray report of the ulna

   c. uric acid test results

6. If a physician telephoned and asked for a copy of the last H&P to be faxed, what is being requested?

   a. heart and pulmonary findings

   b. H_2 antagonist test results

   c. a history and physical

7. If a hospital nurse telephoned and asked you to read the results of the patient's last CBC, what would you be searching for?

   a. carcinoma basal cell report

   b. complete blood count

   c. congenital blindness, complete report

8. If you were asked to make a photocopy of the patient's last CT, what would you be searching for?

   a. chemotherapy record

   b. connective tissue report

   c. computed tomography scan

ASSIGNMENT 4-3 ▸ CRITICAL THINKING: SOLVE AN OFFICE
PROBLEM

Performance Objective

Task: Answer questions after reviewing the case study using critical thinking skills.

Conditions: Use a case study and a pen or pencil.

Standards: Time: _____ minutes

                   Accuracy: _____

Directions. Answer questions after reviewing the case study using your critical thinking skills. Record your answer on the blank lines.

1. A patient comes into the office for treatment. He does not return, because he is dissatisfied with Dr. Practon's treatment. Is it necessary to keep his records when he

   obviously will not return? _____ Why?

   _____

   _____

ASSIGNMENT 4–4 ► ABSTRACT SUBJECTIVE OBSERVATIONS AND OBJECTIVE FINDINGS FROM PATIENT RECORDS

Performance Objective

Task: List subjective observations and objective findings after reading each
                    of the case studies.

Conditions: Use a pencil and four case studies.

Standards: Time: _____ minutes

                    Accuracy: _____

                    (Note: The time element and accuracy criteria may be given by your instructor.)

Case Study 1 Mrs. Smith is 25 years old and was brought into the emergency
department of College Hospital with complaints of difficulty breathing and chest pain. *S*
Her vital signs show an elevated temperature of 101° F and pulse rate of 90. Respirations *O*
are labored at 30/min. BP is 140/80. Her skin is warm and diaphoretic (perspiring). She *O*
states, "This condition has been going on for the past 3 days." *S*

Subjective observations: _____

Objective findings: _____

Case Study 2 Mr. Jones is 56 years old and was admitted to the hospital with chest pain
and elevated pulse and blood pressure. His skin is cold and clammy.

Subjective observations: _____

Objective findings: _____

Case Study 3 You are assisting the radiology technician with Sally Salazar, a 6-year-old
Hispanic girl who was brought into the pediatrician's office with a suspected fracture of
the right arm. Sally states she was "running at school, tripped on my shoelace, and fell."
She tells you her "arm hurts," points out how "funny my arm looks," and starts to cry.
You notice her arm looks disfigured and is covered with dirt. Sally is cradling her arm
against her body and is unwilling to let go because "it's going to fall off."

Subjective observations: _____

Objective findings: _____

Case Study 4 You are working in the business office of College Hospital. A former patient
in your hospital comes in complaining of his billing. He states he was never catheterized,
never had any of the medications listed on his itemized bill, and has "never been in this
hospital for that length of time." His face is red, his voice is gradually getting louder, and
you notice he is standing with the aid of crutches because his left leg is in a full cast.

Subjective observations: _____

Objective findings: _____

ASSIGNMENT 4-5 ▸ REVIEW OF A PATIENT RECORD

Performance Objective

Task: Answer questions after reviewing a patient's record.

Conditions: Use a pencil, internal record review sheet, medical dictionary, abbreviation reference list, drug reference book (i.e., *Mosby's MD Consult*), and laboratory reference book.

Standards: Time: _____ minutes

                 Accuracy: _____

                 (Note: The time element and accuracy criteria may be given by your instructor.)

Directions. In many instances, when developing the skill of reviewing a patient record, you may need critical thinking in addition to efficient use of reference books. Answer only those questions you think can be justified by the documentation presented in the patient's record. Because content of each record is variable, you may or may not have answers to all eight questions.

Answer the questions by recording on the blank the documentation found identifying the components from the patient's record.

If your answers vary, perhaps you have a reason for them that may or may not be valid. List your reasons in the response section. Differences may be reviewed with your instructor privately or via class discussion.

Patient Record

10-21-20xx   HPI This new pt is an 80-year-old white male who has had problems with voiding since 9-5-20xx.
During the night the pt had only 50 cc output and was catheterized this morning because of his poor urinary output (200 cc). He was thought to have a distended bladder; he complains of pressure in the suprapubic region. He has not had any gross hematuria. He has voiding difficulty especially lying down and voiding in the supine position. His voiding pattern is improved while standing and sitting.

Gene Ulibarri, MD

mtf

1. Location: In what body system is the sign or symptom occurring?

   Response: _____

2. Quality: Is the symptom or pain burning, gnawing, stabbing, pressure-like, squeezing, fullness?

   Response: _____

3. Severity: In this case, how would you rank the symptom (how was distress relieved) or pain (slight, mild, severe, persistent)?

   Response: _____

4. Duration: How long has symptom been present or how long does it last?

   Response: _____

5. Timing: When does(do) sign(s) or symptom(s) occur (AM, PM, after or before meals)?

   Response: _____

6. Context: Is the pain/symptom associated with big meals, dairy products, etc.?

   Response: _____

7. Modifying factors: What actions make symptoms worse or better?

   Response: _____

8. Associated signs and symptoms: What other system or body area produces complaints when the presenting problem occurs? (Example: chest pain leads to shortness of breath.)

   Response: _____

ASSIGNMENT 4-6 ▸ **KEY A LETTER OF WITHDRAWAL**

Performance Objective

Task: Key letter for physician's signature with envelope, prepare U.S. Postal Service forms, and complete an authorization form.

Conditions: Use one sheet of letterhead (print from CD or Evolve website), U.S. Postal Service forms for certified mail with return receipt requested (Figure 4–1), Authorization for Release of Information form (Figure 4–2), a number 10 envelope, thesaurus, English dictionary, medical dictionary, computer, printer, and pen or pencil.

Standards: Time: _____ minutes

              Accuracy: _____

              (Note: The time element and accuracy criteria may be given by your instructor.)

Directions. Mrs. McLean is negligent about following Dr. Ulibarri's advice after she received surgery. Refer to *Workbook* Assignment 7–2 for information from the patient record of Mrs. Merry M. McLean. Use a letterhead and type in modified block style an appropriate letter to Mrs. Mclean advising her of the doctor's withdrawal from the case (see *Handbook* Figure 4–23). Date the letter June 30 of the current year. Dr. Ulibarri will be available to this patient for 30 days after receipt of this letter.

     This letter must be prepared for Dr. Ulibarri's signature because it is a legal document. Type Mrs. McLean's address on a number 10 envelope, referring to *Workbook* Figure 4–3. Send the letter by certified mail with return receipt requested, referring to *Handbook* Figure 4–24, A–C, and enclose a completed Authorization for Release of Information form (see Figure 4–2).

     After the instructor has returned your work to you, either make the necessary corrections and place it in a three-ring notebook for future reference, or, if you receive a high score, place it in your portfolio for reference when applying for a job.

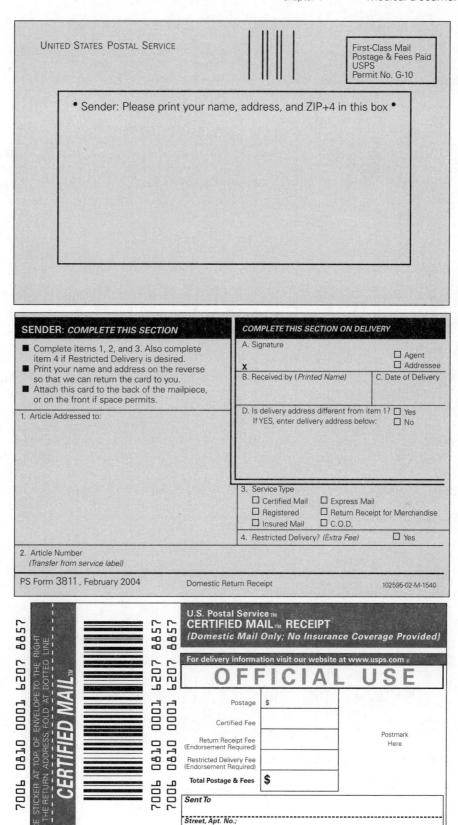

Figure 4–1

AUTHORIZATION FOR RELEASE OF INFORMATION

Section A: Must be completed for all authorizations.

I hereby authorize the use or disclosure of my individually identifiable health information as described below.
I understand that this authorization is voluntary. I understand that if the organization to receive the information is not a health plan or health care provider, the released information may no longer be protected by federal privacy regulations.

Patient name: _____   **ID Number:** _____

Persons/organizations providing information: **Persons/organizations receiving information:**
_____   _____
_____   _____
_____   _____

Specific description of information [including date(s)]: _____
_____

Section B: Must be completed only if a health plan or a health care provider has requested the authorization.

1. The health plan or health care provider must complete the following:
   a. What is the purpose of the use or disclosure? _____
   _____

   b. Will the health plan or health care provider requesting the authorization receive financial or in-kind compensation in exchange for using or disclosing the health information described above? Yes ____ No ____

2. The patient or the patient's representative must read and initial the following statements:
   a. I understand that my health care and the payment of my health care will not be affected if I do not sign this form.

   Initials: _____
   b. I understand that I may see and copy the information described on this form if I ask for it, and that I get a copy of this form after I sign it.

   Initials: _____

Section C: Must be completed for all authorizations.

The patient or the patient's representative must read and initial the following statements:

1. I understand that this authorization will expire on ____/____/____ (DD/MM/YR).

   Initials: _____
2. I understand that I may revoke this authorization at any time by notifying the providing organization in writing, but if I do not it will not have any effect on actions they took before they received the revocation.

   Initials: _____

_____   _____
Signature of patient or patient's representative   **Date**
(Form MUST be completed before signing)

Printed name of patient's representative: _____

Relationship to patient: _____

*YOU MAY REFUSE TO SIGN THIS AUTHORIZATION *
You may not use this form to release information for treatment or payment except when the information to be released is psychotherapy notes or certain research information.

Figure 4–2

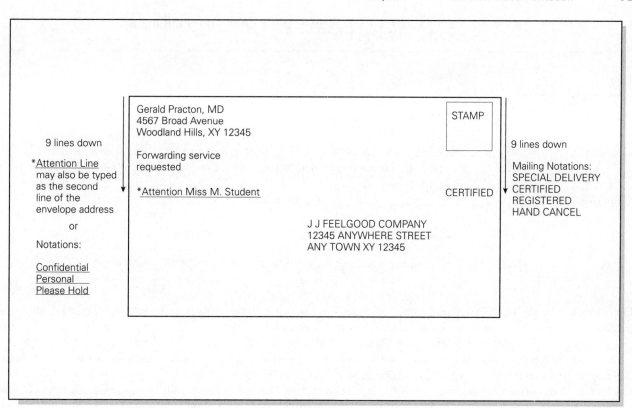

Figure 4–3

ASSIGNMENT **4–7 ▸ KEY A LETTER TO CONFIRM DISCHARGE BY THE PATIENT**

Performance Objective

Task: Key letter for the physician's signature.

Conditions: Use one sheet of letterhead (print from CD or Evolve website), number 10 envelope, and U.S. Postal Service forms for certified mail with return receipt requested (Figure 4–4).

Standards: Time: _____ minutes

                    Accuracy: _____

                    (Note: The time element and accuracy criteria may be given by your instructor.)

Directions. Mr. Walter J. Stone telephones on June 3, sounding extremely upset and irrational. He says that he is unable to return to work on June 22 and that he does not want to be seen by Dr. Input again. Type a letter to confirm this discharge by the patient (see *Handbook* Figure 4–25). Suggest that he contact the local medical society for the names of three internists for further care. This letter must be prepared for Dr. Input's signature because it is a legal document. Refer to Assignment 7–4 for information from the patient record. Use a letterhead and key in modified block style as shown in *Handbook* Figure 4–23. Use current date. Key Mr. Stone's address on a number 10 envelope, referring to *Workbook* Figure 4–3. Send the letter by certified mail with return receipt requested, referring to *Handbook* Figure 4–24, A–C.

After the instructor has returned your work to you, either make the necessary corrections and place it in a three-ring notebook for future reference, or, if you receive a high score, place it in your portfolio for reference when applying for a job.

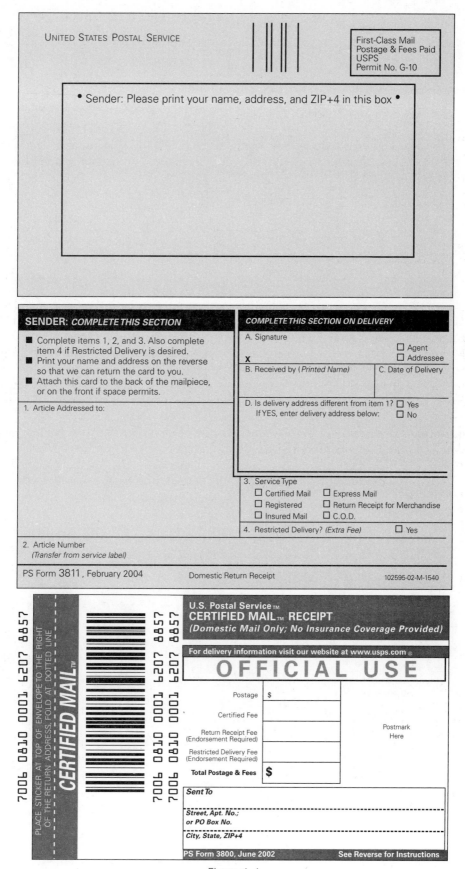

Figure 4–4

ALTAPOINT PRACTICE MANAGEMENT SOFTWARE ASSIGNMENTS

ASSIGNMENT 4-8 ▸ ENTER A NEW PATIENT INTO THE PRACTICE MANAGEMENT SYSTEM

Performance Objective

Task: Enter new patient data into the practice management system.

Conditions: Patient's information and computer

Standards: Time: _____ minutes

                   Accuracy: _____

(Note: The time element and accuracy criteria may be given by your instructor.)

Directions. Before attempting the Practice Management software assignment, refer to Appendix C and follow the instructions provided to familiarize yourself with the software. Then refer to the Practice Management software on the CD that accompanies the *Workbook*. For this assignment, follow the instructions for entering a new patient and enter the information for Denise L. Watson.

1. On page 1 of the patient screen, enter the following information:
   NAME: Denise L. Watson
   ADDRESS: 7229 Brighton Avenue
                  Midvale, UT 84047
   PHONE: (801) 555-7111
   DOB: 08/12/1980
   STATUS: Single
   SEX: Female
   RACE: Black
   PROVIDER: Jeffrey Lyndon, MD
   EMPLOYER: Alta Point Data

2. On the Billing page, enter the following information:
   FEE SCHEDULE: Standard
   INSURANCE COMPANY: United Mutual
   INSURED CODE: Self
   ID#:   8227-38
   GROUP #:   822-DL
   COPAY PER VISIT: $25.00
   DEDUCTIBLE: $500.00

Place a check mark in both "Signature on File" boxes. Place a check mark in the "Accept Assignment" box. Then click the "Accept" button at the bottom of the Billing page.

3. To obtain a grade, either print a hard copy of the patient information and billing page or have your instructor view the data onscreen for approval.

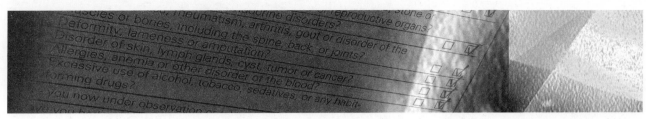

Diagnostic Coding

KEY TERMS

Your instructor may wish to select some words pertinent to this chapter for a test. For definitions of the terms, further study, and/or reference, the words, phrases, and abbreviations may be found in the glossary at the end of the Handbook. *Key terms for this chapter follow.*

adverse effect

benign tumor

chief complaint (CC)

combination code

complication

conventions

E codes

eponym

etiology

in situ

International Classification of Diseases, Ninth Revision, Clinical Modification (ICD-9-CM)

intoxication

italicized code

late effect

malignant tumor

metastasis

neoplasm

not elsewhere classifiable (NEC)

not otherwise specified (NOS)

physician's fee profile

poisoning

primary diagnosis

principal diagnosis

secondary diagnosis

slanted brackets

syndrome

V codes

KEY ABBREVIATIONS

AHA _____

AHIMA _____

ASCVD _____

ASHD _____

CC _____

CM _____

CMS _____

CPT _____

DRG _____

DSM-IV _____

E codes _____

ICD-9-CM _____

ICD-10-CM _____

ICD-10-PCS _____

IDDM (type 1 diabates) _____

LMRP _____

MRI _____

NCHS _____

NEC _____

NIDDM _____

NOS _____

SNOMED _____

V codes _____

PERFORMANCE OBJECTIVES

The student will be able to:

■ Define and spell the key terms and key abbreviations for this chapter, given the information from the *Handbook* glossary, within a reasonable time period and with enough accuracy to obtain a satisfactory evaluation.

■ Answer the fill-in-the-blank, multiple choice, and true/false review questions after reading the chapter, with enough accuracy to obtain a satisfactory evaluation.

■ Assignment 5–2: Indicate main terms, subterms, subterms to subterms, and carryover lines, given a section of a page from the ICD-9-CM code book, with enough accuracy to obtain a satisfactory evaluation.

■ Assignment 5–3: Answer questions given a section of a page from the ICD-9-CM code book, with enough accuracy to obtain a satisfactory evaluation.

■ Assignment 5–4: Select the correct diagnostic code numbers, given diagnoses, and locate the conditions using Volumes 1 and 2 of the ICD-9-CM code book, with enough accuracy to obtain a satisfactory evaluation.

■ Assignments 5–5 through 5–12: Select the correct diagnostic code numbers, given a series of scenarios and diagnoses using Volumes 1 and 2 of the ICD-9-CM code book, with enough accuracy to obtain a satisfactory evaluation.

ALTAPOINT PRACTICE MANAGEMENT SOFTWARE OBJECTIVES

The student will be able to:

● Add new diagnostic codes into the practice management system.

STUDY OUTLINE

The Diagnostic Coding System
 Sequencing of Diagnostic Codes
 Reasons for the Development and Use of
  Diagnostic Codes
 Physician's Fee Profile
History of Coding Diseases
International Classification of Diseases
 History
 Organization and Format
 Contents
Diagnostic Code Book Conventions
 General Coding Guidelines

Rules for Coding
 Signs, Symptoms, and Ill-Defined Conditions
 Sterilization
 Neoplasms
 Circulatory System Conditions
 Diabetes Mellitus
 Pregnancy, Delivery, or Abortion
 Admitting Diagnoses
 Burns
 Injuries and Late Effects
ICD-10-CM Diagnosis and Procedure Codes
Procedure: Basic Steps in Selecting Diagnostic Codes

 A S S I G N M E N T 5–1 ▸ **REVIEW QUESTIONS**

Part I Fill in the Blank on ICD-9-CM

  Review the objectives, key terms, and chapter information before completing the following review questions.

1. When submitting insurance claims for patients seen in a physician's office or in an outpatient hospital setting, the ___primary___ diagnosis is listed first but in the inpatient hospital setting, the ___principal___ diagnosis is used.

2. For retrieving types of diagnoses related to pathology by an institution within an institution, the coding system is found in a book entitled

   ___ICD-9-CM___.

3. The system for coding and billing diagnoses is found in a book entitled

   ___ICD-9-CM___.

4. The abbreviation ICD-9-CM means

   ___International Classification of Diseases, 9th Edition Revision clinical Modification___

5. Volume 1, Diseases, is a/an ___Tabular___ listing of code numbers.

6. Volume 2, Diseases, is a/an ___Alphabetic___ index or listing of code numbers.

7. The coding in ICD-9-CM varies from ___3___ to ___5___ digits.

8. The abbreviation *NEC* appearing in the ICD-9-CM code book means

   ___Not Elsewhere classified___.

9. To code using Volume 2, the Alphabetic Index, the main term, the

    <u>Disease</u> is looked up rather than the anatomic part.

10. E codes are a supplementary classification of coding for <u>External Cause</u>

    rather than disease and of coding for <u>Poisonings</u>.

Part II Multiple Choice on ICD-10

Directions: Choose the best answer.

11. ICD-10-PCS (Procedure Coding System) was developed by 3M Health Information systems under contract with the

    a. National Center for Health Statistics

     b. World Health Organization

    c. Centers for Disease Control

    d. Centers for Medicare and Medicaid Services

12. The disease codes in ICD-10-CM have a maximum of

    a. three digits

    b. four digits

    c. five digits

     d. six digits

    e. seven digits

13. One of the reasons for ICD-10-PCS is that

     a. ICD-9-CM was not capable of necessary expansion

    b. ICD-9-CM was not as comprehensive as it should be

    c. ICD-9-CM included diagnostic information

    d. all of the above

14. Certain conditions are classified according to the cause of the disorder, which is called the

    a. pathology

    b. etiology

    c. etymology

    d. histology

15. When two diagnoses are classified with a single code number, this is called a

    a. code set

    b. complication code

    c. combination code

    d. category code

Part III True/False

Write "T" or "F" in the blank to indicate whether you think the statement is true or false.

___T___ 16. It is permissible to use a zero as a filler character when listing a diagnostic code number on a claim form.

___T___ 17. When a person who is not currently sick encounters health services for some specific purpose, such as to receive a vaccination, then a V code is used.

P133

___F___ 18. Code conventions are rules or principles for determining a diagnostic code when using a diagnostic code book.

P133

___F___ 19. Because there are annual ICD-9-CM code revisions, there is a 3-month grace period to implement these changes and revisions.

P140

___T___ 20. An E code may never be sequenced as the primary diagnosis in the first position.

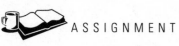

A S S I G N M E N T   5–2 ▶ **IDENTIFY FORMAT COMPONENTS OF ICD-9-CM, VOLUME 2**

Performance Objective

Task: Identify seven format components of ICD-9-CM, Volume 2.

Conditions: Use the abstracted section from ICD-9-CM, Volume 2, and pen or pencil.

Standards: Time: _____ minutes

                   Accuracy: _____

                   (Note: The time element and accuracy criteria may be given by your instructor.)

Directions. Label the line indicated as either main term, subterm, subterm of subterm, or carryover line. Refer to Chapter 5 in the *Handbook*, section on "Diabetes Mellitus," and locate Figure 5–3, which graphically illustrates the format components.

1. *main* ──────────▶ **Saccharomyces** infection (*see also*
2. *Carryover line* ──────▶ Candidiasis) 112.9
   Sacroiliitis NEC 720.2
   Sacrum—*see* condition
   Saddle
3. *subterm* ──────────▶ back 737.8
   embolus, aorta 444.0
   nose 738.0
4. *subterm of subterm* ──────▶ congenital 754.0
   due to syphilis 090.5
5. *subterm* ──────▶ Salicylism
   correct substance properly administered
   535.4
   Salmonella choleraesuis (enteritidis)
6. *Carryover line* ──────▶ (gallinarum) (suipestifer)
   (typhimurium) (see also Infection Salmonella) 003.9
7. *subterm* ──────────▶ arthritis 003.23
   carrier (suspected) of V02.3

ASSIGNMENT 5–3 ▸ LOCATING INFORMATION IN ICD-9-CM, VOLUME 2

Performance Objective

Task: Answer questions pertaining to categories **320** and **321** of ICD-9-CM, Volume 2.

Conditions: Use abstracted section from ICD-9-CM, Volume 2 (Figure 5–1) and pen or pencil.

on other side→

Standards: Time: _____ minutes

Accuracy: _____

(Note: The time element and accuracy criteria may be given by your instructor.)

Directions. Refer to a section from a page of ICD-9-CM, Volume 2 (see Figure 5–1), and answer questions pertaining to categories 320 and 321.

1. Locate the section title *Inflammatory Diseases of the Central Nervous System*

2. Refer to the INCLUSION TERMS listed under category code 320, entitled "Bacterial meningitis." Place an "X" in front of each of the following diagnostic statements that are included in category 320.

   _____ purulent meningitis

   X_____ bacterial meningomyelitis ✓

   X_____ meningitis

   X_____ meningoencephalitis ✓

   _____ pyogenic meningitis

   _____ meningococcal

3. Refer to the EXCLUSION TERMS located under code 320.7, entitled "Meningitis in other bacterial diseases classified elsewhere." Place an "X" in front of the following code number(s) which are excluded.

   _____X_____ secondary syphilis 091.81

   _____ acquired syphilis 097.9

   _____X_____ gonococcal meningitis 098.82

   _____X_____ congenital syphilis 090.42

   _____ primary syphilis 091.2

   _____ gram-negative anaerobes 320.81

6. NERVOUS SYSTEM
AND SENSE ORGANS (320-389)

INFLAMMATORY DISEASES OF THE CENTRAL
NERVOUS SYSTEM (320-326)

320 Bacterial meningitis
Includes: arachnoiditis
leptomeningitis
meningitis   } bacterial
meningoencephalitis
meningomyelitis
pachymeningitis

320.0 *Haemophilus* meningitis
Meningitis due to *Haemophilus
influenzae* [*H. Influenzae*]

320.1 Pneumococcal meningitis

320.2 Streptococcal meningitis

320.3 Staphylococcal meningitis

**320.7 Meningitis in other bacterial
diseases classified elsewhere**

Code first underlying diseases as:
actinomycosis (039.8)
listeriosis (027.0)
typhoid fever (002.0)
whooping cough (033.0-033.9)
Excludes: *meningitis (in):*
epidemic (036.0)
gonococcal (098.82)
meningococcal (036.0)
salmonellosis (003.21)
syphilis:
NOS (094.2)
congenital (090.42)
meningovascular (094.2)
secondary (091.81)
tuberculous (013.0)

320.8 Meningitis due to other specified bacteria

320.81 Anaerobic meningitis
Bacteroides (fragilis)
Gram-negative anaerobes

**320.82 Meningitis due to gram-
negative bacteria, not elsewhere
classified**
*Aerobacter   Klebsiella
aerogenes   pneumoniae
Escherichia coli   Proteus
[E. coli]   morganii
Friedländer   Pseudomonas
bacillus*

Excludes: *gram-negative
anaerobes (320.81)*

**320.89 Meningitis due to other specified
bacteria**
Bacillus pyocyaneus

**320.9 Meningitis due to unspecified
bacterium**
Meningitis:
bacterial NOS
purulent NOS
pyogenic NOS
suppurative NOS

321 Meningitis due to other organisms
Includes: arachnoiditis   }
leptomeningitis   } due to organisms
meningitis   } other than bacteria
pachymeningitis   }

321.0 Cryptococcal meningitis
Code first underlying disease (117.5)

Figure 5–1

4. Place an "X" in front of each of the following diagnostic statements included in category code 320 and its subcategories.

_____X_____ leptomeningitis

_____X_____ meningitis resulting from *E. coli*

_____X_____ pyogenic meningitis

_____ epidemic meningitis ✓

_____ tuberculous meningitis ✓

5. Write the code numbers for category 320 that require fifth digits.

_____

DIAGNOSTIC CODING ASSIGNMENTS

In this chapter, the points awarded for assignments that require diagnostic codes are 1 point for each correct digit.

A S S I G N M E N T 5 – 4 ▸ **OBTAIN GENERAL DIAGNOSTIC CODES FOR CONDITIONS**

Performance Objective

Task: Locate the correct diagnostic code for each diagnosis listed.

Conditions: Use pen or pencil and ICD-9-CM diagnostic code book.

Standards: Time: _____ minutes

                   Accuracy: _____

                   (Note: The time element and accuracy criteria may be given by your instructor.)

Directions. Using the *International Classification of Diseases, Ninth Revision, Clinical Modification* (ICD-9-CM) code book, read each diagnosis and locate the condition in Volume 2, the alphabetical index. Then go to Volume 1, to the Tabular List of Diseases. Match the definition to the written description as close as possible and assign the correct code, entering it on the blank line.

Problems

1. Breast mass   611.72

2. *Klebsiella* pneumonia   482.0

3. Acute lateral wall myocardial infarction; initial episode   410.5

4. Acute cerebrovascular accident   434.91

5. Arteriosclerotic cardiovascular disease   429.2

6. Dyspnea, R/O cystic fibrosis   300.11

7. Ileitis   558.9

8. Arthritis of elbow   716.9

9. Ringing in the ears   388.30

10. Acute exacerbation of chronic asthmatic bronchitis   493.9

ASSIGNMENT **5-5** ▸ **CODE DIAGNOSES FROM MEDICAL RECORDS**

Performance Objective

Task: Locate the correct diagnostic code for each case scenario.

Conditions: Use pen or pencil and ICD-9-CM diagnostic code book.

Standards: Time: _____ minutes

                Accuracy: _____

                (Note: The time element and accuracy criteria may be given by your instructor.)

Directions. This exercise will give you experience in basic diagnostic coding for physicians' insurance claims. First list the ICD-9-CM code for the diagnosis, condition, problem, or other reason for the admission and/or encounter (visit) shown in the medical record to be chiefly responsible for the services provided. Then list additional diagnostic codes that describe any coexisting conditions that affect patient care. Always assign codes to their highest level of specificity—the more digits, the more specific. Do not code probable, rule out, suspected, or questionable conditions. Assign the correct code(s), entering it (them) on the blank line.

Problems:

Problem 1. A patient, Mrs. Jennifer Hanson, calls Dr. Input's office stating she has blood in her stool. Dr. Input suspects a GI bleed and tells Mrs. Hanson to come in immediately. It is discovered that the reason for the blood in the stool is a bleeding duodenal ulcer. Code the diagnosis to be listed on the insurance claim for the office visit.

                _____

Problem 2. a. Jason Belmen comes in with a fractured humerus. He also has chronic obstructive pulmonary disease (COPD), which is not treated. Code the diagnosis.

                a. _____

b. Assume Mr. Belmen needs general anesthesia for open reduction of the fractured humerus. The COPD could now be considered a risk factor. List the diagnostic code in the second part of this scenario.

                b. _____

Problem 3. Margarita Sanchez came into the office for removal of sutures. Code the diagnosis.

                _____

Problem 4. A patient, George Martin, has benign prostatic hypertrophy (BPH). He is seen for catheterization because of urinary retention. Code the primary and secondary diagnoses for the office visit. (Note: BPH is an enlargement of the prostate gland, due to overgrowth of androgen-sensitive glandular elements, which occurs naturally with aging.)

                a. _____

                b. _____

Problem 5. Mia Bartholomew is seen in the office complaining of a sore throat. A throat culture is done and the specimen is sent to an outside laboratory for a culture and sensitivity study to determine the presence of *Streptococcus*. List the diagnostic code the physician would use if the insurance claim is submitted before the results are known.

                a. _____

List the diagnostic code if the physician submits the insurance claim after the laboratory report is received indicating *Streptococcus* is present.

                b. _____

ASSIGNMENT 5-6 ▸ CODE DIAGNOSES USING V CODES

Performance Objective

Task: Locate the correct diagnostic code for each case scenario.

Conditions: Use pen or pencil and ICD-9-CM diagnostic code book.

Standards: Time: _____ minutes

                      Accuracy: _____

                      (Note: The time element and accuracy criteria may be given by your instructor.)

Directions. In this exercise you will be reviewing V codes in the ICD-9-CM code book. Assign the correct code, entering it on the blank line. These are some key words under which V codes may be located in Volume 2:

admission	checking/checkup	donor	insertion of	status post
aftercare	conflict	evaluation	maintenance	vaccination
attention to	contact	examination	observation	
border	contraception	fitting of	person with	
care of	counseling	follow-up	problem with	
carrier	dialysis	history of	screening	

Problems:

1. Kathy Osborn, a patient, is seen in the office for an annual checkup.   _____.

2. Daniel Matsui is seen in the office for adjustment of a lumbosacral corset.   _____.

3. Philip O'Brien comes into the office to receive a prophylactic flu shot.   _____.

4. Bernadette Murphy is seen in the office for a pregnancy test.   _____.

5. Michiko Fujita is seen in the office for a fractured rib.   a. _____
   No x-rays are taken because Mrs. Fujita thinks she
   is pregnant.   b. _____

6. Dr. Perry Cardi sees Kenneth Pickford in the office for cardiac
   pacemaker adjustment. The pacemaker was implanted because
   of sick sinus syndrome.   _____

7. Frank Meadows returns for follow-up, postoperative transurethral   a. _____
   prostatic resection (TURP) for prostate cancer after treatment
   has been completed.   b. _____

ASSIGNMENT **5-7** ▸ **CODE NEOPLASTIC DIAGNOSES**

___

Performance Objective

Task: Locate the correct diagnostic code for each diagnosis listed.

Conditions: Use pen or pencil and ICD-9-CM diagnostic code book.

Standards: Time: _____ minutes

                   Accuracy: _____

                   (Note: The time element and accuracy criteria may be given by your instructor.)

Directions. In this exercise, you will be reviewing diagnostic codes in the ICD-9-CM code book involving neoplasms. The morphology of neoplasm is found in Appendix A of Volume 1. Neoplasms are classified according to their histology. Morphology (M) codes are sometimes used to supplement a diagnostic code. M codes are not used on insurance forms when submitting claims by physicians; therefore, they will not be used in this assignment. M codes are never used as a primary diagnostic code. Assign the correct code, entering it on the blank line.

1. Leiomyoma, uterus   _____

2. Ewing's sarcoma, forearm   _____

3. Adenocarcinoma, right breast, central portion   _____

4. Dyspnea resulting from carcinoma of the breast with metastasis   a. _____
   to the lung
                                                                       b. _____

5. Patient is seen for a yearly examination 1 year after a mastectomy   a. _____
   for breast cancer; she is disease-free at this time.
                                                                       b. _____

6. Patient comes in for chemotherapy because of lymphosarcoma   a. _____
   of the intrathoracic lymph nodes
                                                                       b. _____

ASSIGNMENT 5-8 ▸ CODE DIAGNOSES FOR PATIENTS WITH DIABETES

Performance Objective

Task: Locate the correct diagnostic code for each diagnosis listed.

Conditions: Use pen or pencil and ICD-9-CM diagnostic code book.

Standards: Time: _____ minutes

Accuracy: _____

(Note: The time element and accuracy criteria may be given by your instructor.)

Directions. In this exercise, you will review diagnostic codes in the ICD-9-CM code book involving cases of patients with diabetes. When coding diabetes, first find out the type of diabetes being treated, type I or type II. Then look to see whether the diabetes is under control. These two answers determine the assignment of the fifth digit.

For diabetic complications, determine whether the complication is due to the diabetes and whether the diabetes is out of control. These points need to be regarded as two distinctly different issues. A patient can have controlled diabetes but still have a complication caused by diabetes. Complications arising from diabetes must be coded. The code for the complication is listed after the subterm in brackets.

Example: If a patient with type II uncontrolled diabetes is treated for a skin ulcer on the lower extremity, look up "diabetes" in Volume 2 and find the subterm "ulcer." The diabetes code listed is 250.8 and under the subterm "ulcer" is a sub-subterm of "lower extremity" with the code 707.1 in brackets. Go to Volume 1 and verify the diabetes code and assign a fifth digit. The correct code is 250.82 (2 for type II, uncontrolled). Now verify the ulcer code in Volume 1. You will see that code 707.1 does not mention diabetes. If diabetes is the cause of the ulcer, code the diabetes first and the ulcer second. If the patient's diabetes is under control and is not being treated at the visit, code the ulcer first and diabetes second as an underlying disease. Other complications, such as bone changes (731.8) may tell you to code the underlying disease first. Therefore, always verify all codes in Volume 1 before assigning them.

Assign the correct code(s) for each case involving diabetes, entering it (them) on the blank line.

1. Diabetes mellitus _____

2. Uncontrolled non–insulin-dependent diabetes mellitus
   with ketoacidosis _____

3. Diabetic gangrene (type I diabetes, out of control) a. _____

   b. _____

4. Controlled type II diabetes with cataract a. _____

   b. _____

5. Type I diabetes with diabetic polyneuropathy and retinopathy a. _____

   b. _____

   c. _____

   d. _____

ASSIGNMENT 5–9 ▸ CODE DIAGNOSES FOR PATIENTS WITH HYPERTENSION

Performance Objective

Task: Locate the correct diagnostic code for each diagnosis listed.

Conditions: Use pen or pencil and ICD-9-CM diagnostic code book.

Standards: Time: _____ minutes

                   Accuracy: _____

(Note: The time element and accuracy criteria may be given by your instructor.)

Directions. In this exercise, you will review diagnostic codes in the ICD-9-CM code book involving patients who have hypertension. To begin coding, look in Volume 2 under "hypertension" and find the Hypertension Table. This is designed to simplify coding conditions caused by, or associated with, hypertension or hypertensive disease. At the beginning of the table, many terms are listed in parentheses. These terms are nonessential modifiers, which means that the absence or presence of one of these terms does not change the meaning of the code. From the table, the codes relating to hypertension begin with 401. Go to this number in Volume 1 and look through this section to become familiar with it.

Assign the correct code(s) for each case, entering it (them) on the blank line.

1. High blood pressure   _____

2. Malignant hypertension   _____

3. Antepartum hypertension complicating pregnancy   _____

4. Hypertension with kidney disease   _____

5. Hypertension due to arteriosclerotic cardiovascular
   disease (ASCVD) and congestive heart failure (CHF)   _____

6. Myocarditis and CHF due to malignant hypertension   a. _____

                                                            b. _____

ASSIGNMENT 5-10 ▸ CODE DIAGNOSES FOR INJURIES, FRACTURES, BURNS, LATE EFFECTS, AND COMPLICATIONS

Performance Objective

Task: Locate the correct diagnostic code for each diagnosis listed.

Conditions: Use pen or pencil and ICD-9-CM diagnostic code book.

Standards: Time: _____ minutes

                     Accuracy: _____

                     (Note: The time element and accuracy criteria may be given by your instructor.)

Directions. In this exercise, you will review diagnostic codes from the ICD-9-CM code book involving patients who have suffered injuries, burns, fractures, and late effects. Some guidelines for coding injuries, fractures, burns, late effects, and complications are:

Injuries

✔ Code injuries separately according to their general type and then by anatomic site. Fifth digits are commonly used in the injury section to specify anatomic sites and severity.
✔ Code injuries separately if they are classifiable to more than one subcategory unless the diagnosis does not support separate injuries or the Alphabetic Index provides instructions to use combination code.

Fractures

✔ Fractures are presumed to be closed unless otherwise specified.
✔ Fracture/dislocations are coded as fractures.
✔ Pathologic fractures are coded first and the cause (disease process) coded second.

Burns

✔ Multiple burns at the same site, but of different degrees, are coded to the most severe degree.

✔ Code the extent of body surface involved (percentage of body surface), when specified, as an additional code.

Late Effects

✔ A residual, late effect is defined as the current condition resulting from a previous acute illness or injury that is no longer the current problem. Late effects are coded using the residual or late effect as the primary diagnosis. The cause of the residual or late effect is coded second.

Complications

✔ For conditions resulting from the malfunction of internal devices, use the subterm "mechanical" found under the main term "complication."
✔ Postoperative complications are sometimes found under the subterm "postoperative," which appears under the main term identifying the condition. If not found there, look for a subterm identifying the type of procedure, type of complication, or surgical procedure under the main term "complication."

Assign the correct code(s) for each case, entering it (them) on the blank line.

1. Supracondylar fracture of right femur   _____

2. Fracture of left humerus and left foot   a. _____

                                                       b. _____

3. Comminuted fracture of left radius and ulna   _____

4. Pathologic fracture of right hip due to drug-induced osteoporosis   a. _____

                                                       b. _____

5. Lacerations of arm, with embedded glass   _____

6. Burns on the face and neck   _____

7. Second- and third-degree burns on chest wall; 20% of body
   involved, 10% third-degree   a. _____

   b. _____

8. Bursitis of the knee resulting from crushing injury to the knee 1 year ago   a. _____

   b. _____

A S S I G N M E N T 5–11 ▸ CODE DIAGNOSES FOR PREGNANCY, DELIVERY,
AND NEWBORN CARE

Performance Objective

Task: Locate the correct diagnostic code for each case scenario.

Conditions: Use pen or pencil and ICD-9-CM diagnostic code book.

Standards: Time: _____ minutes

                       Accuracy: _____

                       (Note: The time element and accuracy criteria may be given by your instructor.)

Directions. In this exercise, you will review diagnostic codes from the ICD-9-CM code book involving patients who have conditions involving pregnancy and delivery, and newborn infants.

For the supervision of a normal pregnancy, turn to Volume 2 and look up "pregnancy." This is a long category. Look up the subterm "supervision" and find the sub-subterm "normal" (NEC V22.1) and "first" (V22.0). Check Volume 1 to verify these codes. Also see code V22.2 "pregnancy state, incidental." This code is used in the second position to tell the insurance carrier that the patient is pregnant in addition to any other diagnosis.

If a patient develops complications, turn to Volume 2 and look under the main term "pregnancy." Find the subterm "complicated by," and find the sub-subterm stating the complication. These are codes from ICD-9-CM Chapter 11: "Complications of Pregnancy, Childbirth, and Puerperium" (630-677).

Delivery in a completely normal case is coded 650 and is listed under the main term "delivery, uncomplicated." Normal is described as "delivery without abnormality or complication and with spontaneous cephalic delivery, without mention of fetal manipulation or instrumentation." A different code must be used to describe any complication or deviation from this description of normal.

When coding deliveries, always include a code for the status of the infant. Look up "outcome of delivery" in Volume 2 and you will find various V27 codes listing possible outcomes. These codes would be listed as secondary codes on the insurance claim form for the delivery.

On the insurance claim form for the newborn, turn to "newborn" in Volume 2. You will find V codes from V30.X to V39.X describing the birth of the newborn. Use these codes in the first position when billing for services for the newborn infant.

Assign the correct code(s) for each case entering it (them) on the blank line.

1. A pregnant patient who is due to deliver in 6 weeks presents in the office with preeclampsia.   _____

2. A patient presents with a chief complaint of severe episodes of pain and vaginal hemorrhage. The physician determines that the patient has an incomplete spontaneous abortion complicated by excessive hemorrhage; she was 6 weeks' pregnant.   _____

3. A patient comes in who is diagnosed with a kidney stone; the patient   a. _____
   is also pregnant.

                                                                              b. _____

4. A patient delivers twins by cesarean section because of   a. _____
   cephalopelvic disproportion, which caused an obstruction.

                                                                              b. _____

                                                                              c. _____

ASSIGNMENT 5-12 ▸ CODE DIAGNOSES USING E CODES

Performance Objective

Task: Locate the correct diagnostic code for each diagnosis listed.

Conditions: Use pen or pencil and the ICD-9-CM diagnostic code book.

Standards: Time: _____ minutes

                   Accuracy: _____

                   (Note: The time element and accuracy criteria may be given by your instructor.)

Directions. In this exercise you will be reviewing diagnostic codes from the ICD-9-CM code book involving patients who may have been in an accident, had an adverse effect from ingesting a toxic substance, or suffered an injury. Read the definitions for poisoning and drug intoxication in the *Handbook*.

✔ E codes are not used to describe the primary reason for a patient's visit but identify external environmental events, circumstances, and conditions as the cause of injury, poisoning, and other adverse effects (unfavorable results).

✔ E codes that identify external environmental events, such as an injury, are used only as supplemental codes to describe how an injury occurred. These codes are listed in the back of Volume 2 and provide a more descriptive clinical picture for the insurance carrier.

They may or may not be required and in some cases may speed up the payment of the claim.

✔ E codes are used for coding adverse effects of drugs and chemicals but are not required when coding a poisoning. Use the Table of Drugs and Chemicals at the back of Volume 2 and go to the column titled "Therapeutic Use." In addition, it is necessary to use a code to describe the adverse effect of using a particular drug or medicine. Find this in Volume 2 and verify it in Volume 1.

Assign the correct code(s) for each case and enter it (them) on the blank line.

1. Light-headedness caused by digitalis intoxication

   a. _____

   b. _____

2. Treatment of a rash after an initial dose of penicillin is given

   a. _____

   b. _____

3. Accidental overdose of meperidine (Demerol)

   a. _____

   b. _____

4. A 20-month-old baby accidentally ingests approximately 15 aspirin and is severely nauseated.

   a. _____

   b. _____

   c. _____

5. A patient presents in the physician's office with a vague complaint of not feeling well. The physician notices that the patient has ataxia (a staggering gait). After reviewing the patient's history, the physician determines the ataxia is due to the meprobamate the patient is taking.

a. _____

b. _____

6. Internal bleeding: abnormal reaction to a combination of chloramphenicol and warfarin (Coumadin)

a. _____

b. _____

c. _____

ALTAPOINT PRACTICE MANAGEMENT SOFTWARE ASSIGNMENTS

ASSIGNMENT 5–13 ▸ ADD DIAGNOSTIC CODES INTO THE PRACTICE MANAGEMENT SYSTEM

Performance Objective

Task: Add diagnostic codes into the practice management system.

Conditions: CPT procedure codes and computer

Standards: Time: _____ minutes

                Accuracy: _____

                (Note: The time element and accuracy criteria may be given by your instructor.)

Directions. Before attempting the Practice Management software assignment, refer to Appendix C and follow the instructions provided to familiarize yourself with the software. Then refer to the Practice Management software on the CD that accompanies the *Workbook*.

1. For this assignment, follow the instructions for adding diagnostic procedure codes to the AltaPoint code list. These codes may possibly be used for assignments that appear in subsequent chapters. Enter the following codes.

599.0	Urinary tract infection
891.0	Laceration/leg
825.25	Closed fracture metatarsus
680.2	Furuncle/back
786.52	Chest pain
724.2	Low back pain
802.0	Fractured nasal septum
V04.85	Encounter for flu shot
V06.1	Need for vaccination
E881.0	Fall from ladder

2. To obtain a grade, either print a hard copy of the diagnostic code list or have your instructor view the data onscreen for approval.

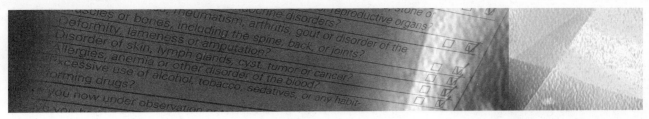

Procedural Coding

KEY TERMS

Your instructor may wish to select some words pertinent to this chapter for a test. For definitions of the terms, further study, and/or reference, the words, phrases, and abbreviations may be found in the glossary at the end of the Handbook. *Key terms for this chapter follow.*

alternative billing codes (ABCs)

bilateral

bundled codes

comprehensive code

conversion factor

Current Procedural Terminology (CPT)

customary fee

downcoding

fee schedule

global surgery policy

Healthcare Common Procedure Coding System (HCPCS)

modifier

procedure code numbers

professional component (PC)

reasonable fee

relative value studies (RVS)

relative value unit (RVU)

resource-based relative value scale (RBRVS)

surgical package

technical component (TC)

unbundling

upcoding

usual, customary, and reasonable (UCR)

KEY ABBREVIATIONS

See how many abbreviations and acronyms you can translate and then use this as a handy reference list. Definitions for the key abbreviations are located near the back of the Handbook *in the glossary.*

ABCs _____

AHA _____

AHIMA _____

CF _____

CPT _____

DME _____

ECG _____

ED _____

E/M services _____

EMTALA _____

EOB _____

FTC _____

GAF _____

GPCIs _____

HCPCS _____

HIPAA _____

NCCI edits _____

PC _____

PPS _____

RVS _____

RVU _____

RBRVS _____

TC _____

UCR _____

PERFORMANCE OBJECTIVES

The student will be able to:

■ Define and spell the key terms and key abbreviations for this chapter, given the information from the *Handbook* glossary, within a reasonable time period and with enough accuracy to obtain satisfactory evaluation.

■ Answer the fill-in-the-blank, mix and match, multiple choice, and true/false review questions after reading the chapter, with enough accuracy to obtain a satisfactory evaluation.

■ Select the 5-digit procedure code numbers, modifiers, and/or descriptors of each service, given

a series of problems relating to various medical procedures and services and using the *Current Procedural Terminology* (CPT) code book or the Mock Fee Schedule in Appendix A of the *Workbook*, with enough accuracy to obtain a satisfactory evaluation.

■ Fill in the correct meaning of each abbreviation given in a list of common medical abbreviations and symbols that appear in chart notes, with enough accuracy to obtain a satisfactory evaluation.

ALTAPOINT PRACTICE MANAGEMENT SOFTWARE OBJECTIVES

The student should be able to:

■ Add new CPT codes to the practice management system.

STUDY OUTLINE

Understanding the Importance of Procedural
  Coding Skills
Coding Compliance Plan
  Current Procedural Terminology
Methods of Payment
  Fee Schedule
  Usual, Customary, and Reasonable
  Developing a Fee Schedule Using Relative Value
    Studies Conversion Factors
Format and Content of the CPT Code Book
  Category I, II, and III Codes
  Code Book Symbols
  Evaluation and Management Section
  Surgery Section

Unlisted Procedures
Coding Guidelines for Code Edits
Code Monitoring
Helpful Hints in Coding
  Office Visits
  Drugs and Injections
  Adjunct Codes
  Basic Life or Disability Evaluation Services
Code Modifiers
  Correct Use of Common CPT Modifiers
  Comprehensive List of Modifier Codes
Procedure: Determine Conversion Factors
Procedure: Choose Correct Procedural Codes for
  Professional Services

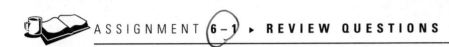

ASSIGNMENT 6–1 ► REVIEW QUESTIONS

Part I Fill in the Blank

Review the objectives, key terms, and chapter information before completing the following review questions.

1. The coding system used for billing professional medical services and procedures is

   found in a book entitled ~~ICD-9-CM~~ *Current Procedural Terminology*

2. The Medicare program uses a system of coding composed of two levels, and this is called ~~Resource Based RVS Relative Value Studies~~ ~~Resource Based~~ (RBRVS) (RBRVS) *Healthcare Common Procedure Coding system (HCPCS)*

3. A medical service or procedure performed that differs in some way from the code

   description may be shown by using a CPT code with a/an *modifier* .

4. A relative value scale or schedule is a listing of procedure codes indicating the relative

   value of services performed, which is shown by ~~RBRVS~~ *CPT Code book*

5. Name three methods for basing payments adopted by insurance companies and by state and federal programs.

   a. *usual fee*

   b. *customary fee*

   c. *reasonable fee*

6. List four situations that can occur in a medical practice when referring to charges and payments from a fee schedule.

   a. Providers participating in the Medicare Program would typically be paid by the fiscal agent an amount from a fee schedule for Medicare Patients

   b. Providers Not Participating in the Medicare Program would Be paid by the fiscal agent an amount based on limiting charges for each service set by Medicare

   c. Providers having a contractual arrangement w/a managed care plan would be paid based on the fee schedule written into the negotiated contract

   d. Providers rendering services to those who have sustained industrial injuries use a seperate workers' comp fee schedule

7. Name the eight main sections of CPT.

   a. CPT section Name

   b. Main Term

   c. Sub term

   d. ~~Subterm~~ SubSubterm

   e. procedure

   f. Condition

   g. description

   h. specialty

8. Name five hospital departments where critical care of a patient may take place.

   a. ER

   b. OR

   c. ICU

   d. neonatal ICU

   e. ~~Delivery~~ Labor /+ Delivery Room

9. A surgical package includes

   a. the operation

   b. local infiltration

   c. subsequent to the decision 4 surgery, 1 related E/M encounter on the date right before or on the date of procedure

d. immediate postop. care

e. writing orders

f. evaluat the patient in the recovery area

g. typical post operative follow-up care

10. Medicare global surgery policy includes

a. preoperative visits

b. Intraoperative services that are a usual & necessary part of the surgical Procedure

c. complications after surgery that don't require additional trips to the OR

d. Postoperative visits including hospital visits, discharge, & office visits for variable Post op. periods of time 0,10, 30, or 90 days

e. Writing orders

f. Evaluating the patient in the recovery area

g. Normal postop. pain management

11. A function of computer software that performs online checking of codes on an insurance claim to detect improper code submission is called a/an

National Correct Coding Initiative

12. A single code that describes two or more component codes bundled together as one unit is known as a/an Comprehensive coding .

13. Two group related codes together is commonly referred to as bundled codes

14. Use of many procedural codes to identify procedures that may be described by one code is termed unbundling .

15. A code used on a claim that does not match the code system used by the third party payer and is converted to the closest code rendering less payment is termed

down coding .

16. Intentional manipulation of procedural codes to generate increased reimbursement is called upcoding .

17. Give eight reasons for using modifiers on insurance claims.

a. A service or procedure has either a professional or technical component

b. A service or procedure was preformed by 1+ Dr's or In 1+ locations

c. A service or procedure has been increased or reduced

d. *A service or procedure has been provided more than once*

e. *only part of the service was provided performed*

f. *An adjunctive service was performed*

g. *A bilateral service was performed*

h. *unusual events occurred*

18. What modifier is usually used when billing for an assistant surgeon who is not in a teaching hospital?

-80

19. Explain when to use the -99 modifier code.

if a procedure requires more than 1 modifier

Part II Mix and Match

20. Match the symbol in the first column with the definitions in the second column. Write the correct letters on the blanks.

____D____ / ►◄   a. New code

____A____ / ●   b. Modifier -51 exempt

____f____ / ⊃   c. Add-on code

____B____ ∅   d. New or revised text

____C____ / +   e. Revised code

____e____ / ▲   f. Reference material

____ABg____ ⊙   g. Conscious sedation

21. Match the two-digit modifier in the first column with the definitions in the second column. Write the correct letters on the blanks.

____F____ -21   a. Unusual procedural services

____A____ -22   b. Multiple procedures

____e____ -25   c. Staged or related procedure

____H____ -26   d. Decision for surgery

____B____ -51   e. Significant, separately identifiable E/M service by the same physician on the same day of the procedure or other service

____g____ -52   f. Prolonged evaluation and management services

____D____ -57   g. Reduced services

____C____ -58   h. Professional component

Part III Multiple Choice Questions

Choose the best answer.

22. The codes used to bill ambulance services, surgical supplies, and durable medical equipment are

    a. CPT codes

    b. alternative billing codes

    c. Level I HCPCS CPT codes

    d. Level II HCPCS national codes

23. A complex reimbursement system in which three fees are considered in calculating payment is known as

    a. usual, customary, and reasonable (UCR)

    b. relative value schedule (RVS)

    c. resource-based relative value scale (RBRVS)

    d. relative value unit (RVU)

24. Medicare defines the postoperative global periods as

    a. 0, 25, 50, or 100 days

    b. 0, 10, 30, or 90 days

    c. 0, 10, 20, or 50 days

    d. 0, 20, 50, or 90 days

25. To code a bilateral procedure as two separate codes that includes the same surgical approach may be referred to as

    a. unbundling

    b. downcoding

    c. bundling

    d. upcoding

26. When two surgeons work together as primary surgeons performing distinct parts of a procedure and each doctor bills for performing their distinct part of the procedure, the CPT surgical code is listed with modifier

    a. -62

    b. -66

    c. -80

    d. -82

Part IV True/False

Write "T" or "F" in the blank to indicate whether you think the statement is true or false.

___T___ 27. Procedure coding is the transformation of written descriptions of procedures and professional services into numeric designations (code numbers).

___T___ 28. Category II codes describe clinical components that may be typically included in evaluation and management services or clinical services.

___F___ 29. When multiple lacerations have been repaired using the same technique and are in the same anatomic category, each repair should be assigned a code when billing an insurance claim.

___T___ 30. When listing a sterile tray for an in-office surgical procedure, the tray is bundled with the procedure unless additional supplies are needed in addition to those usually used.

___F___ 31. HCPCS Level II modifiers consist of only two alphanumeric characters.

ASSIGNMENT 6-2 ▸ **DEFINE MEDICAL ABBREVIATIONS**

To reinforce abbreviations you have learned, let's review some of those encountered during the *Workbook* assignments presented in this chapter. You should be able to decode these abbreviations without a reference. However, if you have difficulty with one or two, simply refer to Appendix A of this *Workbook*.

I & D — incision & drainage

IM — intramuscular (injection)

Pap — Pap smear

ER — emergency room

EEG — electroencephalograph

DPT — diphtheria, pertussis, tetanus

ECG — electrocardiogram

IUD — intrauterine device

OB — obstetrics & gynecology

D & C — dilatation & curettage

OV — office visit

KUB — kidneys, ureters, & bladder

GI — gastrointestinal

Hgb — Hemoglobin

new pt — new pint (?) patient

rt — right

UA — urinalysis

est pt — established patient

ASHD — arteriosclerotic heart disease

tet. tox. — tetanus toxoid

CBC — complete blood count

E/M — evaluation & management

CPT — Current Procedural terminology

Ob-Gyn — obstetrics & gynecology

TURP — transurethral resection of prostate

cm — centimeter

T & A — tonsillectomy & adenoidectomy

mL — milliliter

inj — injection

hx — history

NC — no charge

PROCEDURE CODING ASSIGNMENTS

In this chapter, the points awarded for assignments that require procedure codes are 1 point for each correct digit.

A S S I G N M E N T 6 – 3 ▸ **INTRODUCTION TO CPT AND CODING EVALUATION AND MANAGEMENT SERVICES**

Performance Objective

Task: Locate the correct information and/or procedure code for each question and/or case scenario.

Conditions: Use pen or pencil and the *Current Procedural Terminology* code book.

Standards: Time: _____ minutes

                 Accuracy: _____

                 (Note: The time element and accuracy criteria may be given by your instructor.)

1. To become acquainted with the sections of the *Current Procedural Terminology* code book, match the code number in the left column with the appropriate description in the right column by writing the letters in the blanks. Locate each code number in the *Current Procedural Terminology* code book. As you progress though the assignment, the problems get more difficult and complex.

   99231   _C_   a.   Chest x-ray

   59400   _e_   b.   Anesthesia for procedures on cervical spine and cord

   71010   _A_   c.   Subsequent hospital care

   00600   _B_   d.   Supplies and materials

   85025   _F_   e.   Routine OB care, ante- and postpartum

   99070   _D_   f.   CBC

2. Name the section of the CPT where each of the following codes is located.

   a. 65091 _eye - excision_____

   b. 86038 _antinuclear antibodies_____

   c. 92596 _ear measurements - Ear protector attenuation measurements_

   d. 75982 _Percutaneous placement of drainage catheter_____

   e. 0027T _____

   f. 01320 _Anesthesia 4all procedures on nerves, muscles, tendons, fascia,_

   g. 99321 _PF hx /exam LCDM | + bursae of knee +/or popliteal area_

   h. 0503F _____

3. Evaluation and Management (E/M) codes are used by physicians to report a significant portion of their services. Remember, it is the physician's responsibility to assign E/M codes, and the exercises presented are only for familiarization. The problems will acquaint you with terminology for this section of the CPT code book. Select the appropriate **new patient** office visit codes using the key components:

   a. This is a Level 3 case: Detailed history

      Detailed examination

      Low-complexity decision making   _99203_

   b. This is a Level 1 case: Problem-focused history

      Problem-focused examination

      Straightforward decision making   _99201_

   c. This is a Level 5 case: Comprehensive history

      Comprehensive examination

      High-complexity decision making   _99205_

4. Select the appropriate **established patient** office visit codes using the key components. Coding these cases illustrates consideration of two of three components.

   a. This is a Level 4 case: Detailed history

      Detailed examination

      Low-complexity decision making.   _99213_

   b. This is a Level 5 case: Comprehensive history

      Comprehensive examination

      Moderate-complexity decision making   _99214_

   c. This is a Level 5 case: Detailed history

      Comprehensive examination

      High-complexity decision making   _99215_

5. Evaluation and Management (E/M) codes **99201** to **99239** are used for services provided in the physician's office or in an outpatient or hospital facility. Read the brief statement and then locate the code number in the Current Procedural Terminology code book.

a. Office visit of a 20-year-old patient seen within the past 3 years for instruction in diabetes injection sites by RN (minimal problem). Patient not seen by physician at this brief visit.   99211

b. Office visit of a 30-year-old new patient with allergic rhinitis. This case had an expanded problem-focused hx & exam and straightforward decision making.   99201

c. Discussion of medication with the son of an 80-year-old patient with dementia on discharge from the observation unit.   99238

d. Admission to hospital of 60-year-old established patient in acute respiratory distress with bronchitis. Comprehensive hx & exam and medical decision making of moderate complexity.   99222

e. Hospital visit of a 4-year-old boy, now stable, who will be discharged the next day. This is a problem-focused interval hx & exam and medical decision making of low complexity.   99203

f. New patient seen in the office for chest pain, congestive heart failure, and hypertension. Comprehensive hx & exam and highly complex decision making.   99205

6. Evaluation and Management codes **99241** to **99275** are used for consultations provided in the physician's office or in an outpatient or inpatient hospital facility. A consultation is a service provided by a physician whose opinion about a case is requested by another physician. Read the brief statement and then locate the code number in the *Current Procedural Terminology* code book.

a. Office consultation for a 30-year-old woman complaining of palpitations and chest pains. Her family physician described a mild systolic click. This is an expanded problem-focused hx & exam and straightforward decision making.

99242

b. Follow-up inpatient consultation for a 64-year-old woman, who is now stable, admitted 2 days ago for a bleeding ulcer. This case is a problem-focused hx & exam and low-complexity decision making.

99251

c. Office consultation for a 14-year-old boy with poor grades in school and suspected alcohol abuse. This is a comprehensive hx & exam and medical decision making of moderate complexity.

99244

d. Follow-up inpatient consultation for a 70-year-old man who is diabetic and is suffering with fever, chills, gangrenous heel ulcer, rhonchi, and dyspnea (difficulty breathing), an unstable condition. The patient appears lethargic and tachypneic (rapid breathing). This case is detailed hx & exam with highly complex medical decision making.

99255

e. Initial emergency department consultation for a senior who presents with thyrotoxicosis, exophthalmos, cardiac arrhythmia, and congestive heart failure. This case is a comprehensive hx & exam with highly complex medical decision making.

99255

f. Initial hospital consultation for a 30-year-old woman, postabdominal surgery, who is exhibiting a fever. This case is an expanded problem-focused hx & exam and straightforward medical decision.

99252

7. Evaluation and Management codes **99281** to **99499** are used for emergency department, critical care, nursing facility, rest home, custodial care, home, prolonged, physician standby, and preventive medicine services. Read the brief statement and then locate the code number in the Current Procedural Terminology code book.

a. First hour of critical care of a senior who, following major surgery, suffers a cardiac arrest from a pulmonary embolus.

99291

b. A 40-year-old woman is admitted to the OB unit, and the primary care physician has requested the neonatologist to stand by for possible cesarean section and neonatal resuscitation. Code for a 1-hour standby.

99360

c. A child is seen in the emergency department with a fever, diarrhea, abdominal cramps, and vomiting. This case had an expanded problem-focused hx & exam and a moderately complex medical decision was made.

99283

d. A patient is seen for an annual visit at a nursing facility for detailed hx & comprehensive exam and straightforward medical decision making.

99304

e. An initial visit is made to a domiciliary care facility for a developmentally disabled individual with a mild rash on hands and face. This case had a problem-focused hx & exam and low-complexity medical decision making.

99324

f. A 50-year-old man with a history of asthma comes into the office with acute bronchospasm and moderate respiratory distress. Office treatment is initiated. The case requires intermittent physician face-to-face time with the patient for 2 hours and prolonged services. Assume the appropriate E & M code has been assigned for this case.

99354 x 1
99355 x 2

ASSIGNMENT **6–4 ▸ CODE ANESTHESIA PROBLEMS**

Performance Objective

Task: Locate the correct procedure and modifier, if necessary, for each question and/or case scenario.

Conditions: Use pen or pencil and *Current Procedural Terminology* code book.

Standards: Time: _____ minutes

                    Accuracy: _____

                    (Note: The time element and accuracy criteria may be given by your instructor.)

Directions. Anesthesia codes **00100** to **01999** may be used by anesthesiologists as well as physicians. Some plastic surgeons, other medical specialists, and large clinics may have a room set aside to perform surgical procedures that might be performed in a hospital outpatient surgical department. For Medicare claims, some regions do not use the Anesthesia Section of CPT for billing but use a surgical code with an HCPCS modifier appended. Read the brief statement and then locate the code number in the *Current Procedural Terminology* code book. Special modifiers **P1** through **P6** may be needed when coding for this section, as well as code numbers for cases that have difficult circumstances. Definitions for abbreviations may be found in Appendix A of this *Workbook*.

a. Cesarean delivery following neuraxial labor anesthesia, normal healthy patient   _____ _____
                                                                                     _____ _____

b. Reduction mammoplasty of a woman with mild systemic disease   _____ _____

c. Total right hip replacement, 71-year-old patient, normal healthy patient   _____ _____
                                                                                     _____

d. Repair of cleft palate, newborn infant, normal healthy patient   _____ _____
                                                                                     _____

e. TURP, normal healthy male   _____ _____

ASSIGNMENT 6-5 ▸ CODE SURGICAL PROBLEMS

Performance Objective

Task: Locate the correct procedure code and modifier, if necessary, for each question and/or case scenario.

Conditions: Use pen or pencil and *Current Procedural Terminology* code book.

Standards: Time: _____ minutes

                   Accuracy: _____

                   (Note: The time element and accuracy criteria may be given by your instructor.)

Directions. Surgery codes **10040** to **69979** are used for each anatomic part of the body. Read over each case carefully. It is preferable to use the *Current Procedural Terminology* code book, but if you do not have one then refer to the Mock Fee Schedule found in Appendix A of this *Workbook* to obtain the correct code number for each descriptor given. Full descriptors for services rendered have been omitted in some instances to give you practice in abstracting the correct descriptor from the available information. Indicate the correct two-digit modifier if necessary. The skill of critical thinking enters this section of the assignment, in that you may have to use your own judgment to code because the cases do not contain full details. Definitions for abbreviations may be found in Appendix A of this *Workbook*. Remember to use the index at the back of the CPT code book.

a. Suppose you work in an office that has an encounter form listing code 36530. Check your edition of CPT and see whether you can locate this code number. If the code does not appear, what code number are you directed to use? _____

Integumentary System 10040–19499

b. Removal of benign lesion from the back (1.0 cm) and left foot (0.5 cm) _____

_____ ____

c. Drainage of deep breast abscess _____

d. Laser destruction of two benign facial lesions _____

_____

Musculoskeletal System 20000–29909

e. Aspiration of fluid (arthrocentesis) from right knee joint; not infectious _____

f. Deep tissue biopsy of left upper arm _____

g. Fracture of the left tibia, closed treatment _____

   Does the procedural code include application and removal of the first cast? _____

   If done as an office procedure, may supplies be coded? _____

   If so, what is the code number from the Medicine section? _____

Does the procedural code include subsequent replacement of a cast for follow-up care?   _____

If not, list the code number for application of a walking short leg cast.   _____

Respiratory System 30000–32999

h. Parietal pleurectomy   _____

i. Removal of two nasal polyps, simple   _____

j. Diagnostic bronchoscopy with biopsy   _____

Cardiovascular System 33010–37799

k. Pacemaker insertion with transvenous electrode, atrial   _____

l. Thromboendarterectomy with patch graft   _____

m. Introduction of intracatheter and injection procedure for contrast venography   _____

Hemic/Lymphatic/Diaphragm 38100–39599

n. Repair, esophageal/diaphragmatic hernia transthoracic   _____

o. Partial splenectomy   _____

p. Excision, two deep cervical nodes   _____

Digestive System 40490–49999

q. T & A, 12-year-old boy   _____

r. Balloon dilation of esophagus   _____

Urinary System/Male and Female Genital 50010–55980

s. Removal of urethral diverticulum from female patient   _____

t. Anastomosis of single ureter to bladder   _____

Laparoscopy/Peritoneoscopy/Hysteroscopy/Female Genital/Maternity 56300–59899

u. Routine OB care, ante- and postpartum care   _____

v. Therapeutic D & C, nonobstetric   _____

ASSIGNMENT 6-6 ▸ CODE PROBLEMS FOR RADIOLOGY AND PATHOLOGY

Performance Objective

Task: Locate the correct procedure code and modifier, if necessary, for each question and/or case scenario.

Conditions: Use pen or pencil and *Current Procedural Terminology* code book.

Standards: Time: _____ minutes

                   Accuracy: _____

                   (Note: The time element and accuracy criteria may be given by your instructor.)

Radiologists as well as other physicians in many specialties perform these studies. A physician who interprets, dictates, and signs a report may not bill for the report separately because it is considered part of the radiology procedure.

Some medical practices perform basic laboratory tests under a waived test certificate that complies with the rules of the Clinical Laboratory Improvement Amendments (CLIA) of 1988, implemented in September 1992.

a. Upper GI x-ray study with films and KUB   _____

b. Ultrasound, pregnant uterus after first trimester, multiple gestation   _____

                                                                        _____

c. Routine urinalysis with microscopy, nonautomated   _____

d. Hemoglobin (Hgb), electrophoretic method   _____

ASSIGNMENT 6 - 7 ▸ **PROCEDURE CODE AND MODIFIER PROBLEMS**

Performance Objective

Task: Locate the correct procedure code and modifiers, if necessary, for each case scenario.

Conditions: Use pen or pencil and *Current Procedural Terminology* code book.

Standards: Time: _____ minutes

                       Accuracy: _____

                       (Note: The time element and accuracy criteria may be given by your instructor.)

Directions. Find the correct procedure codes and modifiers, if necessary. This assignment will reinforce what you have already learned about procedural coding, because code numbers for the case scenarios presented are located in all the sections of the CPT code book. Also search for codes in the Medicine Section, if necessary. The CPT list of modifiers may be found in the *Handbook.*

1. A new patient had five benign skin lesions on the right arm destroyed with surgical curettement. Complete the coding for the surgery.

   Code Number   *Description*

   a. _____   Level 3, detailed history and exam with
                                    low-complexity decision making, initial new
                                    pt office visit

   b. _____   Destruction of benign skin lesion rt arm

   c. _____   Destruction of second, third, fourth, and fifth
                                    lesions

2. Mrs. Stayman had four moles on her back. Dr. Davis excised the multiple nevi in one office visit.
   The information on the pathology report stated nonmalignant lesions measuring 2.2 cm, 1.5 cm, 1 cm, and 0.75 cm.

   Code Number   *Description*

   a. _____ _____   Initial OV

   b. _____   Excision, benign lesion 2.2 cm

   c. _____ _____   Excision, benign lesion 1.5 cm

   d. _____ _____   Excision, benign lesion 1 cm

   e. _____ _____   Excision, benign lesion 0.75 cm

   In another case, if a patient required removal of a 1-cm lesion on the back and a 0.5-cm lesion on the neck, the

   procedural codes would be _____ for the back lesion and _____ for the neck

   lesion.

3. Dr. Davis stated on his operative report that Mr. Allen was suffering from a complex, complicated nasal fracture. Dr. Davis debrided the wound, because it was contaminated, and performed an open reduction with internal fixation in a complex and complicated procedure.

Code Number	Description
_____ _____	Initial OV, complex hx & exam, moderate-complexity decision making
_____	Open tx nasal fracture complicated
_____ _____	Debridement, skin, subcutaneous tissue, muscle, and bone

4. An RN, an established patient (est pt), age 40 years, sees the doctor for an annual physical. A Pap (Papanicolaou) smear is obtained and sent to an outside laboratory. The patient also has a furuncle on the right axilla at the time of the visit, which the doctor incises and drains (I & D).

Code Number	Description
_____	Periodic physical examination
_____	Handling of specimen
_____	I & D, furuncle, right axilla
_____	5-mL penicillin inj IM

5. While making his rounds in the hospital during the noon hour, Dr. James sees a new patient in the ED (emergency department) for a laceration of the forehead, 5 cm long. The doctor does a workup for a possible concussion.

Code Number	Description
_____ _____	ED care, expanded problem-focused history, expanded problem-focused examination, low-complexity decision making
_____	Repair of laceration, simple, face

6. The physician sees a new patient in the office with the same condition as the patient in Problem 5; however, an infection has developed and the patient is seen for daily dressing changes. On day 11, the sutures are removed, and on day 12 a final dressing change is made, and the patient is discharged.

Code Number	Description
_____ _____	Level 3, detailed history and exam with low-complexity decision making, initial new patient office visit
_____	Repair of laceration
_____	Tet tox (tetanus toxoid) 0.5 cc
_____	Administration intramuscular injection
_____	Minimal service, OV, dressing change (2 days)
_____	OV, suture removal (4 days)

Note: Some fee schedules allow no follow-up days; Medicare fee schedule allows 10 follow-up days for the procedural code number for repair of laceration.

7. The physician sees 13-year-old Bobby Jones (est pt) for a Boy Scout physical. Bobby is in good health and well groomed. His troop is going for a 1-week camping trip in 12 days. The physician reviewed safety issues with Bobby, talked to him about school, and counseled him about not getting into drugs or alcohol. Bobby denied any problems with that or of being sexually active. He said that he plays baseball. He has no allergies. The physician performed a detailed examination. The physician completed information for scouting papers and cleared him for camping activity.

Code Number   *Description*

_____   Periodic preventive evaluation and management

8. A new patient, David Ramsey, age 15 years, was seen by Dr. Menter for lapses of memory and frequent headaches. The doctor performed an EEG (electroencephalogram) and some psychological tests (including psychodiagnostic assessment of personality and psychopathology tests [Rorschach and MMPI]). Dr. Astro Parkinson was called in as a consultant. All the tests were negative, and the patient was advised to come in for weekly psychotherapy.

Code Number   *Description*

Dr. Menter's bill:

_____   OV, comp hx & exam, moderate-complexity decision making

_____   EEG, extended monitoring (1 hr)

_____   Psychological tests (Rorschach and MMPI)

_____   Psychotherapy (50 min)

Dr. Parkinson's bill:

_____   Consultation, expanded problem-focused hx and exam
                                  straightforward decision making

9. An est pt, age 70 years, requires repair of a bilateral initial inguinal hernia. The code for this initial procedure is

_____ _____.

ASSIGNMENT 6–8 ▸ HCPCS/MODIFIER CODE MATCH

Performance Objective

Task: Locate the correct HCPCS code and modifier, if necessary, for each medical drug, supply item, or service presented.

Conditions: Use pen or pencil and HCPCS code reference list in Appendix B of this *Workbook*.

Standards: Time: _____ minutes

                    Accuracy: _____

                    (Note: The time element and accuracy criteria may be given by your instructor.)

Directions. Match the HCPCS code in the first or second column with the description of the drug, supply item, or service presented in the third or fourth column. Write the correct letters on the blanks.

E1280	_____	J0760	_____	a. Vitamin B12, 1000 mg	k. Blood (whole) for to transfusion/unit
E0141	_____	A9150	_____	b. injection, insulin per 5 units	l. Heavy duty wheelchair with detachable arms
J0290	_____	J2001	_____	c. Rigid walker, wheeled, without seat	m. Ampicillin inj, up to 500 mg
J3420	_____	L0160	_____	d. Waiver of liability statement on file	n. Dimethyl sulfoxide, DMSO inj
J1815	_____	L3100-RT	_____	e. Nonemergency transportation, taxi	o. Urine strips
P9010	_____	A4250	_____	f. Inj of colchicine	p. Vancomycin (Vancocin) inj
J1212	_____	J2590	_____	g. Cervical occipital/ mandibular support	q. Oxytocin (Pitocin) inj
J3370	_____	A4927	_____	h. Inj of lidocaine (Xylocaine)	r. Wide, heavy-duty wheelchair with detachable arms and leg rests
E1092	_____	A0100	_____	i. Gloves, nonsterile	s. Rt hallux valgus night splint
A4211	_____	-GA	_____	j. supplies for self-administered injections	t. Aspirin, nonprescription drug

ASSIGNMENT 6-9 ▸ PROCEDURAL CODING CASE SCENARIOS

Performance Objective

Task: Locate the correct procedure code and modifier, if necessary, for each case scenario.

Conditions: Use pen or pencil and *Current Procedural Terminology* code book.

Standards: Time: _____ minutes

                    Accuracy: _____

                    (Note: The time element and accuracy criteria may be given by your instructor.)

Directions. Find the correct procedure codes and modifiers, if necessary, for each case scenario.

1. The physician sees Horace Hart, a 60-year-old new patient, in the office for bronchial asthma, ASHD (arteriosclerotic heart disease), and hypertension. He performs an ECG (electrocardiogram) and UA (urinalysis) without microscopy, and obtains x-rays. Comprehensive metabolic and lipid panels and a CBC (complete blood count) are done by an outside laboratory.

Code Number   *Description*

Physician's bill:

_____   Initial OV, comp hx & exam, high-complexity decision making

_____   ECG with interpret and report

_____   UA, routine, nonautomated

_____   Chest x-ray, 2 views

_____   Routine venipuncture for handling of specimen

Laboratory's bill:

_____   Comprehensive metabolic panel: albumin, bilirubin, calcium, carbon dioxide, chloride, creatinine, glucose, phosphatase (alkaline), potassium, protein, sodium, ALT, AST, and urea nitrogen

_____   Lipid panel

_____   CBC, completely automated with complete differential

If the doctor decides to have the chest x-rays interpreted by a radiologist, the procedural

code billed by the radiologist would be _____ _____.

2. Mr. Hart is seen again in the office on May 12. On May 25 he is seen at home at 2 AM with asthma exacerbation, possible myocardial infarct, and congestive heart failure. The doctor consulted with a thoracic cardiovascular surgeon by telephone. He also called to make arrangements for hospitalization. These services required 2 hours and 40 minutes of non–face-to-face time to complete the patient care.

Code Number	Description
_____	OV, problem-focused hx & exam, straightforward decision making
_____	Home visit, detailed interval hx & exam, high-complexity decision making
_____	Detention time, prolonged (list time required)

3. On June 9, Horace Hart is seen again in the hospital. The thoracic cardiovascular surgeon who was telephoned the previous day was called in for consultation to formally examine him and says that surgery is necessary, which is scheduled the following day. The patient's physician sees the patient for his asthmatic condition and acts as assistant surgeon. The surgeon does the follow-up care and assumes care in the case.

Code Number	Description

Primary care physician/assistant surgeon's bill:

_____	Hospital visit, problem-focused hx & exam, low-complexity decision making
_____ _____	Pericardiotomy

Thoracic cardiovascular surgeon's bill:

_____ _____	Consultation, comp hx & exam, moderate-complexity decision making
_____	Pericardiotomy

ASSIGNMENT 6–10 ▸ CASE SCENARIO FOR CRITICAL THINKING

Performance Objective

Task: Locate the correct procedure codes and modifiers, if necessary, for a case scenario.

Conditions: Use pen or pencil and *Current Procedural Terminology* code book.

Standards: Time: _____ minutes

                   Accuracy: _____

                   (Note: The time element and accuracy criteria may be given by your instructor.)

Directions. Read through this progress note on Roy A. Takashima. Abstract information from the note about the subjective symptoms, objective findings, and diagnoses. List the diagnostic and procedure codes you think this case would warrant.

Takashima, Roy A.
October 5, 20xx

   Pt. has many things going on. First, he's had no difficulties following the feral cat bite, and the cat was normal on quarantine.

   He seemed to be recovering from the flu but is plagued with a very persisting cough and pain down the center of his chest without fever or grossly discolored phlegm.

   Physical exam shows expiratory rhonchi and gross exacerbation of his cough on forced expiration. Spirometry before and after bronchodilator was remarkably good; nonetheless, it is improved and he is symptomatically improved with a Proventil inhaler, which he is given as a sample. I don't think other antibiotics would help.

   His reflux is under good control with proprietary antacids with a clear exam.

   He has several areas of seborrheic keratoses on his face and head that need attention.

   Finally, in follow-up of all the above, he needs a complete physical exam.

                                                                    Ting Cho, MD

Diagnosis: Influenza and acute bronchitis.

Subjective symptoms   _____

                      _____

Objective findings   _____

                      _____

                      _____

Diagnosis and Dx code _____ _____

_____ _____

_____ _____

_____ _____

E/M code   _____

Spirometry code   _____ _____

ALTAPOINT PRACTICE MANAGEMENT SOFTWARE ASSIGNMENTS

ASSIGNMENT 6-11 ▸ ADD PROCEDURE CODES INTO THE PRACTICE MANAGEMENT SYSTEM AND CHANGE A FEE

Performance Objective

Task: Add procedure codes into the practice management system.

Conditions: CPT procedure codes and computer

Standards: Time: _____ minutes

                 Accuracy: _____

                 (Note: The time element and accuracy criteria may be given by your instructor.)

Directions: Before attempting any Practice Management software assignment, refer to Appendix C and follow the instructions provided to familiarize yourself with the software. Then refer to the Practice Management software on the CD that accompanies the *Handbook*.

1. For this assignment, follow the instructions for adding CPT procedure codes to the AltaPoint code list. These codes will be used for assignments that appear in subsequent chapters. Enter the following codes.

99381	Initial Well Baby Exam	$80.00
99212	Est.Pt. Problem Focused Exam	$60.00
99202	New Pt. Problem Focused Exam	$65.00
90701	DPT	$45.00
90658	Influenza Vaccine	$25.00
90471	Immunization Administration	$15.00
81000	Urinalysis Dipstick	$35.00
10060	Incision and Drainage	$82.00
72100	LS Spine 2 views	$110.00
70160	Nasal bone	$85.00
12002	Suture Repair	$80.00
90703	Tetanus	$25.00
28470	Fracture Repair Foot	$150.00
73620	Foot—2 view	$80.00

2. Following the instructions for changing the fee for an existing code, change the fee for code 93000 from $545 to $125. Change the fee for code 99070 to $95.00. Change the fee for code 99213 to $75.00 and change its description to Est. Pt. Expanded Exam. Change the fee for code 99201 to $50.00 and change its description to New Pt. Low Complexity Exam.

3. To obtain a grade, either print a hard copy of the CPT code list or have your instructor view the data onscreen for approval.

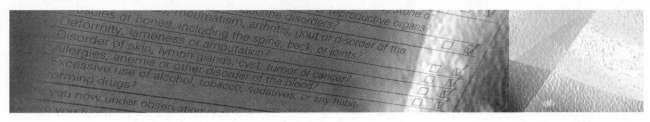

The Paper Claim: CMS-1500 (08-05)

KEY TERMS

Your instructor may wish to select some words pertinent to this chapter for a test. For definitions of the terms, further study, and/or reference, the words, phrases, and abbreviations may be found in the glossary at the end of the Handbook. *Key terms for this chapter follow.*

clean claim

deleted claim

dirty claim

durable medical equipment (DME) number

electronic claim

employer identification number (EIN)

facility provider number

group National Provider Identifier (group NPI)

Health Insurance Claim Form (CMS-1500 [08-05])

incomplete claim

intelligent character recognition (ICR)

invalid claim

National Provider Identifier (NPI)

optical character recognition (OCR)

"other" claims

paper claim

pending claim

physically clean claim

rejected claim

Social Security number (SSN)

state license number

KEY ABBREVIATIONS

See how many abbreviations and acronyms you can translate and then use this as a handy reference list. Definitions for the key abbreviations are located near the back of the Handbook *in the glossary.*

AIDS _____

AMA _____

CLIA _____

CMS-1500 _____

COB _____

DME _____

DNA _____

ECG _____

EIN _____

EMG _____

EOB _____
EPSDT _____
FDA _____
HHA _____
HICN _____
HIPAA _____
HIV _____
HMO _____
ICR _____
IDE _____
LMP _____
MCD _____
MG _____

MSP _____
NA, N/A _____
NOC _____
NPI _____
NPP _____
OCNA key _____
OCR _____
PAYERID _____
PRO _____
SOF _____
SSN _____
TMA _____

PERFORMANCE OBJECTIVES

The student will be able to:

- Define and spell the key terms and key abbreviations, for this chapter, given the information from the *Handbook* glossary, within a reasonable time period and with enough accuracy to obtain a satisfactory evaluation.
- After reading the chapter, answer the fill-in-the-blank, mix and match, multiple choice, and true/false review questions, with enough accuracy to obtain a satisfactory evaluation.
- Given a handwritten CMS-1500 (08-05) form, type a CMS-1500 (08-05) Health Insurance Claim Form and list the reasons why the claim was either rejected or delayed, within a reasonable time period and with enough accuracy to obtain a satisfactory evaluation.

- Given the patients' medical chart notes, ledger cards, encounter forms, and blank insurance claim forms, complete each CMS-1500 (08-05) Health Insurance Claim Form for billing, within a reasonable time period and with enough accuracy to obtain a satisfactory evaluation.
- Using the Mock Fee Schedule in Appendix A in this *Workbook*, correctly post payments, adjustments, and balances to the patients' ledger cards, within a reasonable time period and with enough accuracy to obtain a satisfactory evaluation.
- Given a list of common medical abbreviations and symbols that appear in chart notes, fill in the correct meaning of each abbreviation, within a reasonable time period and with enough accuracy to obtain a satisfactory evaluation.

ALTAPOINT PRACTICE MANAGEMENT SOFTWARE OBJECTIVES

The student should be able to:

- Enter transactions from encounter forms (superbills) and complete, print, and transmit

electronic insurance claims to the insurance company using the practice management system, within a reasonable time period and with enough accuracy to obtain a satisfactory evaluation.

STUDY OUTLINE

History

Compliance Issues Related to Insurance Claim
 Forms

Types of Submitted Claims
 Claim Status

Abstracting from Medical Records
 Cover Letter Accompanying Insurance Claims
 Life or Health Insurance Applications

Health Insurance Claim Form (CMS-1500 [08-05])
 Basic Guidelines for Submitting a Claim
 Completion of Insurance Claim Forms

Common Reasons Why Claim Forms Are Delayed
 or Rejected
 Additional Reasons Why Claim Forms
 Are Delayed

Optical Scanning Format Guidelines
 Optical Character Recognition
 Do's and Don'ts for Optical Character
 Recognition

Procedure: Instructions for the Health Insurance
 Claim Form (CMS-1500 [08-05])
 Insurance Program Templates

 ASSIGNMENT 7–1 ▸ REVIEW QUESTIONS

Part I Fill in the Blank

Review the objectives, key terms, chapter information, glossary definitions
of key terms, and figures before completing the following review questions.

1. Who developed the Standard Form?

   Health Insurance Association of America & American Medical Association

2. State the name of the insurance form approved by the American Medical Association.

   Health Insurance Claim form

3. Does Medicare accept the CMS-1500 (08-05) claim form?

   yes

4. What is dual coverage?

   When 2 insurance policies are involved, 1 primary & other secondary

5. The insurance company with the first responsibility for payment of a bill for medical
   services is known as the

   primary.

6. What important document must you have before an insurance company can photocopy
   a patient's chart?

   patients authorization in writing

7. If the patient brings in a private insurance form that is not group insurance, where do
   you send the form after completion?

   *no Back to the patient if requested or sent to insurance
   company if not*

8. An insurance claim is returned for the reason "diagnosis incomplete." State one or more solutions to this problem on how you would try to obtain reimbursement.

fix it and resubmit as a new claim the mistakes

9. When preparing a claim that is to be optically scanned, birth dates are keyed in with how many digits?

8

10. Define this abbreviation: MG/MCD.

MG = medigap
MCD = medicaid

Part II Mix and Match

11. Match the types of claims listed in the right column with their descriptions, and fill in the blanks with the appropriate letters.

H	Claim missing required information	a. clean claim
F	Phrase used when a claim is held back from payment	b. paper claim
B	Claim that is submitted and then optically scanned by the insurance carrier and converted to electronic form	c. invalid claim
D	Claim that needs manual processing because of errors or to solve a problem	d. dirty claim
G	Claim that needs clarification and answers to some questions	e. electronic claim
I	Claim that is canceled or voided if incorrect claim form is used or itemized charges are not provided	f. pending claim
E	Claim that is submitted via telephone line or computer modem	g. rejected claim
A	Claim that is submitted within the time limit and correctly completed	h. incomplete claim
C	Medicare claim that contains information that is complete and necessary but is illogical or incorrect	i. deleted claim

12. Match the types of numbers listed in the right column with their descriptions, and fill in the blanks with the appropriate letters.

C	A number issued by the federal government to each individual for personal use	a. state license number

___E___ A Medicare lifetime provider number

___D___ A number listed on a claim when submitting insurance claims to insurance companies under a group name

___A___ A number that a physician must obtain to practice in a state

___F___ A number used when billing for supplies and equipment

___G___ A number issued to a hospital

___B___ An individual physician's federal tax identification number issued by the Internal Revenue Service

b. employer identification number

c. Social Security number

d. group national provider number

e. National Provider Identifier

f. durable medical equipment number

g. facility provider number

Part III Multiple Choice

Choose the best answer.

13. A three-part information form that is completed and signed by an insurance agent and an individual to obtain insurance coverage, and requires a medical examination by a physician is known as

    a. CMS-1500 (08-05) claim form

    b. life or health insurance application

    c. universal claim form

    d. Health Insurance Claim Form

14. The insurance claim form required when submitting Medicare claims is

    a. CMS-1500 (08-05) claim form

    b. Attending Physicians Statement

    c. COMB-1

    d. HIPAA form

15. The maximum number of diagnostic codes in the ANSI 837P claim format for transmitting electronic health insurance claims is

    a. four

    b. six

    c. eight

    d. ten

16. If a patient's gender is not indicated in the CMS-1500 (08-05) claim form, the gender block defaults to

    a. male

    b. female

    c. denies the claim

    d. there is no default; it will appear blank

17. If a provider of medical services does not have an NPI number, the characters or digits that must be entered in Block 24I is/are

    a. leave blank

    b. IC

    c. ID

    d. NPI

Part IV True/False

Write "T" or "F" in the blank to indicate whether you think the statement is true or false.

_____F_____   18. A photocopy of a claim form may be optically scanned.

_____F_____   19. Handwriting is permitted on optically scanned paper claims.

_____T_____   20. A CMS-assigned National Provider Identifier (NPI) number consists of 10 characters.

_____F_____   21. When listing a diagnostic code on an insurance claim, insert the decimal points.

_____T_____   22. A diagnosis reference pointer should be entered in Block 24E and not an ICD-9-CM diagnostic code.

ASSIGNMENT 7–2 ▸ COMPLETE A HEALTH INSURANCE CLAIM FORM FOR A PRIVATE CASE

Performance Objective

Task: Complete a health insurance claim form and post the information to the patient's financial account record/statement.

Conditions: Use Merry M. McLean's E/M code slip (Figure 7–1), patient record (Figure 7–2), and financial account record/statement (Figure 7–3); one health insurance claim form (print from CD or Evolve website); a typewriter, computer, or pen; procedural and diagnostic code books; and Appendices A and B in the *Workbook*.

Standards: Claim Productivity Measurement

Time: _____ minutes

Accuracy: _____

(Note: The time element and accuracy criteria may be given by your instructor.)

E/M Code Slip

Patient ___McLean, Merry M.___   Date __5-6-XX__
                                                        CPT Code_____
HISTORY   EXAMINATION   Dx Code_____

☐ Problem Focused   ☐ Problem Focused
  Chief complaint; Brief history of   Exam limited to affected body area or organ system
  present illness

☐ Expanded Problem Focused   ☐ Expanded Problem Focused
  Chief complaint; Brief history of   Exam extended to other symptomatic or related organ
  present illness;   systems
  Problem pertinent system review

☑ Detailed   ☑ Detailed
  Chief complaint: Extended history   Extended exam of affected area(s) and other
  of present illness;   symptomatic or related systems
  Extended system review; Pertinent
  past family, social history

☐ Comprehensive   ☐ Comprehensive
  Chief complaint; Extended history   Complete single system specialty exam or complete
  of present illness;   multi-system exam
  Complete system review; Complete
  past family, social history

MEDICAL DECISION MAKING

Medical Decision	Number of Dx Options	Amount of Data	Risk M and M
☐ Straightforward	minimal 1 dx	minimal	minimal
☑ Low Complexity	limited 1-2 dx	limited	low
☐ Moderate Complexity	multiple 1-2 dx	moderate	moderate
☐ High Complexity	extensive 2-3 dx	extensive	high

☐ Counseling ☐ Time _____
☐ Consult   ☐ Referring Dr. __Emdee Fine__
Diagnosis __See Pt record__

NP ☑   Est pt _____

Figure 7–1

Directions. Complete the Health Insurance Claim Form,* using OCR or ICR guidelines, and send the form to the Prudential Insurance Company for Mrs. Merry M. McLean by referring to her E/M code slip, patient record, and financial account record/statement. Date the claim June 15. Refer to Appendix A in this *Workbook* to fill in the fees on the financial account record/statement.

1. Use your CPT code book or Appendix A in this *Workbook* to determine the correct 5-digit code number and modifiers for each professional service rendered.

2. Record on the financial account record/statement when you have billed the insurance company.

3. A Performance Evaluation Checklist may be reproduced from the "Instruction Guide to the *Workbook*" chapter if your instructor wishes you to submit it to assist with scoring and comments.

4. After the instructor has returned your work to you, either make the necessary corrections and place your work in a three-ring notebook for future reference or, if you received a high score, place it in your portfolio for reference when applying for a job.

Abbreviations pertinent to this record:

NP	LC
UA	MDM
Dx	HV
ptr	PF
Cysto	SF
Pt	RTO
Cont	postop
adm	OV
hosp	lb
C	adv
Hx	retn
exam	est

*See Chapter 7 in the *Handbook* for help in completing this form.

PATIENT RECORD NO. 7-2

McLean	Merry	M.	02-02-48	F	555-486-1859
LAST NAME	FIRST NAME	MIDDLE NAME	BIRTH DATE	SEX	HOME PHONE

4919 Dolphin Way	Woodland Hills,	XY	12345
ADDRESS	CITY	STATE	ZIP CODE

555-430-7709	555-098-3456	555-486-1859	McLean@WB.net
CELL PHONE	PAGER NO.	FAX NO.	E-MAIL ADDRESS

459-XX-9989	M0039857
PATIENT'S SOC. SEC. NO.	DRIVER'S LICENSE

Secretary	Porter Company
PATIENT'S OCCUPATION	NAME OF COMPANY

5490 Wilshire Blvd., Merck, XY 12346	555-446-7781
ADDRESS OF EMPLOYER	PHONE

Harry L. McLean	Computer programmer
SPOUSE OR PARENT	OCCUPATION

IBM Corporation	5616 Wilshire Blvd., Merck, XY 12346	555-664-9023
EMPLOYER	ADDRESS	PHONE

Prudential Insurance Co., 5621 Wilshire Blvd., Merck, XY 12346	Harry L. McLean
NAME OF INSURANCE	INSURED OR SUB SCRIBER

459-XX-9989	8832
POLICY/CERTIFICATE NO.	GROUP NO.

REFERRED BY:Emdee Fine, MD, 5000 Wilshire Blvd., Merck, XY 12346   NPI # 73027175XX

DATE	PROGRESS NOTES	No. 7-2
5-6-xx	NP presents in office with constant dribbling and wetting at night; uses 15 pads/day.	
	Began March 10, 20xx. Pelvic exam done—normal findings. No bladder or uterine	
	prolapse noted. UA dipstick performed (nonautomated with microscopy); few bacteria,	
	few urates. Dx: urinary incontinence. ptr 4 days for cystourethroscopy.	
	GU/llf *Gene Ulibarri, MD*	
5-10-xx	Cysto performed—revealed fistula of bladder with an opening into urinary bladder	
	and copious leakage into vagina. Schedule surgery to repair fistula. Pt cont to work.	
	GU/llf *Gene Ulibarri, MD*	
5-16-xx	Adm to College hosp. C hx/exam LC MDM. Dx: vesicovaginal fistula.	
	GU/llf *Gene Ulibarri, MD*	
5-17-xx	Closure of vesicovaginal fistula; abdominal approach.	
	GU/llf *Gene Ulibarri, MD*	
5-18-xx thru 5-21-xx	Saw patient in hospital (HV) PF hx/exam SF MDM.	
	GU/llf *Gene Ulibarri, MD*	
5-22-xx	Discharge from hospital. RTO 2 weeks.	
	GU/llf *Gene Ulibarri, MD*	
6-5-xx	Post-op OV. Patient presents complaining of pain near operative site. Pt reports she has	
	been walking daily and lifting more than 5 lb objects. Pt adv no excessive walking,	
	no lifting, stooping, or bending until surgical site is completely healed. Retn to clinic in	
	1 wk. Est return to work 7-1-xx. PF hx/exam SF MDM.	
	GU/llf *Gene Ulibarri, MD*	

Figure 7–2

Acct No. _7-2_

STATEMENT
Financial Account
COLLEGE CLINIC
4567 Broad Avenue
Woodland Hills, XY 12345-0001
Tel. 555-486-9002
Fax No. 555-487-8976

Merry McLean
4919 Dolphin Way
Woodland Hills, XY 12345

Phone No. (H)_ (555) 486-1859 _   (W) _ (555) 446-7781 _   Birthdate___02-02-48___

Primary Insurance Co.____Prudential Insurance Co._____   Policy/Group No. __459-XX-9989/8832__

	REFERENCE	DESCRIPTION	CHARGES	CREDITS PYMNTS.	ADJ.	BALANCE
20XX			BALANCE FORWARD →			
05-06-xx		OV NP				
05-06-xx		UA				
05-10-xx		Cystourethroscopy				
5-16-xx		Initial hosp care				
05-17-xx		Repair vesicovaginal fistula				
05-18 to 05-22-xx		HV				
05-22-xx		Discharge				
06-05-xx		PO-OV				

PLEASE PAY LAST AMOUNT IN BALANCE COLUMN ⇧

THIS IS A COPY OF YOUR FINANCIAL ACCOUNT AS IT APPEARS ON OUR RECORDS

Figure 7–3

ASSIGNMENT 7-3 ► **COMPLETE A HEALTH INSURANCE CLAIM FORM FOR A PRIVATE CASE**

Performance Objective

Task: Complete a health insurance claim form and post the information to the patient's financial account record/statement.

Conditions: Use Billy S. Rubin's E/M code slip (Figure 7–4), patient record (Figure 7–5), and financial account record/statement (Figure 7–6); one health insurance claim form (print from CD or Evolve website); a typewriter, computer, or pen; procedural and diagnostic code books; and Appendices A and B in this *Workbook*.

Standards: Claim Productivity Measurement

Time: _____ minutes

Accuracy: _____

(Note: The time element and accuracy criteria may be given by your instructor.)

E/M Code Slip

Patient _Rubin, Billy S._   Date *_____   CPT Code_____   Dx code_____

HISTORY

☑ Problem Focused
Chief complaint; Brief history of present illness

☐ Expanded Problem Focused
Chief complaint; Brief history of present illness; Problem pertinent system review

☐ Detailed
Chief complaint: Extended history of present illness; Extended system review; Pertinent past family, social history

☐ Comprehensive
Chief complaint; Extended history of present illness; Complete system review; Complete past family, social history

EXAMINATION

☑ Problem Focused
Exam limited to affected body area or organ system

☐ Expanded Problem Focused
Exam extended to other symptomatic or related organ systems

☐ Detailed
Extended exam of affected area(s) and other symptomatic or related symptoms

☐ Comprehensive
Complete single system specialty exam or complete multi-system exam

MEDICAL DECISION MAKING

Medical Decision	Number of Dx Options	Amount of Data	Risk M and M
☐ Straightforward	minimal 1 dx	minimal	minimal
☑ Low Complexity	limited 1-2 dx	limited	low
☐ Moderate Complexity	multiple 1-2 dx	moderate	moderate
☐ High Complexity	extensive 2-3 dx	extensive	high

☐ Counseling ☐ Time _____
☐ Consult ☑ Referring Dr. _U.R. Wright_
Diagnosis _see pt. record_

NP _____   Est pt ☑

* For space constraints, this E/M code slip is being used for 8-7-00, 8-14-00, and 8-16-00

Figure 7–4

Directions. Complete the Health Insurance Claim Form* on Mr. Billy S. Rubin for processing and send it to Aetna Life and Casualty Company by referring to Mr. Rubin's E/M code slip, patient record, and financial account record/statement. Date the claim August 30. Refer to Appendix A in this *Workbook* to fill in the fees on the financial statement. Use OCR guidelines.

1. Use your CPT code book or Appendix A in this *Workbook* to determine the correct 5-digit code number and modifiers for each professional service rendered. Do not include no-charge entries on the claim form.

2. Record when you have billed the insurance company on the financial account record/statement.

3. On September 1, Mr. Rubin sends you check No. 421 in the amount of $200 to apply to his account. Post this entry and calculate the balance due.

4. A Performance Evaluation Checklist may be reproduced from the "Instruction Guide to the Workbook" chapter if your instructor wishes you to submit it to assist with scoring and comments.

5. After the instructor has returned your work to you, either make the necessary corrections and place your work in a three-ring notebook for future reference, or, if you received a high score, place it in your portfolio for reference when applying for a job.

Abbreviations pertinent to this record:

est	_____	TURP	_____
pt	_____	wks	_____
CC	_____	HV	_____
BC	_____	PF	_____
diff	_____	hx	_____
PSA	_____	exam	_____
bx	_____	SF	_____
STAT	_____	MDM	_____
PTR	_____	Disch	_____
CA	_____	hosp	_____
adm	_____	postop	_____
surg	_____		

*See Chapter 7 in the *Handbook* for help in completing this form.

Additional Coding

1. Determine CPT codes that you would use to bill for College Hospital from the following services mentioned in the patient's progress notes.

CPT code

A. Blood draw (venipuncture) _____

B. Complete blood cell (CBC) count (automated) with differential _____

C. Prostate-specific antigen (PSA) (total) _____

D. Ultrasonography with guided fine-needle biopsy _____

_____

PATIENT RECORD NO. 7-3

Rubin	Billy	S.	11-09-53	M	555-893-5770
LAST NAME	FIRST NAME	MIDDLE NAME	BIRTH DATE	SEX	HOME PHONE

547 North Oliver Rd.	Woodland Hills	XY	12345	
ADDRESS	CITY	STATE	ZIP CODE	

555-430-9080	555-987-7790	555-893-5770		Rubin@WB.net
CELL PHONE	PAGER NO.	FAX NO.		E-MAIL ADDRESS

505-XX-1159	R0398056
PATIENT'S SOC. SEC. NO.	DRIVER'S LICENSE

salesman	Nate's Clothier's
PATIENT'S OCCUPATION	NAME OF COMPANY

7786 East Chabner Blvd., Dorland, XY 12347	555-449-6605
ADDRESS OF EMPLOYER	PHONE

Lydia B. Rubin (wife)
SPOUSE OR PARENT

EMPLOYER	ADDRESS	PHONE

Aetna Life and Casualty Co., 3055 Wilshire Blvd., Merck, XY 12345	Billy S. Rubin
NAME OF INSURANCE	INSURED OR SUB SCRIBER

42107	2641
POLICY/CERTIFICATE NO.	GROUP NO.

REFERRED BY: U. R. Wright, MD, 5010 Wrong Road, Torres, XY 12349   555-907-5440   NPI # 271385554XX

DATE	PROGRESS NOTES	No. 7-3
8-7-xx	Office exam est pt. CC: urinary hesitancy, frequency and posturinary dribbling since	
	July 15 of this year. Exam revealed hard nodule in prostate. Sent pt to College Hospital for	
	laboratory work; CBC (automated with diff) and PSA (total). PTR in 1 wk.	
	GU/llf	*Gene Ulibarri, MD*
8-14-xx	Office exam. PSA elevated (5.6), CBC normal. Explained to pt that biopsy is needed at this	
	point; may be done as outpatient at College Hospital. Pt elected to have immediate	
	bx;arrangements made for stat. ultrasound with guided fine needle bx. PTR in 2 days for	
	results.	
	GU/llf	*Gene Ulibarri, MD*
8-16-xx	Pt returns for bx report; positive for CA in situ of prostate. Advised patient that an	
	operation is necessary and explained surgical procedure, risks, and complications.	
	Arranged for adm to College Hospital on 8/22/xx.	
	GU/llf	*Gene Ulibarri, MD*
8-22-xx	Admit to College Hospital. Surg: TURP, complete Pt tolerated surg well and is comfortable	
	in the recovery room. Pt last worked 8/21/xx; est disability 6 to 8 wks. Est return to work	
	on 10/22/xx.	
	GU/llf	*Gene Ulibarri, MD*
8-23-xx thru	HV (PF hx/exam SF MDM)	
8-26-xx	GU/llf	*Gene Ulibarri, MD*
8-27-xx	Disch from hosp. Pt confined at home for 1 week at which time patient will return to	
	office for postop check.	
	GU/llf	*Gene Ulibarri, MD*

Figure 7–5

STATEMENT
Financial Account
COLLEGE CLINIC
4567 Broad Avenue
Woodland Hills, XY 12345-0001
Tel. 555-486-9002
Fax No. 555-487-8976

Acct No. 7-3

Billy S. Rubin
547 North Oliver Road
Woodland Hills, XY 12345

Phone No. (H) (555) 893-5770   (W) (555) 449-6605   Birthdate 11-09-53

Primary Insurance Co. Aetna Life and Casualty Co.   Policy/Group No. 421074/2641

	REFERENCE	DESCRIPTION	CHARGES	PYMNTS.	ADJ.	BALANCE
20XX			BALANCE FORWARD →			
08-07-xx		OV Est Pt				
08-14-xx		OV Est Pt				
08-16-xx		OV Est Pt				
08-22-xx		TURP				
08-23 to 08-26-xx		HV				
08-27-xx		Discharge				

PLEASE PAY LAST AMOUNT IN BALANCE COLUMN ⇧

THIS IS A COPY OF YOUR FINANCIAL ACCOUNT AS IT APPEARS ON OUR RECORDS

Figure 7–6

ASSIGNMENT 7-4 ▸ COMPLETE TWO HEALTH INSURANCE CLAIM FORMS
FOR A PRIVATE CASE

Performance Objective

Task: Complete two health insurance claim forms and post the information to the patient's
                   financial account record/statement.

Conditions: Use Walter J. Stone's E/M code slip (Figure 7–7), patient record (Figure 7–8), and financial
                   account record/statement (Figure 7–9); one health insurance claim form (print from CD or
                   Evolve website) and a photocopy of this form to use for the second claim; a typewriter,
                   computer, or pen; procedural and diagnostic code books; and Appendices A and B in
                   this *Workbook*.

Standards: Claim Productivity Measurement

                   Time: _____ minutes

                   Accuracy: _____

                   (Note: The time element and accuracy criteria may be given by your instructor.)

Directions. You will be billing for all services listed on the patient's progress notes for Dr. Gaston Input. Note
that the patient was hospitalized twice, which necessitates two claim forms.

E/M Code Slip

Patient _Stone, Walter J._   Date _5/12/XX_
                                                                                  CPT Code _____
HISTORY   EXAMINATION   Dx Code _____

☐ Problem Focused   ☐ Problem Focused
  Chief complaint; Brief history of present illness   Exam limited to affected body area or organ system

☑ Expanded Problem Focused   ☑ Expanded Problem Focused
  Chief complaint; Brief history of present illness;   Exam extended to other symptomatic or related organ
  Problem pertinent system review   systems

☐ Detailed   ☐ Detailed
  Chief complaint: Extended history of present illness;   Extended exam of affected area(s) and other
  Extended system review; Pertinent past family, social history   symptomatic or related systems

☐ Comprehensive   ☐ Comprehensive
  Chief complaint; Extended history of present illness;   Complete single system specialty exam or complete
  Complete system review; Complete past family, social history   multi-system exam

MEDICAL DECISION MAKING

Medical Decision	Number of Dx Options	Amount of Data	Risk M and M
☐ Straightforward	minimal 1 dx	minimal	minimal
☑ Low Complexity	limited 1-2 dx	limited	low
☐ Moderate Complexity	multiple 1-2 dx	moderate	moderate
☐ High Complexity	extensive 2-3 dx	extensive	high

☐ Counseling ☐ Time _____
☐ Consult   ☐ Referring Dr. _____
Diagnosis _see pt. record_

NP ____   Est pt ☑

Figure 7–7

Complete two Health Insurance Claim Forms,* addressing them to Travelers Insurance Company for Mr. Walter J. Stone by referring to his E/M code slip, patient record, and financial account record/statement. Date the claims June 1. Refer to Appendix A in this *Workbook* to fill in the fees on the financial account record/statement. Use OCR guidelines.

1. Use your CPT code book or Appendix A in this *Workbook* to determine the correct 5-digit code number and modifiers for each professional service rendered. The surgeon, Dr. Cutler, is charging $714.99 for the cholecystectomy. You are submitting a claim for the assistant surgeon, Dr. Input, and calculating a standard 20% of the surgeon's fee.

2. On May 14, the insurance company sends the physician a check, number 48572, for $25. Post this entry.

3. Record on the financial account record/statement when you have billed the insurance company.

4. A Performance Evaluation Checklist may be reproduced from the "Instruction Guide to the *Workbook*" chapter if your instructor wishes you to submit it to assist with scoring and comments.

5. After the instructor has returned your work to you, either make the necessary corrections and place your work in a three-ring notebook for future reference or, if you received a high score, place it in your portfolio for reference when applying for a job.

Abbreviations pertinent to this record:

est	_____	exam	_____
pt	_____	LC	_____
ER	_____	MDM	_____
BP	_____	EGD	_____
Dx	_____	bx	_____
GI	_____	ofc	_____
HV	_____	wk	_____
PF	_____	OV	_____
hx	_____	adv	_____

Additional Coding

1. Refer to Mr. Stone's patient record, abstract information, and code the procedures for services that would be billed by the hospital.

Description of Service   *Code*

a. _____   _____

b. _____   _____

c. _____   _____

*See Chapter 7 in the *Handbook* for help in completing this form.

PATIENT RECORD NO. 7-4

Stone	Walter	J.	03-14-49	M	555-345-0776
LAST NAME	FIRST NAME	MIDDLE NAME	BIRTH DATE	SEX	HOME PHONE

2008 Converse Street	Woodland Hills	XY	12345
ADDRESS	CITY	STATE	ZIP CODE

555-980-7750	555-930-5674	555-345-0776	Stone@WB.net
CELL PHONE	PAGER NO.	FAX NO.	E-MAIL ADDRESS

456-XX-9989	H9834706
PATIENT'S SOC. SEC. NO.	DRIVER'S LICENSE

advertising agent	R. V. Black and Associates
PATIENT'S OCCUPATION	NAME OF COMPANY

1267 Broad Street, Woodland Hills, XY 12345	555-345-6012
ADDRESS OF EMPLOYER	PHONE

widower
SPOUSE OR PARENT

EMPLOYER	ADDRESS	PHONE

Travelers Insurance Co. 5460 Olympic Blvd., Woodland Hills, XY 12345	Walter J. Stone
NAME OF INSURANCE	INSURED OR SUB SCRIBER

456-XX-9989	6754
POLICY/CERTIFICATE NO.	GROUP NO.

REFERRED BY: John B. Stone (brother), former patient of Dr. Input

DATE	PROGRESS NOTES	No. 7-4
5-3-xx	Est pt presented in ER after experiencing sudden onset of profuse rectal bleeding with	
	nausea and severe abdominal pains. Elevated BP 180/100. Dr. Input called to ER by	
	Dr. Cutler who recommended pt be admitted for further evaluation and diagnostic workup.	
	Dr. Input performed a comprehensive history and examination with moderate complexity	
	decision making and admitted the pt to College Hospital. Dx: Unspecified GI hemorrhage.	
	Pt disabled from work.	
	GI/llf	*Gaston Input, MD*
5-4-xx	HV (PF hx/exam LC MDM). Pt symptoms have subsided somewhat. Cholecystography	
	with oral contrast and complete abdominal ultrasound confirmed inflammatory gallbladder	
	with stones. EGD with bx confirmed prepyloric gastric ulcer.	
	GI/llf	*Gaston Input, MD*
5-5-xx	Discharged to home. Pt to be seen in ofc in 1 wk.	
	GI/llf	*Gaston Input, MD*
5-12-xx	Pt returns for an OV. Pt complains of ongoing GI distress. Continued elevated	
	BP of 186/98 shows a concern for hypertension. Adv to see Dr. Cutler for further	
	evaluation and possible surgery. DX: Acute prepyloric gastric ulcer with hemorrhage,	
	cholecystitis with cholelithiasis, benign hypertension.	
	GI/llf	*Gaston Input, MD*
5-16-xx	Pt admitted to College Hospital by surgeon, Dr. Cutler. He performed a laparoscopic	
	cholecystectomy in which I assisted. Pt will resume work on 6/22/xx.	
	GI/llf	*Gaston Input, MD*

Figure 7–8

Acct No. _7-4_

STATEMENT
Financial Account
COLLEGE CLINIC
4567 Broad Avenue
Woodland Hills, XY 12345-001
Tel. 555-486-9002
Fax No. 555-487-8976

Walter J. Stone
2008 Converse Street
Woodland Hills, XY 12345

Phone No. (H) _(555) 345-0776_   (W) _(555) 345-6012_   Birthdate _03-14-49_

Primary Insurance Co. _Travelers Insurance Co,_   Policy/Group No. _456-XX9989/6754_

	REFERENCE	DESCRIPTION	CHARGES		CREDITS PYMNTS.		ADJ.		BALANCE	
20XX					BALANCE FORWARD ➔					
01-03-xx	99214	OV	61	51					61	51
01-15-xx	01-03-xx	Billed Travelers Ins.							61	51
03-02-xx	Ck 95268	ROA Travelers Ins.			49	21			12	30
03-03-xx	99213	OV	40	20					52	50
04-03-xx	3-3-xx	Billed Travelers Ins.							52	50
05-03-xx		Initial hosp care								
05-04-xx		HV								
05-05-xx		Discharge								
05-12-xx		OV								
05-16-xx		Cholecystectomy Asst.								

PLEASE PAY LAST AMOUNT IN BALANCE COLUMN ⬆

THIS IS A COPY OF YOUR FINANCIAL ACCOUNT AS IT APPEARS ON OUR RECORDS

Figure 7–9

ASSIGNMENT **7–5** ▸ **LOCATE ERRORS ON A COMPLETED HEALTH INSURANCE CLAIM FORM**

Performance Objective

Task: Complete a health insurance claim form and post the information to the patient's ledger card.

Conditions: Use Tom N. Parkinson's completed insurance claim (Figure 7–10), one health insurance claim form (print from CD or Evolve website), and either a typewriter and/or computer or a pen.

Standards: Time: _____ minutes

                 Accuracy: _____

                 (Note: The time element and accuracy criteria may be given by your instructor.)

Guidance. To alleviate frustration and ease the process of completing a claim form for the first time, you will be editing a claim and then taking the correct information and inserting it on a blank CMS-1500 (08-05) form. Refer to Chapter 7 in the *Handbook* for block-by-block private payer instructions for completing the CMS-1500 (08-05) insurance claim form. Refer to Figure 7–5 in the *Handbook* for visual placement of data. Refer to Appendix A in this *Workbook* for the physician/clinic information and the clinic's mock fee schedule. The billing physician is Gerald Practon. The name of the insurance carrier is ABC Insurance Company at 111 Main Street in Denver, CO, 80210.

Directions. Study the completed claim form (see Figure 7–10) and search for missing or incorrect information. If possible, verify all information. Highlight or circle in red all incorrect or missing information. Insert the correct information on the claim form. Now transfer all the data to a blank CMS-1500 (08-05) claim form. If mandatory information is missing, insert the word "NEED" in the corresponding block of the claim form.

     A Performance Evaluation Checklist may be reproduced from the "Instruction Guide to the *Workbook*" chapter if your instructor wishes you to submit it to assist with scoring and comments.

Optional. List, in block-by-block order, the reasons why the claim may be either rejected or delayed according to the errors found.

General Directions for Claim Form Completion

Assume that the Health Insurance Claim Form* CMS-1500 (08-05) is printed in red ink for processing by OCR or ICR. Complete the form using OCR/ICR guidelines pertinent to the type of carrier that you are billing (e.g., private, Medicare, TRICARE) and send it to the proper insurance carrier. Refer to Chapter 7 in the *Handbook* for block instructions for each major type of insurance carrier. All blocks are clearly labeled, and each major carrier has an icon that is color coded for easy reference. Claim form templates have been completed to use as visual examples for placement of data; they may be found at the end of Chapter 7 in the *Handbook*. Screened areas on each form do not apply to the insurance program example shown and should be left blank.

     Many physicians complete an evaluation and management (E/M) code slip for each patient encounter. Chapter 7 assignments feature this form as a reference for part of each exercise and are used to assist you with E/M CPT code selection. In future assignments, you identify key components for E/M services in the medical record. All physicians in College Clinic accept assignment of benefits for all types of insurance that you will be billing for; indicate this by checking "yes" in Block 27. For each claim completed, be sure to insert your initials at the lower left corner of the claim form. When coding services from the Surgery Section of CPT, be sure to check the Mock Fee Schedule in Appendix A in this *Workbook* to determine how many follow-up days are included in the surgical or global package. Services provided during the surgical/global package time frame should not be included on the claim form; however, such services should be documented on the financial accounting record, referenced with code 99024

---

*See Chapter 7 in the *Handbook* for help in completing this form.

(postoperative follow-up visit; included in global service), and listed as no charge (N/C). Refer to the *Handbook* for detailed information about surgical/global package and follow-up days.

A list of abbreviations pertinent to the medical record have been provided as an exercise to reinforce learning. Not all medical offices use abbreviations in medical record documentation. In the College Clinic scenario, abbreviations are used in patient progress notes to give you an opportunity to practice reading and interpreting them.

1500

HEALTH INSURANCE CLAIM FORM

APPROVED BY NATIONAL UNIFORM CLAIM COMMITTEE 08/05

☐☐ PICA | | | | | | | | | PICA ☐☐

1. MEDICARE ☐ (Medicare #)	MEDICAID ☐ (Medicaid #)	TRICARE CHAMPUS ☐ (Sponsor's SSN)	CHAMPVA ☐ (Member ID#)	GROUP HEALTH PLAN ☐ (SSN or ID)	FECA BLK LUNG ☐ (SSN)	OTHER ☐ (ID)	1a. INSURED'S I.D. NUMBER (For Program in Item 1) PX4278A

2. PATIENT'S NAME (Last Name, First Name, Middle Initial) PARKINSON TOM N	3. PATIENT'S BIRTH DATE MM DD YY 04 06 1993 SEX M ☒ F ☐	4. INSURED'S NAME (Last Name, First Name, Middle Initial) PARKINSON JAMIE B

5. PATIENT'S ADDRESS (No., Street) 4510 SOUTH A STREET	6. PATIENT RELATIONSHIP TO INSURED Self ☐ Spouse ☐ Child ☒ Other ☐	7. INSURED'S ADDRESS (No., Street) 4510 SOUTH A STREET
CITY WOODLAND HILLS STATE XY	8. PATIENT STATUS Single ☒ Married ☐ Other ☐	CITY WOODLAND HILLS STATE XY
ZIP CODE 12345 TELEPHONE (Include Area Code) (555) 74221580	Employed ☐ Full-Time Student ☐ Part-Time Student ☒	ZIP CODE 12345 TELEPHONE (INCLUDE AREA CODE) (555) 742 1560

9. OTHER INSURED'S NAME (Last Name, First Name, Middle Initial)	10. IS PATIENT'S CONDITION RELATED TO:	11. INSURED'S POLICY GROUP OR FECA NUMBER
a. OTHER INSURED'S POLICY OR GROUP NUMBER	a. EMPLOYMENT? (CURRENT OR PREVIOUS) YES ☐ NO ☒	a. INSURED'S DATE OF BIRTH MM DD YY SEX M ☐ F ☐
b. OTHER INSURED'S DATE OF BIRTH MM DD YY SEX M ☐ F ☐	b. AUTO ACCIDENT? PLACE (State) YES ☐ NO ☒	b. EMPLOYER'S NAME OR SCHOOL NAME
c. EMPLOYER'S NAME OR SCHOOL NAME	c. OTHER ACCIDENT? YES ☐ NO ☒	c. INSURANCE PLAN NAME OR PROGRAM NAME
d. INSURANCE PLAN NAME OR PROGRAM NAME	10d. RESERVED FOR LOCAL USE	d. IS THERE ANOTHER HEALTH BENEFIT PLAN? YES ☐ NO ☒ *If yes*, return to and complete item 9 a-d.

READ BACK OF FORM BEFORE COMPLETING & SIGNING THIS FORM.

12. PATIENT'S OR AUTHORIZED PERSON'S SIGNATURE I authorize the release of any medical or other information necessary to process this claim. I also request payment of government benefits either to myself or to the party who accepts assignment below.

SIGNED _____ DATE _____

13. INSURED'S OR AUTHORIZED PERSON'S SIGNATURE I authorize payment of medical benefits to the undersigned physician or supplier for services described below.

SIGNED _____

14. DATE OF CURRENT: MM DD YY ◄ ILLNESS (First symptom) OR INJURY (Accident) OR PREGNANCY(LMP)	15. IF PATIENT HAS HAD SAME OR SIMILAR ILLNESS. GIVE FIRST DATE MM DD YY	16. DATES PATIENT UNABLE TO WORK IN CURRENT OCCUPATION MM DD YY MM DD YY FROM TO
17. NAME OF REFERRING PHYSICIAN OR OTHER SOURCE	17a. 17b. NPI	18. HOSPITALIZATION DATES RELATED TO CURRENT SERVICES MM DD YY MM DD YY FROM TO
19. RESERVED FOR LOCAL USE		20. OUTSIDE LAB? YES ☐ NO ☒ $ CHARGES

21. DIAGNOSIS OR NATURE OF ILLNESS OR INJURY. (RELATE ITEMS 1,2,3 OR 4 TO ITEM 24E BY LINE)

1. ∟___ . ___   3. ∟___ . ___
2. ∟___ . ___   4. ∟___ . ___

22. MEDICAID RESUBMISSION CODE ORIGINAL REF. NO.
23. PRIOR AUTHORIZATION NUMBER

24. A. DATE(S) OF SERVICE From MM DD YY	To MM DD YY	B. PLACE OF SERVICE	C. EMG	D. PROCEDURES, SERVICES, OR SUPPLIES (Explain Unusual Circumstances) CPT/HCPCS	MODIFIER	E. DIAGNOSIS POINTER	F. $ CHARGES	G. DAYS OR UNITS	H. EPSDT Family Plan	I. ID. QUAL.	J. RENDERING PROVIDER ID. #
1 07 14 20XX				99242			80 24	1		NPI	
2 07 14 20XX				71020		1	38 96	1		NPI	4627889700
3										NPI	
4										NPI	
5										NPI	
6										NPI	

25. FEDERAL TAX I.D. NUMBER SSN EIN 7034597 ☐	26. PATIENT'S ACCOUNT NO.	27. ACCEPT ASSIGNMENT? (For govt. claims, see back) ☒ YES ☐ NO	28. TOTAL CHARGE $ 119 20	29. AMOUNT PAID $	30. BALANCE DUE $

31. SIGNATURE OF PHYSICIAN OR SUPPLIER INCLUDING DEGREES OR CREDENTIALS (I certify that the statements on the reverse apply to this bill and are made a part thereof.) GERALD PRACTON 07/14/20XX SIGNED DATE	32. SERVICE FACILITY LOCATION INFORMATION a. NPI b.	33. BILLING PROVIDER INFO & PH # (555) 486 9002 COLLEGE CLINIC 4567 BROAD AVENUE WOODLAND HILLS XY 12345 0001 a. 3664021CC NPI b.

NUCC Instruction Manual available at: www.nucc.org   **PLEASE PRINT OR TYPE**   APPROVED OMB-0938-0999 FORM CMS-1500 (08-05)

Figure 7–10

ASSIGNMENT 7-6 ▸ REVIEW PATIENT RECORD ABBREVIATIONS

Performance Objective

Task: Insert meanings of abbreviations.

Conditions: Use a pencil or pen.

Standards: Time: _____ minutes

                   Accuracy: _____

                   (Note: The time element and accuracy criteria may be given by your instructor.)

Directions. After completing all the patient records in the *Workbook* that are pertinent to this chapter, you will be able to answer the next two questions.

1. What do these abbreviations mean?

   a. PTR _____

   b. TURP _____

   c. HX _____

   d. IVP_____

   e. c̄ _____

   f. Dx _____

   g. BP _____

   h. CC _____

   i. UA _____

   j. PE _____

2. Give the abbreviations for the following terms.

   A. return _____

   B. cancer, carcinoma _____

   C. patinent _____

   D. established _____

   E. discharged _____

   F. gallbladder _____

   G. initial _____

ALTAPOINT PRACTICE MANAGEMENT SOFTWARE ASSIGNMENTS

ASSIGNMENT 7-7 ▸ ENTER TRANSACTIONS FROM AN ENCOUNTER FORM (SUPERBILL) INTO THE PRACTICE MANAGEMENT SYSTEM

Performance Objective

Task: Enter transactions from Teri E. Simpson's encounter from (superbill) into the practice management system.

Conditions: Encounter form (superbill) Figure 7-11 and computer

Standards: Time:_____ minutes

                    Accuracy:_____

                    (Note: The time element and accuracy criteria may be given by your instructor.)

Directions. Before attempting the Practice Management software assignment, refer to Appendix C and follow the instructions provided to familiarize yourself with the software. Then refer to the Practice Management software on the CD that accompanies the *Workbook*.

1. For this assignment, follow the instructions for entering transactions from an encounter form (superbill) and enter the charges for Teri E. Simpson's office visit on February 9.

2. To obtain a grade, either print a hard copy of the patient's financial account record or have your instructor view the data onscreen for approval.

Assignment 7-7

College Clinic

4567 Broad Avenue
Woodlands Hills, XY
12345-0001
Tel (555) 486-9002
Fax (555) 487-8976

Doctors No. _____

☒ PRIVATE   ☐ MANAGED CARE   ☐ MEDICAID   ☐ MEDICARE   ☐ TRICARE   ☐ W/C

ACCOUNT #	PATIENT'S LAST NAME	FIRST	INITIAL	TODAY'S DATE
SIMPS00001	Simpson	Teri	E.	02/09/2007

ASSIGNMENT: I hereby assign payment directly to College Clinic of the surgical and/or medical benefits, if any, otherwise payable to me for his/her services as described below.
SIGNED (Patient, or Parent, if Minor)   DATE:

DESCRIPTION	CPT-4/MD	FEE	DESCRIPTION	CPT-4/MD	FEE	DESCRIPTION	CPT-4/MD	FEE
OFFICE VISIT-NEW PATIENT			**WELL BABY EXAM**			**LABORATORY**		
Level 1	99201		Intial	99381		Glucose	82951	
Level 2	99202		Periodic	99391		Heamatocrit	85013	
Level 3	99203		**OFFICE PROCEDURES**			Occult Blood	82270	
Level 4	99204		Anscopy	46600		Urine Dip	81000	
Level 5	99205		ECG 24-hr	93000		**X-RAY**		
OFFICE VISIT-ESTAB, PATIENT			Fracture Rpr Foot	28470		Foot - 2 View	73620	
Level 1	99211		I & D	10060		Forearm - 2 View	73090	
✓ Level 2	99212	60.00	Suture Repair			Nasal Bone - 3	70160	
Level 3	99213					Spine LS - 2 view	72100	
Level 4	99214		**INJECTIONS/VACCINATIONS**					
Level 5	99215		DPT	90701		**MISCELLANEOUS**		
OFFICE CONSULT-NP/EST			IM-Antibiotic	90788		Handling of Spec	99000	
Level 3	99243		✓ Influenza Vac	90658	25.00	Supply	99070	
Level 4	99244		Tetanus	90703		Venipuncture	36415	
Level 5	99245		✓ Immun Admin	90471	15.00			

COMMENTS:

Physician:

RETURN APPOINTMENT

_____ Week(s)   _____ Month(s)

DIAGNOSIS:
Primary: DESCRIPTION   CODE
Encounter for flu shot   V04.85
Secondary: _____ _____
_____ _____

REC'D BY:
☐ BANK CARD
☐ CASH
☐ CHECK
  # _____

PREVIOUS BALANCE *267.50*
TODAY'S FEE *100.00*
AMOUNT REC'D/CO-PAY
BALANCE *367.50*

Figure 7–11

ASSIGNMENT **7–8** ▸ **ENTER TRANSACTIONS FROM AN ENCOUNTER FORM (SUPERBILL) INTO THE PRACTICE MANAGEMENT SYSTEM**

Performance Objective

Task: Enter transactions from Michael Lee's encounter from (superbill) into the practice management system.

Conditions: Encounter form (superbill) Figure 7-12 and computer

Standards: Time:_____ minutes

Accuracy:_____

(Note: The time element and accuracy criteria may be given by your instructor.)

Directions. Before attempting the Practice Management software assignment, refer to Appendix C and follow the instructions provided to familiarize yourself with the software. Then refer to the Practice Management software on the CD that accompanies the *Workbook*.

1. For this assignment, follow the instructions for entering transactions from an encounter form (superbill) and enter the charges for Michael Lee's office visit on March 14.

2. To obtain a grade, either print a hard copy of the patient's financial account record or have your instructor view the data onscreen for approval.

Assignment 7-8

College Clinic
4567 Broad Avenue
Woodlands Hills, XY
12345-0001
Tel (555) 486-9002
Fax (555) 487-8976

Doctors No. _____

☒ PRIVATE ☐ MANAGED CARE ☐ MEDICAID ☐ MEDICARE ☐ TRICARE ☐ W/C

ACCOUNT #	PATIENT'S LAST NAME	FIRST	INITIAL	TODAY'S DATE
SIMPSO0002	*Lee*	*Michael*		*03/14/2007*

ASSIGNMENT: I hereby assign payment directly to College Clinic of the surgical and/or medical benefits, if any, otherwise payable to me for his/her services as described below.
SIGNED (Patient, or Parent, if Minor)   DATE:

DESCRIPTION	CPT-4/MD	FEE		DESCRIPTION	CPT-4/MD	FEE		DESCRIPTION	CPT-4/MD	FEE
OFFICE VISIT-NEW PATIENT				**WELL BABY EXAM**				**LABORATORY**		
Level 1	99201			Intial	99381			Glucose	82951	
Level 2	99202			Periodic	99391			Heamatocrit	85013	
Level 3	99203			**OFFICE PROCEDURES**				Occult Blood	82270	
Level 4	99204			Anscopy	46600			Urine Dip	81000	
Level 5	99205			ECG 24-hr	93000			**X-RAY**		
OFFICE VISIT-ESTAB, PATIENT				Fracture Rpr Foot	28470			Foot - 2 View	73620	
Level 1	99211			I & D	10060			Forearm - 2 View	73090	
Level 2	99212		✓	Suture Repair	12002	*80.00*		Nasal Bone - 3	70160	
✓ Level 3	99213	*75.00*						Spine LS - 2 view	72100	
Level 4	99214			**INJECTIONS/VACCINATIONS**						
Level 5	99215			DPT	90701			**MISCELLANEOUS**		
OFFICE CONSULT-NP/EST				IM-Antibiotic	90788			Handling of Spec	99000	
Level 3	99243			Influenza Vac	90658			Supply	99070	
Level 4	99244		✓	Tetanus	90703	*25.00*		Venipuncture	36415	
Level 5	99245		✓	Immun Admin	90471	*15.00*				

COMMENTS:

Physician:

RETURN APPOINTMENT

_____ Week(s)   _____ Month(s)

DIAGNOSIS:	DESCRIPTION	CODE
Primary:	*Laceration Leg*	*891.0*
Secondary:	*Fall from Ladder*	*E881.0*

REC'D BY:
☐ BANK CARD
☐ CASH
☐ CHECK
_____

PREVIOUS BALANCE *55.00*
TODAY'S FEE *195.00*
AMOUNT REC'D/CO-PAY
BALANCE *250.00*

Figure 7–12

ASSIGNMENT **7-9** ▸ **STUDENT SOFTWARE CHALLENGE**

ASSIGNMENTS FOR CASES 1 THROUGH 6 ONSCREEN COMPLETION OF CMS-1500 (08-05) INSURANCE CLAIM FORMS FOR PRIVATE INSURANCE

Performance Objective

Task: Enter transactions from patients' onscreen encounter forms (superbills) and complete block-by-block onscreen health insurance claim forms

Conditions: Onscreen encounter forms (superbills) and computer

Standards: Time:_____ minutes

                          Accuracy:_____

                          (Note: The time element and accuracy criteria may be given by your instructor.)

Directions. Before attempting the assignments, refer to *Workbook* Appendix C and follow the instructions provided to familiarize yourself with the Student Software Challenge section of the software. Then insert the CD that accompanies the *Workbook* into the computer disk drive.

1. For these assignments, follow the instructions for entering data into the onscreen CMS-1500 (08-05) health insurance claim form completing blocks 1 through 33 for Cases 1 through 6.

2. Use your CPT code book or Appendix A in this *Workbook* to determine the correct five-digit code number and modifiers for each professional service rendered.

3. Print a hard copy of the completed health insurance claim form for each case.

4. After the instructor has returned your work to you, either make the necessary corrections and place your work in a three-ring notebook for future reference, or, if you received a high score, place it in your portfolio for reference when applying for a job.

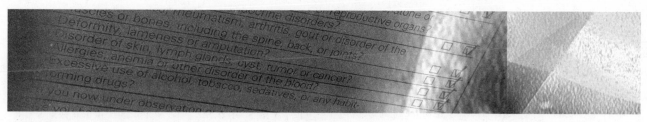

Electronic Data Interchange: Transactions and Security

KEY TERMS

Your instructor may wish to select some words pertinent to this chapter for a test. For definitions of the terms, further study, and/or reference, the words, phrases, and abbreviations may be found in the glossary at the end of the Handbook. *Key terms for this chapter follow.*

Accredited Standards Committee X12 (ASC X12)

application service provider (ASP)

back up

batch

business associate agreement

cable modem

clearinghouse

code sets

covered entity

data elements

digital subscriber line (DSL)

direct data entry (DDE)

electronic data interchange (EDI)

electronic funds transfer (EFT)

electronic remittance advice (ERA)

encoder

encryption

HIPAA Transaction and Code Set (TCS) Rule

National Standard Format (NSF)

password

real time

standard transactions

T-1

taxonomy codes

trading partner agreement

KEY ABBREVIATIONS

See how many abbreviations and acronyms you can translate and then use this as a handy reference list. Definitions for the key abbreviations are located near the back of the Handbook *in the glossary.*

ANSI _____

ASC X12 _____

ASET _____

ASP _____

ATM _____

CMS _____

COB _____

DDE _____

DSL _____

EDI _____

EFT _____

EHR _____

EIN _____

EMC _____

EOB _____

EOMB _____

ePHI _____

ERA _____

HHS _____

HIPAA _____

IRS _____

LMP _____

MTS _____

NPI _____

NPP _____

NSF _____

P&P _____

PHI _____

PMS _____

R _____

RA _____

S _____

TCS rule _____

UPS _____

PERFORMANCE OBJECTIVES

The student will be able to:

- Define and spell the key terms and key abbreviations for this chapter, given the information from the *Handbook* glossary, within a reasonable time period and with enough accuracy to obtain a satisfactory evaluation.
- After reading the chapter, answer the fill-in-the-blanks, multiple choice, and true/false review questions with enough accuracy to obtain a satisfactory evaluation.
- Decide whether keyed medical and nonmedical data elements are required, situational, or not used when electronically submitting the 837P health care claim.
- Decide which medical and nonmedical code sets for 837P electronic claims are required, situational, or not used.

- Input data into the element for place of service codes for 837P electronic claims submission.
- Indicate the patient's relationship to the insured by using the individual relationship code numbers for 837P electronic claims submission.
- Select the correct individual relationship code number for 837P electronic claims submission.
- Select the correct taxonomy codes for the specialists for submission of 837P electronic claims submission.
- Locate errors, given computer-generated insurance forms, within a reasonable time period and with enough accuracy to obtain a satisfactory evaluation.
- Fill in the correct meaning of each abbreviation, given a list of common medical abbreviations and symbols that appear in chart notes, with enough accuracy to obtain a satisfactory evaluation.

ALTAPOINT PRACTICE MANAGEMENT SOFTWARE OBJECTIVES

The student will be able to:

■ Transmit electronic insurance claims for private cases using practice management software, within a reasonable time period and with enough accuracy to obtain a satisfactory evaluation.

STUDY OUTLINE

Electronic Data Interchange

Electronic Claims

Advantages of Electronic Claim Submission

Clearinghouses

Transaction and Code Set Regulations: Streamlining Electronic Data Interchange
  Transaction and Code Set Standards

Transition from Paper CMS-1500 (08-05) to Electronic Standard HIPAA 837
  Levels of Information for 837P Standard Transaction Format

Claims Attachments Standards
  Standard Unique Identifiers

Practice Management System

Building the Claim
  Encounter or Multipurpose Billing Forms
  Scannable Encounter Form
  Keying Insurance Data for Claim Transmission
  Encoder
  Clean Electronic Claims Submission

Putting HIPAA Standard Transactions to Work
  Interactive Transactions

Electronic Remittance Advice

Driving the Data

Methods for Sending Claims

Computer Claims Systems
  Payer or Carrier-Direct
  Clearinghouse

Transmission Reports
  Electronic Processing Problems
  Billing and Account Management Schedule
  Administrative Simplification Enforcement Tool (ASET)
  The Security Rule: Administrative, Physical, and Technical Safeguards

HIPAA: Application to the Practice Setting

Computer Confidentiality
  Confidentiality Statement
  Prevention Measures

Records Management
  Data Storage
  Data Disposal
  Electronic Power Protection

 ASSIGNMENT **8-1** ▸ REVIEW QUESTIONS

Part I Fill in the Blank

Review the objectives, key terms, glossary definitions of key terms, chapter information, and figures before completing the following review questions.

1. Exchange of data in a standardized format through computer systems is a technology

   known as _____.

2. The act of converting computerized data into a code so that unauthorized users are

   unable to read it is a security system known as _____.

3. Payment to the provider of service of an electronically submitted insurance claim

   may be received in approximately _____.

4. List benefits of using HIPAA standard transactions and code sets.

   a. _____

   b. _____

   c. _____

   d. _____

   e. _____

   f. _____

5. Dr. Morgan has 10 or more full-time employees and submits insurance claims for his
   Medicare patients. Is his medical practice subject to the HIPAA transaction rules? _____

6. Dr. Maria Montez does not submit insurance claims electronically and has five
   full-time employees. Is she required to abide by HIPAA transaction rules? _____

7. Name the standard code sets used for the following:

   a. physician services

   _____

   b. diseases and injuries

   _____

   c. pharmaceuticals and biologics

   _____

8. Refer to Table 8–3 in the *Handbook* to complete these statements.

   a. The staff at College Clinic submits professional health care claims for each of their

   providers and must use the industry standard electronic format called _____
   to transmit them electronically.

b. The billing department at College Hospital must use the industry standard

   electronic format called _____

   to transmit health care claims electronically.

c. The Medicare fiscal intermediary (insurance carrier) uses the industry standard

   electronic format called _____

   to transmit payment information to the College Clinic and College Hospital.

d. It has been 3 weeks since Gordon Marshall's health care claim was transmitted
   to the XYZ insurance company and you wish to inquire about the status of the
   claim. The industry standard electronic format that must be used to transmit

   this inquiry is called _____

e. Dr. Practon's insurance billing specialist must use the industry standard electronic

   format called _____ to obtain information

   about Beatrice Garcia's health policy benefits and coverage from the insurance plan.

9. The family practice taxonomy code is _____.

10. A Medicare patient, Charles Gorman, signed a signature authorization form, which is

    on file. The patient's signature source code for data element #1351 is _____.

11. Name the levels for data collected to construct and submit an electronic claim.

    a. _____

    b. _____

    c. _____

    d. _____

    e. _____

    f. _____

12. The most important function of a practice management system is

    _____.

13. To look for and correct all errors before the health claim is transmitted to the insurance carrier, you may

_____

or _____.

14. Add-on software to a practice management system that can reduce the time it takes

to build or review a claim before batching is known as a/an _____.

15. Software that is used in a network that serves a group of users working on a related

project allowing access to the same data is called a/an _____.

Part II Multiple Choice

Choose the best answer.

16. An alert feature that may be incorporated into the software in a physician's office that finds errors so they may be corrected before transmitting an insurance claim is called a/an

   a. online error-edit process

   b. encoder

   c. clearing transactions

   d. edit code sets

17. Under HIPAA, data elements that are used uniformly to document why patients are seen (diagnosis) and what is done to them during their encounter (procedure) are known as

   a. medical code sets

   b. information elements

   c. TCS standards

   d. National Standard Format (NSF)

18. The standard transaction that replaces the paper CMS-1500 (08-05) claim form and more than 400 versions of the electronic National Standard Format is called the

   a. 270

   b. 837I

   c. 837P

   d. 837D

19. A paperless computerized system that enables payments automatically to be transferred to a physician's bank account by a third-party payer may be done via

   a. electronic savings account

   b. electronic remittance advice (ERA)

   c. electronic funds transfer (EFT)

   d. electronic data interchange (EDI)

20. An electronic Medicare remittance advice that takes the place of a paper Medicare explanation of benefits (EOB) is referred to as

   a. ANSI 277

   b. ANSI 820

   c. ANSI 830

   d. ANSI 835

Part III True/False

Write "T" or "F" in the blank to indicate whether you think the statement is true or false.

_____   21. When transmitting electronic claims, inaccuracies that violate the HIPAA standard transaction format are known as syntax errors.

_____   22. An organization may file a complaint online against someone whose actions impact the ability of a transaction to be accepted or efficiently processed by using the Administration Simplification Enforcement Tool (ASET).

_____   23. Incidental uses and disclosures of protected health information (PHI) are permissible under HIPAA when reasonable safeguards have been used to prevent inappropriate revelation of PHI.

_____   24. Deleting files or formatting the hard drive is sufficient to keep electronic protected health information from being accessed.

_____   25. Employees that handle sensitive computer documents should sign an annual confidentiality statement.

_____   26. When an insurance billing specialist e-mails a colleague to ask a coding question, it is permissible to refer to the case using the patient's name.

ASSIGNMENT 8-2 ▸ CRITICAL THINKING FOR MEDICAL
AND NONMEDICAL CODE SETS FOR 837P
ELECTRONIC CLAIMS SUBMISSION

Performance Objective

Task: Decide whether keyed medical and nonmedical data elements are required, situational, or
                      not used when electronically submitting the 837P health care claim.

Conditions: List of keyed data elements (Table 8-6 in *Handbook*) and pen or pencil.

Standards: Time: _____ minutes

                      Accuracy: _____

                      (Note: The time element and accuracy criteria may be given by your instructor.)

Directions. When submitting the 837P health care claim, supporting code sets of medical and nonmedical data
are composed of "Required" and "Situational" data elements. Read each keyed data element and answer whether
you think it is **R** for required, **S** for situational, or **N** for not used.

a. Patient's last menstrual period   _____

b. Patient's telephone number   _____

c. Insured's name   _____

d. Diagnosis code   _____

e. Provider's PIN   _____

f. Procedure code   _____

g. Provider's signature   _____

h. Employer's name   _____

i. Type of service   _____

j. Procedure modifier   _____

ASSIGNMENT 8-3 ▸ INPUT DATA INTO ELEMENT FOR PLACE OF SERVICE CODES FOR 837P ELECTRONIC CLAIMS SUBMISSIONS

Performance Objective

Task: Insert the correct place of service code for each location description where medical professional service was rendered.

Conditions: Place of service codes reference (Figure 8–1), list of places where medical care was rendered, and pen or pencil.

Standards: Time: _____ minutes

Accuracy: _____

(Note: The time element and accuracy criteria may be given by your instructor.)

Directions. When submitting the 837P electronic claim, place of service codes must be entered in data element 1331. Refer to the place of service codes reference list and insert the correct code for each place of service for the following locations.

a. Inpatient psychiatric facility   _____

b. Doctor's office   _____

c. Outpatient hospital   _____

d. Intermediate nursing facility   _____

e. Independent clinic   _____

f. Independent laboratory   _____

g. Birthing center   _____

h. End-stage renal disease treatment facility _____

i. Inpatient hospital   _____

j. Hospice   _____

PLACE OF SERVICE CODES	
Codes	**Place of Service**
01	Pharmacy
02	Unassigned
03	School
04	Homeless shelter
05	Indian health service free-standing facility
06	Indian health service provider-based facility
07	Tribal 638 free-standing facility
08	Tribal 638 provider-based facility
09	Prison/correctional facility
10	Unassigned
11	Doctor's office
12	Patient's home
13	Assisted living facility
14	Group home
15	Mobile unit
16-19	Unassigned
20	Urgent care facility
21	Inpatient hospital
22	Outpatient hospital
23	Emergency department—hospital
24	Ambulatory surgical center
25	Birthing center
26	Military treatment facility/uniformed service treatment facility
27-30	Unassigned
31	Skilled nursing facility (swing bed visits)
32	Nursing facility (intermediate/long-term care facilities)
33	Custodial care facility (domiciliary or rest home services)
34	Hospice (domiciliary or rest home services)
35	Adult living care facility
36-40	Unassigned
41	Ambulance—land
42	Ambulance—air or water
43-48	Unassigned
49	Independent clinic
50	Federally qualified health center
51	Inpatient psychiatric facility
52	Psychiatric facility—partial hospitalization
53	Community mental health care (outpatient, 24-hours-a-day services, admission screening, consultation, and educational services)
54	Intermediate care facility/mentally retarded
55	Residential substance abuse treatment facility
56	Psychiatric residential treatment center
57	Nonresidential substance abuse treatment facility
58-59	Unassigned
60	Mass immunization center
61	Comprehensive inpatient rehabilitation facility
62	Comprehensive outpatient rehabilitation facility
63-64	Unassigned
65	End-stage renal disease treatment facility
66-70	Unassigned
71	State or local public health clinic
72	Rural health clinic
73-80	Unassigned
81	Independent laboratory
82-98	Unassigned
99	Unlisted facility

Figure 8–1

ASSIGNMENT 8–4 ▸ SELECT THE CORRECT INDIVIDUAL RELATIONSHIP CODE NUMBER FOR 837P ELECTRONIC CLAIMS SUBMISSION

Performance Objective

Task: Insert the correct individual relationship code for the patient's relationship to the insured.

Conditions: Individual relationship code number reference (Figure 8–2), list of individuals or entities, and pen or pencil.

Standards: Time: _____ minutes

                    Accuracy: _____

                    (Note: The time element and accuracy criteria may be given by your instructor.)

Directions. Refer to the individual relationship code number list, choose the correct code for the patient's relationship to the insured for the following persons, and insert it on the lines.

a. Mother _____

b. Spouse _____

c. Child _____

d. Father _____

e. Stepdaughter _____

f. Emancipated minor _____

g. Adopted child _____

h. Handicapped dependent _____

i. Stepson _____

j. Sponsored dependent _____

Individual Relationship Code	
Code	**Relationship**
01	Spouse
04	Grandfather or grandmother
05	Grandson or granddaughter
07	Nephew or niece
09	Adopted child
10	Foster child
15	Ward
17	Stepson or stepdaughter
19	Child
20	Employee
21	Unknown
22	Handicapped dependent
23	Sponsored dependent
24	Dependent of a minor dependent
29	Significant other
32	Mother
33	Father
34	Other adult
36	Emancipated minor
39	Organ donor
40	Cadaver donor
41	Injured plaintiff
43	Child where insured has no financial responsibility
53	Life partner
G8	Other relationship

Figure 8–2

ASSIGNMENT 8–5 ▸ SELECT THE CORRECT TAXONOMY CODES FOR
MEDICAL SPECIALIST FOR 837P
ELECTRONIC CLAIMS SUBMISSION

Performance Objective

Task: Choose the correct taxonomy code for each specialist for submission of 837P electronic claims by
                     referring to the Healthcare Provider Taxonomy code list.

Conditions: Healthcare Provider Taxonomy code list (Figure 8–3), list of providers of service, and pen or
                     pencil.

Standards: Time: _____ minutes

                     Accuracy: _____

                     (Note: The time element and accuracy criteria may be given by your instructor.)

Directions. Refer to the Health Care Provider Taxonomy code list, choose the correct code for each of the following
specialists, and insert the code numbers on the lines.

    a. Raymond Skeleton, MD, orthopedist   _____

    b. Gaston Input, MD, gastroenterologist   _____

    c. Vera Cutis, MD, dermatologist   _____

    d. Gene Ulibarri, MD, urologist   _____

    e. Bertha Caesar, MD, obstetrician/gynecologist   _____

    f. Gerald Practon, MD, general practitioner   _____

    g. Pedro Atrics, MD, pediatrician   _____

    h. Astro Parkinson, MD, neurosurgeon   _____

    i. Brady Coccidioides, MD, pulmonary disease   _____

    j. Max Gluteus, RPT, physical therapist   _____

Name	Speciality	Taxonomy Code
College Clinic Staff		
Health Care Provider Taxonomy Codes		
Name	**Speciality**	**Taxonomy Code**
Concha Antrum, MD	Otolaryngologist	207Y00000X
Pedro Atrics, MD	Pediatrician	208000000X
Bertha Caesar, MD	Obstetrician/Gynecologist	207V00000X
Perry Cardi, MD	Cardiologist	207RC0000X
Brady Coccidioides, MD	Pulmonary disease	207RP1001X
Vera Cutis, MD	Dermatologist	207N00000X
Clarence Cutler, MD	General surgeon	208600000X
Dennis Drill, DDS	Dentist	122300000X
Max Gluteus, RPT	Physical therapist	208100000X
Cosmo Graff, MD	Plastic surgeon	208200000X
Malvern Grumose, MD	Pathologist	207ZP0105X
Gaston Input, MD	Gastroenterologist	207RG0100X
Adam Langerhans, MD	Endocrinologist	207RE0101X
Cornell Lenser, MD	Ophthalmologist	207W00000X
Michael Menter, MD	Psychiatrist	2084P0800X
Arthur O. Dont, DDS	Orthodontist	1223X0400X
Astro Parkinson, MD	Neurosurgeon	207T00000X
Nick Pedro, MD	Podiatrist	213E00000X
Gerald Practon, MD	General practitioner	208D00000X
Walter Radon, MD	Radiologst	2085R0202X
Rex Rumsey, MD	Proctologist	208C00000X
Sensitive E. Scott, MD	Anesthesiologist	207L00000X
Raymond Skeleton, MD	Orthopedist	207X00000X
Gene Ulibarri, MD	Urologist	208800000X

Figure 8–3

ASSIGNMENT 8-6 ▸ COMPOSE ELECTRONIC MAIL MESSAGES

Performance Objective

Task: Compose brief messages for electronic mail transmission after reading each scenario.

Conditions: List of scenarios, one sheet of 8½- × 11-inch plain typing paper, and either a typewriter
                         and/or computer or a pen.

Standards: Time: _____ minutes

                         Accuracy: _____

                         (Note: The time element and accuracy criteria may be given by your instructor.)

Directions. Read each scenario. Compose polite, effective, and brief messages that, on the job, would be transmitted via electronic mail (e-mail). Use the guidelines presented in the *Handbook*. Be sure to list a descriptive subject line as the first item in each composition. Single-space the message. Insert a short signature at the end of the message to include your name and affiliation, and create an e-mail address for yourself if you do not have one.

Scenario 1:

Ask an insurance biller, Mary Davis, in a satellite office to locate and fax you a copy of the billing done on account number 43500 for services rendered to Margarita Sylva on March 2, 20xx. Explain that you must telephone the patient about her account. Mary Davis' e-mail address is mdavis@aal.com.

Scenario 2:

Patient Ellen Worth was recently hospitalized; her hospital number is 20-9870-11. Compose an e-mail message to the medical record department at College Hospital (collegehospmedrecords@rrv.net) for her final diagnosis and the assigned diagnostic code needed to complete the insurance claim form.

Scenario 3:

You are working for a billing service and receive an encounter form that is missing the information about the patient's professional service received on August 2, 20xx. The patient's account number is 45098. You have the diagnosis data. Compose an e-mail message to Dr. Mason (pmason@email.mc.com) explaining what you must obtain to complete the billing portion of the insurance claim form.

Scenario 4:

A new patient, John Phillips, has e-mailed your office to ask what the outstanding balance is on his account. The account number is 42990. You look up the financial record and note the service was for an office visit on June 14, 20xx. The charge was $106.11. Compose an e-mail response to Mr. Phillips, whose e-mail address is: bphillips@hotmail.com.

Scenario 5:

You are having difficulty deciding whether the codes 13101, 13102, and 13132 with modifier -51 selected for a case are appropriate. Compose an e-mail message that will be posted on the Part B News Internet listserv (PartB-L@usa.net) asking for comments. The case involves a 12-year-old boy who fell against a bicycle, lacerating the left side of his chest to the pectoralis muscle through a 12-cm gaping wound. He also sustained a 5-cm laceration to his left cheek. Complex repairs were required for these two wounds and totaled 17 cm. Find out whether modifier -15 should be appended to the second code or to the third code.

　　After the instructor has returned your work to you, either make the necessary corrections and place your work in a three-ring notebook for future reference or, if you received a high score, place it in your portfolio for use when applying for a job.

ASSIGNMENT 8–7 ▸ PROOFREAD A COMPUTER-GENERATED HEALTH INSURANCE CLAIM FORM AND LOCATE INCORRECT AND MISSING DATA

Performance Objective

Task: Locate and designate blocks on the computer-generated insurance claim form that have incorrect information or need completion; correct or add data before submission to the insurance company.

Conditions: Use Brad E. Diehl's patient record (Figure 8–4), completed insurance claim (Figure 8–5), and a highlighter and a red ink pen.

Standards: Time: _____ minutes

               Accuracy: _____

               (Note: The time element and accuracy criteria may be given by your instructor.)

Directions. Proofread the insurance claim form (Figure 8–5) and locate blocks that need correction or completion before submission to the insurance company. Highlight all errors you discover. Refer to the patient's record (Figure 8–4) to verify pertinent demographic and insurance information. Refer to the progress notes to verify procedures and determine diagnoses. Verify all entries on the claim form, including dates, codes, rounded out fees, and physician identification numbers. Insert all corrections and missing information in red. If you cannot locate the necessary information but know it is mandatory, write "NEED" in the corresponding block.

Optional. Retype a blank CMS-1500 (08-05) claim form with all corrections and changes. Or if you have access to a computer, use the CD that accompanies the *Workbook* and go to the Handouts folder and print a blank CMS-1500 (08-05) claim form for manual completion.

Additional Coding

1. Assume that Mr. Diehl followed Dr. Input's treatment plan. Refer to his record, abstract information, and locate procedure codes that would be billed by providers outside of the office and the surgeon.

Site	*Description of Service*	*Code*
a. ABC Radiology	_____	_____
b. College Hospital	_____	_____
c. Surgeon	_____	_____

2. Code the symptoms Mr. Diehl was complaining about when he presented for the January 5, 20xx, office visit.

Symptom	*Code*
a. _____	_____
b. _____	_____
c. _____	_____
d. _____	_____
e. _____	_____

PATIENT RECORD NO. 8-7

Diehl	Brad	E.	09-21-46	M	555-222-0123
LAST NAME	FIRST NAME	MIDDLE NAME	BIRTH DATE	SEX	HOME PHONE

3975 Hills Road	Woodland Hills	XY	12345
ADDRESS	CITY	STATE	ZIP CODE

555-703-6600	555-321-0988	555-222-0123	Diehl@WB.net
CELL PHONE	PAGER NO.	FAX NO.	E-MAIL ADDRESS

561-XX-1501	M0983457
PATIENT'S SOC. SEC. NO.	DRIVER'S LICENSE

radio advertising salesman	KACY Radio
PATIENT'S OCCUPATION	NAME OF COMPANY

4071 Mills Road, Woodland Hills, XY 12335	555-201-6666
ADDRESS OF EMPLOYER	PHONE

Tak E. Diehl (birthdate 4-7-45)	legal secretary
SPOUSE OR PARENT	OCCUPATION

Attys. Dilman, Forewise & Gilson,	12 West Dix Street, Woodland Hills, XY 12345	555-222-6432
EMPLOYER	ADDRESS	PHONE

Aetna Insurance Co., 2412 Main Street, Woodland Hills, XY 12345	Brad E. Diehl
NAME OF INSURANCE	INSURED OR SUB SCRIBER

403119	
POLICY/CERTIFICATE NO.	GROUP NO.

REFERRED BY: Raymond Skeleton, MD

DATE	PROGRESS NOTES	No. 8-7
1-6-20xx	NP pt comes in complaining of coughing and sneezing; some difficulty breathing.	
	Occasional dizziness and epigastric abdominal pain with cramping. Symptoms started in	
	July of last year. Performed a detailed history and physical examination with low	
	complexity medical decision making. AP & lat chest x-rays taken; neg findings. BP 178/98.	
	Pt to have cholecystography with oral contrast at ABC Radiology. Diagnostic colonoscopy	
	(flexible) to be scheduled at College Hospital. Dx: hypertension and respiratory distress;	
	R/O irritable colon. No disability at this time.	
	GI/llf *Gaston Input, MD*	
1-20-xx	Pt retns for a EPF hx/exam LC MDM. Oral cholecystography reveals a single 1.5 cm	
	radiolucent calculus within the cholecyst. Colonoscopy confirmed irritable bowel	
	syndrome. Blood drawn and CBC (auto with diff) performed in office indicates	
	WBC 10,000. DX: cholecistitis with cholelithiasis. Adv. cholecystectomy	
	(abdominal approach) as soon as possible; to be scheduled at College Hospital.	
	GI/llf *Gaston Input, MD*	

Figure 8–4

Figure 8–5

ASSIGNMENT 8-8 ▸ PROOFREAD A COMPUTER-GENERATED HEALTH INSURANCE CLAIM FORM AND LOCATE INCORRECT AND MISSING DATA

Performance Objective

Task: Locate and designate blocks on the computer-generated insurance claim form that have incorrect information or need completion; correct or add data before submission to the insurance company.

Conditions: Use Evert I. Strain's patient record (Figure 8–6), completed insurance claim (Figure 8–7), and a highlighter and a red ink pen.

Standards: Time: _____ minutes

Accuracy: _____

(Note: The time element and accuracy criteria may be given by your instructor.)

Directions. Proofread the insurance claim form (Figure 8–7) and locate blocks that need correction or completion before submission to the insurance company. Highlight all errors you discover. Refer to the patient's record (Figure 8–6) to verify pertinent demographic and insurance information. Refer to the progress notes to verify procedures and determine diagnoses. Verify all entries on the claim form, including dates, codes, rounded out fees, and physician identification numbers. Insert all corrections and missing information in red. If you cannot locate the necessary information but know it is mandatory, write "NEED" in the corresponding block.

Optional. Retype a blank CMS-1500 (08-05) claim form with all corrections and changes. Or if you have access to a computer, use the CD that accompanies the *Workbook* and go to the Handouts folder and print a blank CMS-1500 (08-05) claim form for manual completion.

Additional Coding

1. Refer to Mr. Strain's medical record, abstract information, and code procedures that would be billed by outside providers.

Site	Description of Service	Code
a. ABC Laboratory	_____	_____
b. ABC Radiology	_____	_____

PATIENT RECORD NO. 8-8

Strain,	Evert	I	09-11-46	M	555-678-0211
LAST NAME	FIRST NAME	MIDDLE NAME	BIRTH DATE	SEX	HOME PHONE

7650 None Such Road	Woodland Hills	XY	12345
ADDRESS	CITY	STATE	ZIP CODE

555-430-2101	555-320-9980	555-678-0211	Strain@WB.net
CELL PHONE	PAGER NO.	FAX NO.	E-MAIL ADDRESS

453-XX-4739	Y0923658
PATIENT'S SOC. SEC. NO.	DRIVER'S LICENSE

mechanical engineer	R & R Company
PATIENT'S OCCUPATION	NAME OF COMPANY

2400 Davon Road, Woodland Hills, XY 12345	555-520-8977
ADDRESS OF EMPLOYER	PHONE

Ester I. Strain (wife)	administrative assistant
SPOUSE OR PARENT	OCCUPATION

University College, 4021 Book Road, Woodland Hills, XY 12345	555-450-9908
EMPLOYER	ADDRESS	PHONE

ABC Insurance Co., P.O.Box 130, Woodland Hills, XY 12345	Evert I. Strain
NAME OF INSURANCE	INSURED OR SUBSCRIBER

453-XX-4739	96476A
POLICY/CERTIFICATE NO.	GROUP NO.

REFERRED BY: Gerald C. Jones, MD, 1403 Haven Street, Woodland Hills, XY 12345   NPI # 54754966XX

DATE	PROGRESS NOTES	No. 8-8
1-8-20xx	Est pt comes in complaining of frequent urination, headaches, polyphagia; unable to	
	remember current events. These problems have been present for almost a year.	
	A comprehensive history is taken and compared to his last H & P 2 years ago.	
	A com PX is performed. BP 160/110; pt was prescribed antihypertensive medication but	
	discontinued it when the prescription ran out. Lab report, hand carried by pt from an	
	urgent care center indicates SGOT in normal range and cholesterol elevated. Fasting blood	
	sugar extremely high. Dx: diabetes mellitus, malignant hypertensive, and ASCVD.	
	Pt to have 3 hour GTT tomorrow a.m. at ABC laboratory. STAT CT scan of head s⁻ contrast	
	ordered at ABC radiology to follow lab work. Arrangement will be made for pt to be	
	admitted to College Hospital. Disability 1/9 through 1/31.	
	GI/llf *Gerald Practon, MD*	
1-9-xx	Admit to College Hospital (C hx/exam MC MDM).	
	GI/llf *Gerald Practon, MD*	
1-10-xx	Hosp visit (PF hx/exam SF MDM). CT scan of head reviewed, neg. findings. Pt alert and	
	comfortable. If blood sugar and BP remain stable, discharge planned for tomorrow.	
	BP 130/85.	
	GI/llf *Gerald Practon, MD*	
1-11-xx	DC from hosp. Pt to be seen in one week in ofc.	
	GI/llf *Gerald Practon, MD*	

Figure 8–6

(1500) HEALTH INSURANCE CLAIM FORM

APPROVED BY NATIONAL UNIFORM CLAIM COMMITTEE 08/05

☐☐ PICA   PICA ☐☐

1. MEDICARE (Medicare #)	MEDICAID (Medicaid #)	TRICARE CHAMPUS (Sponsor's SSN)	CHAMPVA (Member ID#)	GROUP HEALTH PLAN (SSN or ID) [X]	FECA BLK LUNG (SSN)	OTHER (ID)	1a. INSURED'S I.D. NUMBER (For Program in Item 1)

453 XX 4739   96476A

2. PATIENT'S NAME (Last Name, First Name, Middle Initial)
STRAIN EVERT I

3. PATIENT'S BIRTH DATE MM DD YY   **SEX** M [X] F ☐

4. INSURED'S NAME (Last Name, First Name, Middle Initial)
SAME

5. PATIENT'S ADDRESS (No., Street)
7650 NONE SUCH ROAD

6. PATIENT RELATIONSHIP TO INSURED
Self ☐ Spouse ☐ Child ☐ Other ☐

7. INSURED'S ADDRESS (No., Street)

CITY WOODLAND HILLS   **STATE** XY

8. PATIENT STATUS
Single ☐ Married [X] Other ☐

CITY   **STATE**

ZIP CODE   **TELEPHONE (Include Area Code)** ( )

Employed [X] Full-Time Student ☐ Part-Time Student ☐

ZIP CODE   **TELEPHONE (INCLUDE AREA CODE)** ( )

9. OTHER INSURED'S NAME (Last Name, First Name, Middle Initial)

10. IS PATIENT'S CONDITION RELATED TO:

11. INSURED'S POLICY GROUP OR FECA NUMBER

a. OTHER INSURED'S POLICY OR GROUP NUMBER

a. EMPLOYMENT? (CURRENT OR PREVIOUS)
YES ☐ [X] NO

a. INSURED'S DATE OF BIRTH MM DD YY   **SEX** M ☐ F ☐

b. OTHER INSURED'S DATE OF BIRTH MM DD YY   **SEX** M ☐ F ☐

b. AUTO ACCIDENT?   PLACE (State)
YES ☐ [X] NO

b. EMPLOYER'S NAME OR SCHOOL NAME

c. EMPLOYER'S NAME OR SCHOOL NAME

c. OTHER ACCIDENT?
YES ☐ [X] NO

c. INSURANCE PLAN NAME OR PROGRAM NAME

d. INSURANCE PLAN NAME OR PROGRAM NAME

10d. RESERVED FOR LOCAL USE

d. IS THERE ANOTHER HEALTH BENEFIT PLAN?
YES ☐ NO ☐   *If yes*, return to and complete item 9 a-d.

READ BACK OF FORM BEFORE COMPLETING & SIGNING THIS FORM.
12. PATIENT'S OR AUTHORIZED PERSON'S SIGNATURE I authorize the release of any medical or other information necessary to process this claim. I also request payment of government benefits either to myself or to the party who accepts assignment below.

SIGNED _____   DATE _____

13. INSURED'S OR AUTHORIZED PERSON'S SIGNATURE I authorize payment of medical benefits to the undersigned physician or supplier for services described below.

SIGNED _____

14. DATE OF CURRENT: MM DD YY ◄ ILLNESS (First symptom) OR INJURY (Accident) OR PREGNANCY(LMP)

15. IF PATIENT HAS HAD SAME OR SIMILAR ILLNESS. GIVE FIRST DATE MM DD YY

16. DATES PATIENT UNABLE TO WORK IN CURRENT OCCUPATION
FROM MM DD YY   TO MM DD YY

17. NAME OF REFERRING PHYSICIAN OR OTHER SOURCE
GERALD C JONES

17a.
17b. NPI 54754966XX

18. HOSPITALIZATION DATES RELATED TO CURRENT SERVICES
FROM 01 09 20XX   TO 01 11 20XX

19. RESERVED FOR LOCAL USE

20. OUTSIDE LAB? YES ☐ [X] NO $ CHARGES

21. DIAGNOSIS OR NATURE OF ILLNESS OR INJURY. (RELATE ITEMS 1,2,3 OR 4 TO ITEM 24E BY LINE)

1. 250.00
2. 401.0
3. ___.___
4. ___.___

22. MEDICAID RESUBMISSION CODE 1   ORIGINAL REF. NO.

23. PRIOR AUTHORIZATION NUMBER

24. A. DATE(S) OF SERVICE From MM DD YY To MM DD YY	B. PLACE OF SERVICE	C. EMG	D. PROCEDURES, SERVICES, OR SUPPLIES (Explain Unusual Circumstances) CPT/HCPCS MODIFIER	E. DIAGNOSIS POINTER	F. $ CHARGES	G. DAYS OR UNITS	H. EPSDT Family Plan	I. ID. QUAL.	J. RENDERING PROVIDER ID. #
1	01 08 20XX	11		99215		96 97	1		NPI	46278897XX
2	01 09 20XX	21		99222		120 80	1		NPI	46278897XX
3	1 10 20XX	21		99231		37 74	1		NPI	46278897XX
4	01 11 20XX	21		99231		65 26	1		NPI	46278897XX
5									NPI	
6									NPI	

25. FEDERAL TAX I.D. NUMBER 7034597   SSN ☐ EIN [X]

26. PATIENT'S ACCOUNT NO. 8

27. ACCEPT ASSIGNMENT? (For govt. claims, see back)
[X] YES NO ☐

28. TOTAL CHARGE $ 320 77

29. AMOUNT PAID $

30. BALANCE DUE $ 320 77

31. SIGNATURE OF PHYSICIAN OR SUPPLIER INCLUDING DEGREES OR CREDENTIALS (I certify that the statements on the reverse apply to this bill and are made a part thereof.)

GERALD PRACTON MD   01/25/20XX
SIGNED   DATE

32. SERVICE FACILITY LOCATION INFORMATION
a. NPI   b.

33. BILLING PROVIDER INFO & PH # (555) 4869002
COLLEGE CLINIC
4567 BROAD AVENUE
WOODLAND HILLS XY 12345 0001
a. 3664021CC NPI   b.

NUCC Instruction Manual available at: www.nucc.org   **PLEASE PRINT OR TYPE**   APPROVED OMB-0938-0999 FORM CMS-1500 (08-05)

Figure 8–7

ASSIGNMENT 8–9 ▸ DEFINE PATIENT RECORD ABBREVIATIONS

Performance Objective

Task: Insert definitions of abbreviations.

Conditions: Use pencil or pen.

Standards: Time: _____ minutes

                   Accuracy: _____

                   (Note: The time element and accuracy criteria may be given by your instructor.)

Directions. After completing the assignments in this chapter, you will be able to define the abbreviations shown here.

Abbreviations pertinent to the record of Brad E. Diehl:

NP	_____	R/O	_____
LC	_____	auto	_____
pt	_____	retn	_____
MDM	_____	diff	_____
AP	_____	EPF	_____
cm	_____	WBC	_____
lat	_____	hx	_____
neg	_____	DX	_____
BP	_____	exam	_____
CBC	_____	adv	_____

Abbreviations pertinent to the record of Evert I. Strain:

est	_____	exam	_____
CT	_____	PX	_____
pt	_____	MC	_____
C	_____	BP	_____
H & P	_____	MDM	_____
hx	_____	lab	_____
comp	_____	hosp	_____

SGOT _____   neg _____

PF _____   GTT _____

Dx _____   DC _____

SF _____   STAT _____

ASCVD _____   ofc _____

ALTAPOINT PRACTICE MANAGEMENT SOFTWARE ASSIGNMENTS

ASSIGNMENT 8–10 ▸ TRANSMIT AN ELECTRONIC INSURANCE CLAIM TO A PRIVATE INSURANCE COMPANY USING THE PRACTICE MANAGEMENT SYSTEM

Performance Objective

Task: Transmit an electronic insurance claim using the practice management system.

Conditions: Patient computer data and computer

Standards: Time:_____ minutes

                 Accuracy:_____

                 (Note: The time element and accuracy criteria may be given by your instructor.)

Directions. Before attempting the Practice Management software assignment, refer to Appendix C and follow the instructions provided to familiarize yourself with the software. Then refer to the Practice Management software on the CD that accompanies the *Workbook*.

1. For this assignment, follow the instructions for transmitting and insurance claim electronically and transmit the claim for Teri E. Simpson's February 9 charges.

2. Print a hard copy of the insurance claim to hand in to your instructor to receive a score.

3. A Performance Evaluation Checklist may be reproduced from the " Instruction Guide to the *Workbook*" chapter if your instructor wishes you to submit it to assist with scoring and comments.

After the instructor has returned your work to you, either make the necessary corrections and place your work in a three-ring notebook for future reference or, if you received a high score, place it in your portfolio for reference when applying for a job.

ASSIGNMENT 8-11 ▶ ENTER A NEW PATIENT INTO THE PRACTIC E MANAGEMENT SYSTEM AND TRANSMIT AN INSURANCE CLAIM ELECTONICALLY

Performance Objective

Task:
Enter new patient data into the practice management system and transmit an insurance claim electronically

Conditions:
Encounter form (Figure 8-8) and computer

Standards:
Time:_____ minutes

Accuracy:_____

(Note: The time element and accuracy criteria may be given by your instructor.)

Directions. Before attempting the Practice Management software assignment, refer to Appendix C and follow the instructions provided to familiarize yourself with the software. Then refer to the Practice Management software on the CD that accompanies the *Workbook*.

1. For this assignment, follow the instructions for entering a new patient and enter the information and fee for Luisa Garcia's first office visit on May 7 from the encounter form (superbill).

2. After the information has been entered, transmit the insurance claim to Luisa Garcia's insurance company by following the instructions for transmitting a claim electronically.

3. Print a hard copy of the insurance claim to hand in to your instructor to receive a score.

4. A Performance Evaluation Checklist may be reproduced form the "Instruction Guide to the *Workbook*" chapter if your instructor wishes you to submit it to assist with scoring and comments.

After the instructor has returned your work to you, either make the necessary corrections and place your work in a three-ring notebook for future reference or, if you received a high score, place it in your portfolio for reference when applying for a job.

Assignment 8-11

College Clinic
4567 Broad Avenue
Woodlands Hills, XY
12345-0001
Tel (555) 486-9002
Fax (555) 487-8976

Doctors No. _____

☒ PRIVATE   ☐ MANAGED CARE   ☐ MEDICAID   ☐ MEDICARE   ☐ TRICARE   ☐ W/C

ACCOUNT #: GARC000001	TODAY'S DATE: 05-07-2007		

LAST NAME: Garcia	FIRST NAME: Luisa	MIDDLE INITIAL: M	DOB: 11/23/2006 SEX: F

HOME PHONE: (801) 555-1237	CELL PHONE: / PAGER:	PATIENT EMAIL:

ADDRESS: 2163 Main St. Midvale, UT 84047   EMPLOYER NAME:

SSN: 555-33-8798   DRIVER'S LICENSE: EMPLOYER ADDRESS:

NAME OF SPOUSE OR PARENT: Manuel Garcia   PATIENT OCCUPATION:

NAME OF INSURANCE CO.: United Western Benefits   EMPLOYER PHONE:

ADDRESS OF INSURANCE CO.: 151 S. Market Street Salt Lake City, UT   POLICY NUMBER: A555-66-1111   GROUP NUMBER: AL-106

ASSIGNMENT: I hereby assign payment directly to College Clinic of the surgical and/or medical benefits, if any, otherwise payable to me for his/her services as described below.
SIGNED (Patient, or Parent, if Minor)   DATE:

DESCRIPTION	CPT-4/MD	FEE		DESCRIPTION	CPT-4/MD	FEE	DESCRIPTION	CPT-4/MD	FEE
OFFICE VISIT-NEW PATIENT				**WELL BABY EXAM**			**LABORATORY**		
Level 1	99201		X	Intial	99381	80.00	Glucose	82951	
Level 2	99202			Periodic	99391		Heamatocrit	85013	
Level 3	99203			**OFFICE PROCEDURES**			Occult Blood	82270	
Level 4	99204			Anscopy	46600		Urine Dip	81000	
Level 5	99205			ECG	93000		**X-RAY**		
OFFICE VISIT-ESTAB. PATIENT				Fracture Rpr Foot	28470		Foot - 2 View	73620	
Level 1	99211			I & D	10060		Forearm - 2 View	73090	
Level 2	99212			Suture Repair	12002		Nasal Bone - 3	70160	
Level 3	99213						Spine LS - 2 view	72100	
Level 4	99214			**INJECTIONS/VACCINATIONS**					
Level 5	99215		X	DPT	90701	45.00	**MISCELLANEOUS**		
OFFICE CONSULT-NP/EST				IM-Antibiotic	90788		Handling of Spec	99000	
Level 3	99243			Influenza Vac	90658		Supply	99070	
Level 4	99244			Tetanus	90703		Venipuncture	36415	
Level 5	99245		X	Immun Admin	90471	15.00			

COMMENTS:

Physician:

RETURN APPOINTMENT
_____ Week(s)   _____ Month(s)

DIAGNOSIS:
Primary: Routine Health Check   CODE V20.2
Secondary: Vaccination   V06.1

REC'D BY:
☐ BANK CARD
☐ CASH
☐ CHECK
#_____

PREVIOUS BALANCE 0
TODAY'S FEE 140.00
AMOUNT REC'D/CO-PAY
BALANCE

Figure 8–8

ASSIGNMENT 8-12 ▸ ENTER A NEW PATIENT INTO THE PRACTICE MANAGEMENT SYSTEM AND TRANSMIT AN INSURANCE CLAIM ELECTRONICALLY

Performance Objective

Task: Enter new patient data into the practice management system and transmit an insurance claim electronically

Conditions: Encounter form (Figure 8-9) and computer

Standards: Time:_____ minutes

Accuracy:_____

(Note: The time element and accuracy criteria may be given by your instructor.)

Directions. Before attempting the Practice Management software assignment, refer to Appendix C and follow the instructions provided to familiarize yourself with the software. Then refer to the Practice Management software on the CD that accompanies the *Workbook*.

1. For this assignment, follow the instructions for entering a new patient and enter the information and fee for Jane R. Maywood's first office visit on May 10 from the encounter form (superbill).

2. After the information has been entered, transmit the insurance claim to Jane R. Maywood's insurance company by following the instructions for transmitting a claim electronically.

3. Print a hard copy of the insurance claim to hand in to your instructor to receive a score.

4. A Performance Evaluation Checklist may be reproduced from the "Instruction Guide to the *Workbook*" chapter if your instructor wishes you to submit it to assist with scoring and comments.

After the instructor has returned your work to you, either make the necessary corrections and place your work in a three-ring notebook for future reference or, if you received a high score, place it in your portfolio for reference when applying for a job.

Assignment 8-12a

College Clinic

4567 Broad Avenue
Woodlands Hills, XY
12345-0001
Tel (555) 486-9002
Fax (555) 487-8976

Doctors No. _____

[X] PRIVATE   [ ] MANAGED CARE   [ ] MEDICAID   [ ] MEDICARE   [ ] TRICARE   [ ] W/C

ACCOUNT #: MAYW000001	TODAY'S DATE: 05-10-2007		

LAST NAME: Maywood	FIRST NAME: Jane	MIDDLE INITIAL: R	DOB: 3/14/1968 SEX: F

HOME PHONE: (801) 555-6868	CELL PHONE: PAGER:	PATIENT EMAIL:

ADDRESS: 9218 W. Daisy Av. Midvale, UT 84047	EMPLOYER NAME: Altadata Systems

SSN: 555-11-XXXX	DRIVER'S LICENSE: T738625	EMPLOYER ADDRESS: 1100 East South Union Ave Midvale, UT 84047

NAME OF SPOUSE OR PARENT: John Maywood	PATIENT OCCUPATION: Programmer

NAME OF INSURANCE CO.: United Western Benefits	EMPLOYER PHONE: (801) 555-2313

ADDRESS OF INSURANCE CO.: 151 S. Market St. Salt Lake City, UT 84131	POLICY NUMBER: A555-66-1212	GROUP NUMBER: AL-119

ASSIGNMENT: I hereby assign payment directly to College Clinic of the surgical and/or medical benefits, if any, otherwise payable to me for his/her services as described below.
SIGNED (Patient, or Parent, if Minor)   DATE:

DESCRIPTION	CPT-4/MD	FEE	DESCRIPTION	CPT-4/MD	FEE	DESCRIPTION	CPT-4/MD	FEE
OFFICE VISIT-NEW PATIENT			**WELL BABY EXAM**			**LABORATORY**		
Level 1	99201		Intial	99381		Glucose	82951	
X Level 2	99202	65.00	Periodic	99391		Heamatocrit	85013	
Level 3	99203		**OFFICE PROCEDURES**			Occult Blood	82270	
Level 4	99204		Anscopy	46600		X Urine Dip	81000	35.00
Level 5	99205		ECG	93000		**X-RAY**		
OFFICE VISIT-ESTAB, PATIENT			Fracture Rpr Foot	28470		Foot - 2 View	73620	
Level 1	99211		I & D	10060		Forearm - 2 View	73090	
Level 2	99212		Suture Repair	12002		Nasal Bone - 3	70160	
Level 3	99213					Spine LS - 2 view	72100	
Level 4	99214		**INJECTIONS/VACCINATIONS**					
Level 5	99215		DPT	90701		**MISCELLANEOUS**		
OFFICE CONSULT-NP/EST			IM-Antibiotic	90788		Handling of Spec	99000	
Level 3	99243		Influenza Vac	90658		Supply	99070	
Level 4	99244		Tetanus	90703		Venipuncture	36415	
Level 5	99245		Immun Admin	90471				

COMMENTS: RETURN APPOINTMENT
Physician: ____ Week(s) ____ Month(s)

DIAGNOSIS: DESCRIPTION CODE
Primary: Urinary Tract Inf. 599.0
Secondary: _____

REC'D BY:
[ ] BANK CARD
[ ] CASH
[ ] CHECK
_____

PREVIOUS BALANCE 0
TODAY'S FEE 100.00
AMOUNT REC'D/CO-PAY
BALANCE

Figure 8–9

ASSIGNMENT **8–13** ▸ **ENTER A NEW PATIENT INTO THE PRACTICE MANAGEMENT SYSTEM AND TRANSMIT AN INSURANCE CLAIM ELECTONICALLY**

Performance Objective

Task: Enter new patient data into the practice management system and transmit an insurance claim electronically

Conditions: Encounter form (Figure 8-10) and computer

Standards: Time:_____ minutes

                Accuracy:_____

                (Note: The time element and accuracy criteria may be given by your instructor.)

Directions. Before attempting the Practice Management software assignment, refer to Appendix C and follow the instructions provided to familiarize yourself with the software. Then refer to the Practice Management software on the CD that accompanies the *Workbook*.

1. For this assignment, follow the instructions for entering new patient information on Glen Waxman.

2. Then follow the instructions for entering charges from an encounter form (superbill) and enter the fees for Glen Waxman's new patient office visit on July 30 from the encounter form (superbill).

3. After the information has been entered, transmit the insurance claim to Mr. Waxman's insurance company by following the instructions for transmitting a claim electronically.

4. Print a hard copy of the insurance claim to hand in t o your instructor to receive a score.

5. A Performance Evaluation Checklist may be reproduced form the "Instruction Guide to the *Workbook*" chapter if your instructor wishes you to submit it to assist with scoring and comments.

After the instructor has returned your work to you, either make the necessary corrections and place your work in a three-ring notebook for future reference or, if you received a high score, place it in your portfolio for reference when applying for a job.

Assignment 8-12b

College Clinic
4567 Broad Avenue
Woodlands Hills, XY
12345-0001
Tel (555) 486-9002
Fax (555) 487-8976

Doctors No. _____

☒ PRIVATE   ☐ MANAGED CARE   ☐ MEDICAID   ☐ MEDICARE   ☐ TRICARE   ☐ W/C

ACCOUNT #:	TODAY'S DATE:
WAXM000001	07/30/2007

LAST NAME:	FIRST NAME:	MIDDLE INITIAL:	DOB:	SEX:
Waxman	Glen	R	10/19/1948	M

HOME PHONE:	CELL PHONE:	PATIENT EMAIL:
(801) 555-1191	PAGER:	

ADDRESS:	EMPLOYER NAME:
3691 Thomson Drive Midvale, UT 84047	Altadata Systems

SSN:	DRIVER'S LICENSE:	EMPLOYER ADDRESS:
555-88-4444	S911026	1100 East South Union Ave Midvale, UT 84047

NAME OF SPOUSE OR PARENT:	PATIENT OCCUPATION:
Marjorie Waxman	Programmer

NAME OF INSURANCE CO.:	EMPLOYER PHONE:
United Western Benefits	

ADDRESS OF INSURANCE CO.:	POLICY NUMBER:	GROUP NUMBER:
151 S. Market St. Salt Lake City, UT 84131	A555-77-1193	AL-271

ASSIGNMENT: I hereby assign payment directly to College Clinic of the surgical and/or medical benefits, if any, otherwise payable to me for his/her services as described below.
SIGNED (Patient, or Parent, if Minor)   DATE:

DESCRIPTION	CPT-4/MD	FEE	DESCRIPTION	CPT-4/MD	FEE	DESCRIPTION	CPT-4/MD	FEE
OFFICE VISIT-NEW PATIENT			**WELL BABY EXAM**			**LABORATORY**		
Level 1	99201		Intial	99381		Glucose	82951	
X Level 2	99202	65.00	Periodic	99391		Heamatocrit	85013	
Level 3	99203		**OFFICE PROCEDURES**			Occult Blood	82270	
Level 4	99204		Anscopy	46600		Urine Dip	81000	
Level 5	99205		X ECG	93000	125.00	**X-RAY**		
OFFICE VISIT-ESTAB, PATIENT			Fracture Rpr Foot	28470		Foot - 2 View	73620	
Level 1	99211		I & D	10060		Forearm - 2 View	73090	
Level 2	99212		Suture Repair	12002		Nasal Bone - 3	70160	
Level 3	99213					Spine LS - 2 view	72100	
Level 4	99214		**INJECTIONS/VACCINATIONS**					
Level 5	99215		DPT	90701		**MISCELLANEOUS**		
OFFICE CONSULT-NP/EST			IM-Antibiotic	90788		Handling of Spec	99000	
Level 3	99243		Influenza Vac	90658		Supply	99070	
Level 4	99244		Tetanus	90703		Venipuncture	36415	
Level 5	99245		Immun Admin	90471				

COMMENTS:

Physician:

RETURN APPOINTMENT

_____ Week(s)   _____ Month(s)

DIAGNOSIS: DESCRIPTION   CODE
Primary: Chest Pain   786.52
Secondary: _____   _____

REC'D BY:
☐ BANK CARD
☐ CASH
☐ CHECK
_____

PREVIOUS BALANCE 0
TODAY'S FEE 190.00
AMOUNT REC'D/CO-PAY
BALANCE 190.00

Figure 8–10

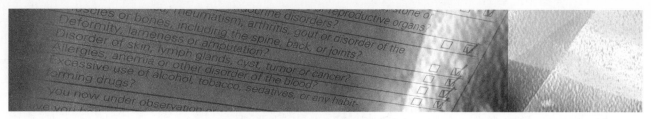

Receiving Payments and Insurance Problem Solving

KEY TERMS

Your instructor may wish to select some words pertinent to this chapter for a test. For definitions of the terms, further study, and/or reference, the words, phrases, and abbreviations may be found in the glossary at the end of the Handbook. *Key terms for this chapter follow.*

appeal

delinquent claim

denied paper or electronic claim

explanation of benefits (EOB)

inquiry

lost claim

overpayment

peer review

rebill (resubmit)

rejected claim

remittance advice (RA)

review

suspended claim

suspense

tracer

KEY ABBREVIATIONS

See how many abbreviations and acronyms you can translate and then use this as a handy reference list. Definitions for the key abbreviations are located near the back of the Handbook *in the glossary.*

ALJ _____

CMS _____

DAB _____

EOB _____

ERISA _____

FTC _____

HIPAA _____

HMO _____

HO _____

NPI _____

RA _____

UPIN _____

PERFORMANCE OBJECTIVES

The student will be able to:

■ Define and spell the key terms and key abbreviations for this chapter, given the information from the *Handbook* glossary, within a reasonable time period and with enough accuracy to obtain a satisfactory evaluation.
■ After reading the chapter, answer the fill-in-the-blanks, multiple choice, and true and false review questions with enough accuracy to obtain a satisfactory evaluation.
■ Complete the insurance claim tracer form, given a request for an insurance claim trace and the patient's insurance claim, within a reasonable time period and with enough accuracy to obtain a satisfactory evaluation.

■ Locate the errors on each claim, given three returned insurance claims, within a reasonable time period and with enough accuracy to obtain a satisfactory evaluation.
■ Complete form CMS-1965, Request for Hearing, Part B, Medicare Claim, within a reasonable time period and with enough accuracy to obtain a satisfactory evaluation.
■ File an appeal by composing and typing a letter with envelope, within a reasonable time period and with enough accuracy to obtain a satisfactory evaluation.

ALTAPOINT PRACTICE MANAGEMENT SOFTWARE OBJECTIVES

The student will be able to:

■ Post payments from an explanation of benefits document to a patient's account and print patients' financial accounting records using practice

management software, within a reasonable time period and with enough accuracy to obtain a satisfactory evaluation.

STUDY OUTLINE

Follow-Up after Claim Submission
Claim Policy Provisions
  Insured
  Payment Time Limits
Explanation of Benefits
  Components of an EOB
  Interpretation of an EOB
  Posting an EOB
Claim Management Techniques
  Insurance Claims Register
  Tickler File
  Insurance Company Payment History
Claim Inquiries
Problem Paper and Electronic Claims
  Types of Problems

Rebilling
Review and Appeal Process
Filing an Official Appeal
  Medicare Review and Redetermination Process
  TRICARE Review and Appeal Process
State Insurance Commissioner
  Commission Objectives
  Types of Problems
  Commission Inquiries
Procedure: Trace an Unpaid Insurance Claim
Procedure: File an Official Appeal

ASSIGNMENT (9-1)▸ REVIEW QUESTIONS

Part I Fill in the Blank

Review the objectives, key terms, and chapter information before completing
the following review questions.

1. Name provisions seen in health insurance policies.

   a. Payment time limits   inso. Co to claiment

   b. notification time limits claiment to ins. co.

   c. if caiment is in disagreement then claiment has 3yrs after claim is submitted to take legal action

   d. Claiment can't bring legal action against a co. until 60 days after claim is submitted

2. After an insurance claim is processed by the insurance carrier (paid, suspended,

   rejected, or denied), a document known as a/an __EOB__
   is sent to the patient and to the provider of professional medical services.

3. Name other items that indicate the patient's responsibility to pay that may appear on
   the document explaining the payment and check issued by the insurance carrier.

   a. Amount not covered

   b. Copayment amount

   c. deductable

   d. Co insurance

   e. Other insurance payment

   f. the patients total responsibility

4. After receiving an explanation of benefits (EOB) document and posting insurance

   payment, the copy of the insurance claim form is put into a file marked clearly in patients folder

5. To locate delinquent insurance claims on an insurance claims register quickly, which
   column should be looked at first?

   tickler File

   Would it appear blank or completed? Completed

6. Name some of the principal procedures that should be followed in good bookkeeping and record-keeping practice when a payment has been received from an insurance company.

① Keep a 3x5 card or 8x11 piece of paper in patients file & when payment comes in mark it it patients file as well as the accounting books.
② use a good check & balance & that'll help you find any mistakes if there are any

7. In good office management, a manual method used to track submitted pending or resubmitted insurance claims, a/an ___claim inquiry___ is used.

8. Two procedures to include in a manual reminder system to track pending claims are:

   a. ___inquiry___

   b. ___tracer___

9. In making an inquiry about a claim by telephone, efficient secretarial procedure would be to

   ___ID Yourself___
   ___ID Your Boss + office___
   ___ID the Patient and claim in question___

10. Denied paper or electronic claims are those denied because of

    P.352 ___selected diagnoses not covered___
    or ___frequency limitations ir restrictions per payperiod___.

11. State the solution if a claim has been denied because the professional service rendered was for an injury that is being considered as compensable under workers' compensation.

    ↑ = entitled to Compensation

    ___= Best Pay it___
    ___I didn't know what tment dog looked it up on the Net.___

12. At the time of his first office visit, Mr. Doi signed an Assignment of Benefits, and Dr. James' office submitted a claim to ABC Insurance Company. Mr. Doi received, in error, a check from the insurance company and cashed it. What steps should be taken by Dr. James' office after this error is discovered?

    a. ___Call Doi & tell him thats your $___

    b. ___Call insurance Co & tell them of the mistake___

    c. ___Collect $ from Doi___

13. If an appeal of an insurance claim is not successful, the next step to proceed with is a/an

P. 345

Peer Review .

14. Name the five levels for appealing a Medicare claim.

a. _Re determination_

b. _Hearing officer_

P. 346

c. _Administrative law judge_

d. _Departmental appeal Board review_

e. _Judicial review in US District Court_

15. Medicare reconsideration by the insurance carrier is usually completed

P. 349

within ____30____ to ____45____ days.

16. A Medicare patient has insurance with United American (a Medigap policy), and payment has not been received from the Medigap insurer within a reasonable length of time. State the action to take in this case.

P. 349

1st try the paper or electronic claim solutions for delinquent claims

17. A TRICARE EOB is received stating that the allowable charge for Mrs. Dayton's office visit is $30. Is it possible to appeal this for additional payment? Answer "yes" or "no," and explain.

yes if the Dr's office is registered w/ TRICARE

18. A state department or agency that helps resolve complaints about insurance policies, medical claims, or insurance agents or brokers and that verifies that insurance contracts are carried out in good faith is known as a/an

State insurance Commissioner .

19. When an insurance company consistently pays slowly on insurance claims, it may help speed up payments if a formal written complaint is made to the

insurance Commissioner .

Part II Multiple Choice

Choose the best answer.

20. If the insurance carrier is a self-insured plan, a Medicaid or Medicare health maintenance organization, or an Employee Retirement Income Security Act (ERISA)–based plan, the insurance commissioner

    a. is able to assist with carrier issues.

    b. is not able to assist with carrier issues.

    c. is able to assist on specific problem issues related to payment.

    d. is able to give help on denied insurance claims.

21. A written request made to an insurance company to locate the status of an insurance claim is often referred to as

    a. inquiry

    b. follow-up

    c. tracer

    d. all of the above

22. An insurance claim transmitted to the third-party payer that is rejected because it contains a technical error, such as missing insured's birth date, is also known as a/an

    a. soft denial

    b. suspended claim

    c. delinquent claim

    d. downcoded claim

23. When an electronic claim is transmitted for several services and one service is rejected for incomplete information, the solution is to

    a. resubmit a paper claim with the needed data for the rejected services only

    b. add the required information in Field 19 that it is a retransmission

    c. add the required information and retransmit the rejected claim

    d. not retransmit a rejected claim

24. A request for payment to a third-party payer asking for a review of an insurance claim that has been denied is referred to as a/an

    a. review

    b. appeal

    c. request

    d. demand

Part III True/False

Write "T" or "F" in the blank to indicate whether you think the statement is true or false.

 25. If the provider has no contract with the insurance carrier, the provider is not obligated to the carrier's deadline.

 26. A patient should be asked to sign an Advance Beneficiary Notice if he or she has decided to undergo plastic surgery that is not related to a medical condition.

 27. An *overpayment* is receipt of less than the contract rate from a managed care plan for a patient who has received medical services.

 28. In the Medicare reconsideration Level 2 process, the request must be within 9 months from the date of the original determination shown on the remittance advice.

F 29. A decision to appeal a claim should be based on whether there is sufficient data to back up the claim and if there is a large amount of money in question.

ASSIGNMENT **9–2 ▸ CRITICAL THINKING: LOCATE AND EXPLAIN CHOICE OF DIAGNOSTIC CODES**

Performance Objective

Task: Locate the correct diagnostic code for the case scenario presented.

Conditions: Use a pen or pencil and the *International Classification of Diagnoses, Ninth Revision, Clinical Modification* (ICD-9-CM) diagnostic code book.

Standards: Time: _____ minutes

                    Accuracy: _____

                    (Note: The time element and accuracy criteria may be given by your instructor.)

Directions. Using your critical thinking skills, answer question after reading the scenario. Record your answer on the blank lines. This question is presented to enhance your skill in critical thinking.

Scenario. Using your diagnostic code book, look up the ICD-9-CM diagnostic code for a patient being treated for bacillary dysentery. How would you code this case and why?

1. Locate the main term or condition in the Alphabetic Index, Volume 2. What is the main term or condition?   _____

2. Refer to any notes under the main term. What is the subterm?   _____

3. Read any notes or terms enclosed in parentheses after the main term. What is the code number listed after the main term and subterm?   _____

4. What is the appropriate subterm after that?   _____

5. Look for appropriate sub-subterm and follow any cross-reference instructions. What does it say?

_____

_____

6. What is the generic code?   _____

7. Verify the code number in the Tabular List, Volume 1, and list it here.   _____

8. Read and be guided by any instructional terms in the Tabular List. It reads: _____

9. Read complete description and then code to the highest specificity. (Assign the code and write it here.)   _____

10. Write justification of chosen code(s). _____

_____

ASSIGNMENT 9-3 ▸ **POST TO A FINANCIAL ACCOUNTING RECORD (LEDGER) FROM AN EXPLANATION OF BENEFITS DOCUMENT**

Performance Objective

Task: Post data from an EOB document to a patient's financial accounting record (ledger).

Conditions: Use a blank financial accounting record (ledger) (Figure 9–1), an EOB document (Figure 9–2), and a pen or typewriter.

Standards: Time: _____ minutes

Accuracy: _____

(Note: The time element and accuracy criteria may be given by your instructor.)

Directions. Post in ink the payment received and preferred provider organization (PPO) adjustment to a patient's financial accounting record (ledger) (Figure 9–1) by referring to an EOB document (Figure 9–2). An example of financial accounting record (ledger) entries is shown in Figure 3–16 in the *Handbook*. An EOB document is defined in Figure 9–1 in the *Handbook*.

After the instructor has returned your work to you, either make the necessary corrections and place your work in a three-ring notebook for future reference or, if you received a high score, place it in your portfolio for reference when applying for a job.

1. Locate patient's financial accounting record (ledger) and EOB.

   Note: Refer to the step-by-step procedures at the end of Chapter 3 in the *Handbook* and graphic examples Figures 3–16 and 10–3.

2. Ledger lines 6 and 7: Insert date of service (DOS), reference (CPT code number, check number, or dates of service for posting adjustments or when insurance was billed), description of the transaction, charge amounts, payments, adjustments, and running current balance. The posting date is the actual date the transaction is recorded. If the DOS differs from the posting date, list the DOS in the reference or description column.

   Note: A good bookkeeping practice is to take a red pen and draw a line across the financial accounting record (ledger) from left to right to indicate the last entry billed to the insurance company.

Acct No. 9-3

STATEMENT
Financial Account
COLLEGE CLINIC
4567 Broad Avenue
Woodland Hills, XY 12345-0001
Tel. 555-486-9002
Fax No. 555-487-8976

Mr. Jabe Bortolussi
989 Moorpark Road
Woodland Hills, XY 12345

Phone No. (H) (555) 230-8870 (W) (555) 349-6689 Birthdate 04-07-71

Primary Insurance Co. ABC Insurance Company Policy/Group No. 4206/010

DATE	REFERENCE	DESCRIPTION	CHARGES		CREDITS				BALANCE	
					PYMNTS.		ADJ.			
		BALANCE FORWARD →								
6-3-xx	99204	E/M NP Level 4	250	00					250	00
6-3-xx	94375	Respiratory flow vol loop	40	00					290	00
6-3-xx	94060	Spirometry	75	00					365	00
6-3-xx	94664	Aerosol inhalation	50	00					415	00
6-3-xx	94760	Pulse oximetry	50	00					465	00

PLEASE PAY LAST AMOUNT IN BALANCE COLUMN

THIS IS A COPY OF YOUR FINANCIAL ACCOUNT AS IT APPEARS ON OUR RECORDS

Figure 9–1

ABC Insurance Company
P.O. Box 4300
Woodland Hills, XY 12345-0001

Claim No.:	1-00-16987087-00-zmm
Group Name:	COLLEGE CLINIC
Group No.:	010
Employee:	JABE V. BORTOLUSSI
Patient:	JABE V. BORTOLUSSI
SSN:	554-XX-8876
Plan No.:	4206
Prepared by:	M. SMITH
Prepared on:	07/04/20XX

GERALD PRACTON MD
4567 BROAD AVENUE
WOODLAND HILLS XY 12345

Patient Responsibility	
Amount not covered:	00
Co-pay amount:	00
Deductible:	00
Co-insurance:	64.61
Patient's total responsibility:	64.61
Other insurance payment:	00

EXPLANATION OF BENEFITS

Treatment Dates	Service Code	CPT Code	Charge Amount	Not Covered	Reason Code	PPO Discount	Covered Amount	Deductible Amount	Co-pay Amount	Paid At	Payment Amount
06/03/xx	200	99204	250.00	00	48	136.00	114.00	00	00	80%	91.20
06/03/xx	540	94375	40.00	00	48	00	40.00	00	00	80%	32.00
06/03/xx	540	94060	75.00	00	48	00	75.00	00	00	80%	60.00
06/03/xx	200	94664	50.00	00	48	1.55	48.45	00	00	80%	38.76
06/03/xx	540	94760	50.00	00	48	4.40	45.60	00	00	80%	36.48
		TOTAL	465.00	00		141.95	323.05	00	00		258.44

Other Insurance Credits or Adjustments   00

Total Payment Amount   258.44

CPT Code
99204 OFFICE/OUTPT VISIT E&M NEW MOD-HI SEVERIT
94375 RESPIRATORY FLOW VOLUM LOOP
94060 BRONCHOSPSM EVAL SPIROM PRE & POST BRON
94664 AEROSOL/VAPOR INHALA; INIT DEMO & EVAL
94760 NONINVASIVE EAR/PULSE OXIMETRY-02 SAT

Reason Code
48 CON DISCOUNT/PT NOT RESPONSIBLE

Participant GERALD PRACTON MD	Date 07-04-xx
Patient JABE V. BORTOLUSSI	ID Number 554-XX-8876
Plan Number 4206	Patient Number	Office No. 010

GC 1234567890

258.44

PAY
TO THE
ORDER
OF

COLLEGE CLINIC
4567 BROAD AVENUE
WOODLAND HILLS XY 12345

J M Smith
_____
ABC Insurance Company

Figure 9–2

ASSIGNMENT **9-4** ▸ **TRACE AN UNPAID INSURANCE CLAIM**

Performance Objective

Task: Complete an insurance claim tracer form and attach to this document a photocopy of the claim.

Conditions: Use an Insurance Claim Tracer form (Figure 9–3), an insurance claim form from the *Handbook* (Figure 7–5), and a computer or typewriter.

Standards: Time: _____ minutes

                   Accuracy: _____

                   (Note: The time element and accuracy criteria may be given by your instructor.)

Directions. You discover that the insurance claim you submitted to Blue Shield, 146 Main Street, Woodland Hills, XY 12345, on Harry N. Forehand 3 months ago was never paid. Complete an insurance claim tracer form (Figure 9–3). Make a photocopy of Harry Forehand's insurance claim form from the *Handbook* in Chapter 7 to attach to the tracer form. Mr. Forehand's employer is Acme Electrical Company at 450 South Orange Street, Woodland Hills, XY 12345. Place your name on the tracer form as the person to contact at Dr. Antrum's office.

   After the instructor has returned your work to you, either make the necessary corrections and place your work in a three-ring notebook for future reference or, if you received a high score, place it in your portfolio for reference when applying for a job.

COLLEGE CLINIC
4567 Broad Avenue
Woodland Hills, XY 12345-0001
Telephone (555) 486-9002
Fax (555) 487-8976

INSURANCE CLAIM TRACER

INSURANCE COMPANY NAME _____ DATE: _____ .

ADDRESS _____ .

Patient name: _____

Date of birth: _____

Employer: _____

Insured: _____

Policy/certificate No. _____

Group name/No. _____

Date of initial claim submission: _____

Date(s) of service: _____

Total charges submitted: _____

An inordinate amount of time has passed since submission of our original claim. We have not received a request for additional information and still await payment of this assigned claim. Please review the attached duplicate and process for payment within 7 days.

DETAILS OF INQUIRY

Please check the claim status and return this letter to our office. Thank you.

☐ No record of claim.
☐ Claim received and payment is in process.
☐ Claim is in suspense (comment please).
☐ Claim is in review (comment please).
☐ Additional information needed (comment please).
☐ Applied to deductible. Amount: $ _____
☐ Patient not eligible for benefits.
☐ Determination issued to beneficiary.
☐ Claim paid. Date: _____ Amount: $ _____ To whom: _____
☐ Claim denied (comment please).

Comments: _____

_____

Thank you for your assistance in this important matter. Please contact the insurance specialist named below if you have any questions regarding this claim.

Insurance Specialist: _____ (555) 486-9002 Ext. _____ .

Treating Physician: _____ State license number _____ .

Provider Number: _____ Provider's IRS number _____ .

Figure 9–3

A S S I G N M E N T **9–5** ▸ **L O C A T E   E R R O R S   O N   A   R E T U R N E D   I N S U R A N C E   C L A I M**

Performance Objective

Task: Highlight the blocks on the insurance claim form where errors are discovered.

Conditions: Use an insurance claim form (Figure 9–4) and a highlighter or red pen.

Standards: Time: _____ minutes

                             Accuracy: _____

                             (Note: The time element and accuracy criteria may be given by your instructor.)

Directions. An insurance claim (Figure 9–4) was returned by the Prudential Insurance Company. Highlight or circle in red all blocks on the claim form where errors are discovered.

Option 1. Retype the claim and either insert the correction if data are available to fix the error or insert the word "NEED" in the block of the claim form.

Option 2. On a separate sheet of paper, list the blocks from 1 to 33 and state where errors occur.

A Performance Evaluation Checklist may be reproduced from the "Instruction Guide to the *Workbook*" chapter if your instructor wishes you to submit it to assist with scoring and comments.

After the instructor has returned your work to you, either make the necessary corrections and place your work in a three-ring notebook for future reference or, if you received a high score, place it in your portfolio for reference when applying for a job.

(1500)

HEALTH INSURANCE CLAIM FORM

APPROVED BY NATIONAL UNIFORM CLAIM COMMITTEE 08/05

PRUDENTIAL INSURANCE COMPANY
500 SOUTH BEND STREET
WOODLAND HILLS XY 12345

CARRIER

PICA		PICA

1. MEDICARE ▢ (Medicare #)   MEDICAID ▢ (Medicaid #)   TRICARE CHAMPUS ▢ (Sponsor's SSN)   CHAMPVA ▢ (Member ID#)   GROUP HEALTH PLAN ▢ (SSN or ID)   FECA BLK LUNG ▢ (SSN)   OTHER ☒ (ID)

1a. INSURED'S I.D. NUMBER   (For Program in Item 1)

2. PATIENT'S NAME (Last Name, First Name, Middle Initial)
JOHNSON EMILY B.

3. PATIENT'S BIRTH DATE: MM 02 DD 12 YY 1963   SEX M ☐ F ☐

4. INSURED'S NAME (Last Name, First Name, Middle Initial)
JOHNSON ERRON T.

5. PATIENT'S ADDRESS (No., Street)
4391 EVERETT STREET

6. PATIENT RELATIONSHIP TO INSURED: Self ☐ Spouse ☒ Child ☐ Other ☐

7. INSURED'S ADDRESS (No., Street)
SAME

CITY WOODLAND HILLS   STATE XY

8. PATIENT STATUS: Single ☐ Married ☒ Other ☐

CITY   STATE

ZIP CODE 12345   TELEPHONE (Include Area Code) ( )

Employed ☐ Full-Time Student ☐ Part-Time Student ☐

ZIP CODE   TELEPHONE (INCLUDE AREA CODE) ( )

9. OTHER INSURED'S NAME (Last Name, First Name, Middle Initial)

10. IS PATIENT'S CONDITION RELATED TO:

11. INSURED'S POLICY GROUP OR FECA NUMBER

a. OTHER INSURED'S POLICY OR GROUP NUMBER

a. EMPLOYMENT? (CURRENT OR PREVIOUS) YES ☐ NO ☐

a. INSURED'S DATE OF BIRTH MM DD YY   SEX M ☐ F ☐

b. OTHER INSURED'S DATE OF BIRTH MM DD YY   SEX M ☐ F ☐

b. AUTO ACCIDENT? PLACE (State) YES ☐ NO ☐

b. EMPLOYER'S NAME OR SCHOOL NAME

c. EMPLOYER'S NAME OR SCHOOL NAME

c. OTHER ACCIDENT? YES ☐ NO ☐

c. INSURANCE PLAN NAME OR PROGRAM NAME

d. INSURANCE PLAN NAME OR PROGRAM NAME

10d. RESERVED FOR LOCAL USE

d. IS THERE ANOTHER HEALTH BENEFIT PLAN? YES ☐ NO ☒ *If yes, return to and complete item 9 a-d.*

READ BACK OF FORM BEFORE COMPLETING & SIGNING THIS FORM.

12. PATIENT'S OR AUTHORIZED PERSON'S SIGNATURE I authorize the release of any medical or other information necessary to process this claim. I also request payment of government benefits either to myself or to the party who accepts assignment below.
SIGNED *Emily B. Johnson*   DATE 1/4/2020

13. INSURED'S OR AUTHORIZED PERSON'S SIGNATURE I authorize payment of medical benefits to the undersigned physician or supplier for services described below.
SIGNED *Emily B. Johnson*

14. DATE OF CURRENT: MM DD YY ILLNESS (First symptom) OR INJURY (Accident) OR PREGNANCY(LMP)

15. IF PATIENT HAS HAD SAME OR SIMILAR ILLNESS. GIVE FIRST DATE MM DD YY

16. DATES PATIENT UNABLE TO WORK IN CURRENT OCCUPATION FROM MM DD YY TO MM DD YY

17. NAME OF REFERRING PHYSICIAN OR OTHER SOURCE
17a.
17b. NPI 67805027XX

18. HOSPITALIZATION DATES RELATED TO CURRENT SERVICES FROM MM DD YY TO MM DD YY

19. RESERVED FOR LOCAL USE

20. OUTSIDE LAB? YES ☐ NO ☒ $ CHARGES

21. DIAGNOSIS OR NATURE OF ILLNESS OR INJURY. (RELATE ITEMS 1,2,3 OR 4 TO ITEM 24E BY LINE)
1. ⌞__.__   3. ⌞__.__
2. ⌞__.__   4. ⌞__.__

22. MEDICAID RESUBMISSION CODE   ORIGINAL REF. NO.

23. PRIOR AUTHORIZATION NUMBER

24. A. DATE(S) OF SERVICE From MM DD YY	To MM DD YY	B. PLACE OF SERVICE	C. EMG	D. PROCEDURES, SERVICES, OR SUPPLIES CPT/HCPCS	MODIFIER	E. DIAGNOSIS POINTER	F. $ CHARGES	G. DAYS OR UNITS	H. EPSDT Family Plan	I. ID. QUAL.	J. RENDERING PROVIDER ID. #
1 01 04 20XX		11		99213		1	25 00	1		NPI	705687717XX
2 01 04 20XX		11		99213		1	25 00			NPI	
3										NPI	
4										NPI	
5										NPI	
6										NPI	

25. FEDERAL TAX I.D. NUMBER 7180561XX   SSN ☐ EIN ☐

26. PATIENT'S ACCOUNT NO. 9

27. ACCEPT ASSIGNMENT? (For govt. claims, see back) YES ☒ NO ☐

28. TOTAL CHARGE $ 60 00

29. AMOUNT PAID $

30. BALANCE DUE $ 60 00

31. SIGNATURE OF PHYSICIAN OR SUPPLIER INCLUDING DEGREES OR CREDENTIALS (I certify that the statements on the reverse apply to this bill and are made a part thereof.)
SIGNED *Vera Cutis, MD*   DATE 01/06/20XX

32. SERVICE FACILITY LOCATION INFORMATION
a. NPI   b.

33. BILLING PROVIDER INFO & PH # (555) 4869002
COLLEGE CLINIC
4567 BROAD AVENUE
WOODLAND HILLS XY 12345
a. 3664021XX NPI   b.

NUCC Instruction Manual available at: www.nucc.org   **PLEASE PRINT OR TYPE**   APPROVED OMB-0938-0999 FORM CMS-1500 (08-05)

PHYSICIAN OR SUPPLIER INFORMATION   PATIENT AND INSURED INFORMATION

Figure 9–4

ASSIGNMENT **9-6 ▸ LOCATE ERRORS ON A RETURNED INSURANCE CLAIM**

Performance Objective

Task: Highlight the blocks on the insurance claim form where errors are discovered.

Conditions: Use an insurance claim form (Figure 9–5) and a highlighter or red pen.

Standards: Time: _____ minutes

                 Accuracy: _____

                 (Note: The time element and accuracy criteria may be given by your instructor.)

Directions. An insurance claim was returned by the Healthtech Insurance Company. Highlight or circle in red all blocks on the claim form where errors are discovered.

Option 1. Retype the claim and either insert the correction if data are available to fix the error or insert the word "NEED" in the block of the claim form.

Option 2. On a separate sheet of paper, list the blocks from 1 to 33 and state where errors occur.

     A Performance Evaluation Checklist may be reproduced from the "Instruction Guide to the *Workbook*" chapter if your instructor wishes you to submit it to assist with scoring and comments.

     After the instructor has returned your work to you, either make the necessary corrections and place your work in a three-ring notebook for future reference or, if you received a high score, place it in your portfolio for reference when applying for a job.

(1500)

HEALTH INSURANCE CLAIM FORM

APPROVED BY NATIONAL UNIFORM CLAIM COMMITTEE 08/05

HEALTHTECH INSURANCE COMPANY
4821 WEST LAKE AVENUE
WOODLAND HILLS XY 12345

CARRIER

| | PICA | | | | | | | | | | PICA | | |

1. MEDICARE	MEDICAID	TRICARE CHAMPUS	CHAMPVA	GROUP HEALTH PLAN	FECA BLK LUNG	OTHER	1a. INSURED'S I.D. NUMBER (For Program in Item 1)
(Medicare #)	[X] (Medicaid #)	[X] (Sponsor's SSN)	(Member ID#)	(SSN or ID)	(SSN)	[X] (ID)	433 12 9870ANC

2. PATIENT'S NAME (Last Name, First Name, Middle Initial)
DUGAN CHARLES C

3. PATIENT'S BIRTH DATE MM 12 DD 24 YY 1968 SEX M [X] F

4. INSURED'S NAME (Last Name, First Name, Middle Initial)
SAME

5. PATIENT'S ADDRESS (No., Street)
5900 ELM STREET

6. PATIENT RELATIONSHIP TO INSURED
Self [X] Spouse Child Other

7. INSURED'S ADDRESS (No., Street)
SAME

CITY WOODLAND HILLS STATE XY

8. PATIENT STATUS
Single Married [X] Other
Employed Full-Time Student Part-Time Student

CITY STATE

ZIP CODE 12345 TELEPHONE (Include Area Code) (555) 559 3300

ZIP CODE TELEPHONE (INCLUDE AREA CODE) ( )

9. OTHER INSURED'S NAME (Last Name, First Name, Middle Initial)

10. IS PATIENT'S CONDITION RELATED TO:

11. INSURED'S POLICY GROUP OR FECA NUMBER

a. OTHER INSURED'S POLICY OR GROUP NUMBER

a. EMPLOYMENT? (CURRENT OR PREVIOUS) YES [X] NO

a. INSURED'S DATE OF BIRTH MM DD YY SEX M F

b. OTHER INSURED'S DATE OF BIRTH MM DD YY SEX M F

b. AUTO ACCIDENT? PLACE (State) YES [X] NO

b. EMPLOYER'S NAME OR SCHOOL NAME

c. EMPLOYER'S NAME OR SCHOOL NAME

c. OTHER ACCIDENT? YES [X] NO

c. INSURANCE PLAN NAME OR PROGRAM NAME

d. INSURANCE PLAN NAME OR PROGRAM NAME

10d. RESERVED FOR LOCAL USE

d. IS THERE ANOTHER HEALTH BENEFIT PLAN? YES NO *If yes,* return to and complete item 9 a-d.

READ BACK OF FORM BEFORE COMPLETING & SIGNING THIS FORM.
12. PATIENT'S OR AUTHORIZED PERSON'S SIGNATURE I authorize the release of any medical or other information necessary to process this claim. I also request payment of government benefits either to myself or to the party who accepts assignment below.

SIGNED _____ DATE _____

13. INSURED'S OR AUTHORIZED PERSON'S SIGNATURE I authorize payment of medical benefits to the undersigned physician or supplier for services described below.

SIGNED _____

PATIENT AND INSURED INFORMATION

14. DATE OF CURRENT: MM DD YY ILLNESS (First symptom) OR INJURY (Accident) OR PREGNANCY(LMP)

15. IF PATIENT HAS HAD SAME OR SIMILAR ILLNESS. GIVE FIRST DATE MM DD YY

16. DATES PATIENT UNABLE TO WORK IN CURRENT OCCUPATION FROM MM DD YY TO MM DD YY

17. NAME OF REFERRING PHYSICIAN OR OTHER SOURCE
17a.
17b. NPI 67805027XX

18. HOSPITALIZATION DATES RELATED TO CURRENT SERVICES FROM MM DD YY TO MM DD YY

19. RESERVED FOR LOCAL USE

20. OUTSIDE LAB? YES [X] NO $ CHARGES

21. DIAGNOSIS OR NATURE OF ILLNESS OR INJURY. (RELATE ITEMS 1,2,3 OR 4 TO ITEM 24E BY LINE)

1. 881.00
2. ___.___
3. ___.___
4. ___.___

22. MEDICAID RESUBMISSION CODE ORIGINAL REF. NO.

23. PRIOR AUTHORIZATION NUMBER

24. A. DATE(S) OF SERVICE From MM DD YY To MM DD YY	B. PLACE OF SERVICE	C. EMG	D. PROCEDURES, SERVICES, OR SUPPLIES (Explain Unusual Circumstances) CPT/HCPCS MODIFIER	E. DIAGNOSIS POINTER	F. $ CHARGES	G. DAYS OR UNITS	H. EPSDT Family Plan	I. ID. QUAL.	J. RENDERING PROVIDER ID. #
1	09 55 20XX	11		99203	1	70 92	1		NPI	46278897XX
2	09 55 20XX	11		12001	1				NPI	46278897XX
3									NPI	
4									NPI	
5									NPI	
6									NPI	

25. FEDERAL TAX I.D. NUMBER SSN EIN
7034597XX [X]

26. PATIENT'S ACCOUNT NO.
9

27. ACCEPT ASSIGNMENT? (For govt. claims, see back) [X] YES NO

28. TOTAL CHARGE $

29. AMOUNT PAID $

30. BALANCE DUE $

31. SIGNATURE OF PHYSICIAN OR SUPPLIER INCLUDING DEGREES OR CREDENTIALS (I certify that the statements on the reverse apply to this bill and are made a part thereof.)
Gerald Practon, MD 09/30/20XX
SIGNED DATE

32. SERVICE FACILITY LOCATION INFORMATION
COLLEGE HOSPITAL
4500 BROAD AVENUE
WOODLAND HILLS XY 12345
a. 937310XX NPI b.

33. BILLING PROVIDER INFO & PH # (555) 4869002
COLLEGE CLINIC
4567 BROAD AVENUE
WOODLAND HILLS XY 12345 0001
a. 3664021XX NPI b.

PHYSICIAN OR SUPPLIER INFORMATION

NUCC Instruction Manual available at: www.nucc.org **PLEASE PRINT OR TYPE** APPROVED OMB-0938-0999 FORM CMS-1500 (08-05)

Figure 9–5

ASSIGNMENT 9–7 ▸ LOCATE ERRORS ON A RETURNED INSURANCE CLAIM

Performance Objective

Task: Highlight the blocks on the insurance claim form where errors are discovered.

Conditions: Use an insurance claim form (Figure 9–6) and a highlighter or red pen.

Standards: Time: _____ minutes

                         Accuracy: _____

                         (Note: The time element and accuracy criteria may be given by your instructor.)

Directions. An insurance claim (Figure 9–6) was returned by an insurance plan. Highlight or circle in red all blocks on the claim form where errors are discovered.

Option 1. Retype the claim and either insert the correction if data are available to fix the error or insert the word "NEED" in the block of the claim form.

Option 2. On a separate sheet of paper, list the blocks from 1 to 33 and state where errors occur.

A Performance Evaluation Checklist may be reproduced from the "Instruction Guide to the *Workbook*" chapter if your instructor wishes you to submit it to assist with scoring and comments.

After the instructor has returned your work to you, either make the necessary corrections and place your work in a three-ring notebook for future reference or, if you received a high score, place it in your portfolio for reference when applying for a job.

1500
HEALTH INSURANCE CLAIM FORM
APPROVED BY NATIONAL UNIFORM CLAIM COMMITTEE 08/05

AMERICAN INSURANCE COMPANY
509 MAIN STREET
WOODLAND HILLS XY 12345

CARRIER

| | | PICA | | | | | | | PICA | | |

1. MEDICARE MEDICAID TRICARE CHAMPUS CHAMPVA GROUP HEALTH PLAN FECA BLK LUNG OTHER [X] (ID)
(Medicare #) (Medicaid #) (Sponsor's SSN) (Member ID#) (SSN or ID) (SSN)

1a. INSURED'S I.D. NUMBER   (For Program in Item 1)

2. PATIENT'S NAME (Last Name, First Name, Middle Initial)
AVERY MARY T

3. PATIENT'S BIRTH DATE MM 05 DD 07 YY 1980   SEX M F

4. INSURED'S NAME (Last Name, First Name, Middle Initial)
SAME

5. PATIENT'S ADDRESS (No., Street)
4309 MAIN STREET

6. PATIENT RELATIONSHIP TO INSURED
Self [X] Spouse Child Other

7. INSURED'S ADDRESS (No., Street)

CITY WOODLAND HILLS   STATE XY

8. PATIENT STATUS
Single Married Other
Employed Full-Time Student Part-Time Student

CITY   STATE

ZIP CODE 12345   TELEPHONE (Include Area Code) (555) 450-9899

ZIP CODE   TELEPHONE (INCLUDE AREA CODE) ( )

9. OTHER INSURED'S NAME (Last Name, First Name, Middle Initial)

10. IS PATIENT'S CONDITION RELATED TO:

11. INSURED'S POLICY GROUP OR FECA NUMBER

a. OTHER INSURED'S POLICY OR GROUP NUMBER

a. EMPLOYMENT? (CURRENT OR PREVIOUS) YES [X] NO

a. INSURED'S DATE OF BIRTH MM DD YY   SEX M F

b. OTHER INSURED'S DATE OF BIRTH MM DD YY SEX M F

b. AUTO ACCIDENT? PLACE (State) YES [X] NO

b. EMPLOYER'S NAME OR SCHOOL NAME

c. EMPLOYER'S NAME OR SCHOOL NAME

c. OTHER ACCIDENT? YES [X] NO

c. INSURANCE PLAN NAME OR PROGRAM NAME

d. INSURANCE PLAN NAME OR PROGRAM NAME

10d. RESERVED FOR LOCAL USE

d. IS THERE ANOTHER HEALTH BENEFIT PLAN?
YES NO *If yes*, return to and complete item 9 a-d.

READ BACK OF FORM BEFORE COMPLETING & SIGNING THIS FORM.
12. PATIENT'S OR AUTHORIZED PERSON'S SIGNATURE I authorize the release of any medical or other information necessary to process this claim. I also request payment of government benefits either to myself or to the party who accepts assignment below.

SIGNED Mary T. Avery   DATE 11/20/2007

13. INSURED'S OR AUTHORIZED PERSON'S SIGNATURE I authorize payment of medical benefits to the undersigned physician or supplier for services described below.

SIGNED Mary T. Avery

14. DATE OF CURRENT: ILLNESS (First symptom) OR INJURY (Accident) OR PREGNANCY(LMP) MM DD YY

15. IF PATIENT HAS HAD SAME OR SIMILAR ILLNESS. GIVE FIRST DATE MM DD YY

16. DATES PATIENT UNABLE TO WORK IN CURRENT OCCUPATION
FROM MM 11 DD 09 YY 20XX   TO MM 11 DD 30 YY 20XX

17. NAME OF REFERRING PHYSICIAN OR OTHER SOURCE
GERALD PRACTON MD

17a.
17b. NPI

18. HOSPITALIZATION DATES RELATED TO CURRENT SERVICES
FROM MM 11 DD 11 YY 20XX   TO MM 11 DD 12 YY 20XX

19. RESERVED FOR LOCAL USE

20. OUTSIDE LAB? YES [X] NO $ CHARGES

21. DIAGNOSIS OR NATURE OF ILLNESS OR INJURY. (RELATE ITEMS 1,2,3 OR 4 TO ITEM 24E BY LINE)
1. 463
2.
3.
4.

22. MEDICAID RESUBMISSION CODE   ORIGINAL REF. NO.

23. PRIOR AUTHORIZATION NUMBER

24. A. DATE(S) OF SERVICE						B. PLACE OF SERVICE	C. EMG	D. PROCEDURES, SERVICES, OR SUPPLIES (Explain Unusual Circumstances) CPT/HCPCS MODIFIER	E. DIAGNOSIS POINTER	F. $ CHARGES	G. DAYS OR UNITS	H. EPSDT Family Plan	I. ID. QUAL.	J. RENDERING PROVIDER ID. #
From MM	DD	YY	To MM	DD	YY									
11	10	20XX				11		99203	1	50 00			NPI	43050047XX
11	11	20XX				21		99222	1	120 80			NPI	43050047XX
11	11	20XX				21		42821	1	410 73			NPI	43050047XX
11	22	20XX				21		99231	1	20 00			NPI	
													NPI	
													NPI	

25. FEDERAL TAX I.D. NUMBER   SSN EIN [X]
715737291XX

26. PATIENT'S ACCOUNT NO.

27. ACCEPT ASSIGNMENT? (For govt. claims, see back) YES NO

28. TOTAL CHARGE $

29. AMOUNT PAID $

30. BALANCE DUE $

31. SIGNATURE OF PHYSICIAN OR SUPPLIER INCLUDING DEGREES OR CREDENTIALS (I certify that the statements on the reverse apply to this bill and are made a part thereof.)
SIGNED   DATE 11/15/20XX

32. SERVICE FACILITY LOCATION INFORMATION
COLLEGE HOSPITAL
4500 BROAD AVENUE
WOODLAND HILLS XY 12345
a. 9507310XX NPI   b.

33. BILLING PROVIDER INFO & PH # (555) 4869002
COLLEGE CLINIC
4567 BROAD AVENUE
WOODLAND HILLS XY 12345
a. 3664021XX NPI   b.

NUCC Instruction Manual available at: www.nucc.org   **PLEASE PRINT OR TYPE**   APPROVED OMB-0938-0999 FORM CMS-1500 (08-05)

PATIENT AND INSURED INFORMATION

PHYSICIAN OR SUPPLIER INFORMATION

Figure 9–6

ASSIGNMENT 9–8 ▸ **REQUEST A HEARING ON A PREVIOUSLY APPEALED CLAIM**

Performance Objective

Task: Insert information on a CMS-1965 Request for Hearing, Part B, Medicare Claim form.

Conditions: Use a Request for Hearing, Part B, Medicare Claim form (Figure 9–7) and a typewriter.

Standards: Time: _____ minutes

                   Accuracy: _____

                   (Note: The time element and accuracy criteria may be given by your instructor.)

Directions. After Medicare processes the tracer on the insurance claim for Bill Hutch, you receive a Medicare EOB and payment check, but the amount is incorrect because of an excessive reduction in the allowed payment. An appeal was made in September and denied; Dr. Brady Coccidioides believes that a mistake has been made and wishes to request a hearing.

Complete the CMS-1965 Request for Hearing, Part B, Medicare Claim form for this case (Figure 9–7) by referring to the tracer form completed for Assignment 9–4 (Figure 9–3) and Figure 7–8 in the *Handbook*. Complete the form as the claimant's representative and do not fill in the claimant's portion. As you will learn in the chapter on Medicare, the Health Insurance Claim Number is the patient's Medicare identification number as shown in Figure 7–8, Block 1a. No additional evidence is to be presented, and the doctor does not wish to appear for the hearing. Date the form December 5, 20xx.

After the instructor has returned your work to you, either make the necessary corrections and place your work in a three-ring notebook for future reference or, if you received a high score, place it in your portfolio for reference when applying for a job.

DEPARTMENT OF HEALTH AND HUMAN SERVICES
CENTERS FOR MEDICARE & MEDICAID SERVICES

REQUEST FOR HEARING
PART B MEDICARE CLAIM
Medical Insurance Benefits - Social Security Act

NOTICE—Anyone who misrepresents or falsifies essential information requested by this form may upon conviction be subject to fine and imprisonment under Federal Law.

CARRIER'S NAME AND ADDRESS	**1** NAME OF PATIENT
	2 HEALTH INSURANCE CLAIM NUMBER

3 I disagree with the review determination on my claim, and request a hearing before a hearing officer of the insurance carrier named above.

MY REASONS ARE: (Attach a copy of the Review Notice. NOTE: If the review decision was made more than 6 months ago, include your reason for not making this request earlier.)

4 CHECK ONE OF THE FOLLOWING

☐ I have additional evidence to submit.
(Attach such evidence to this form or forward it to the carrier within 10 days.)

☐ I do not have additional evidence.

CHECK **ONLY ONE** OF THE STATEMENTS BELOW:

☐ I wish to appear in person before the Hearing Officer.

☐ I do not wish to appear and hereby request a decision on the evidence before the Hearing Officer.

5 EITHER THE CLAIMANT OR REPRESENTATIVE SHOULD SIGN IN THE APPROPRIATE SPACE BELOW

SIGNATURE OR NAME OF CLAIMANT'S REPRESENTATIVE	CLAIMANT'S SIGNATURE	
ADDRESS	ADDRESS	
CITY, STATE, AND ZIP CODE	CITY, STATE, AND ZIP CODE	
TELEPHONE NUMBER	DATE	TELEPHONE NUMBER	DATE

(Claimant should not write below this line)

- -

ACKNOWLEDGMENT OF REQUEST FOR HEARING

Your request for a hearing was received on _____ . You will be notified of the time and place of the hearing at least 10 days before the date of the hearing.

SIGNED	DATE

Form CMS-1965 (05/03)

Figure 9–7

ASSIGNMENT **9–9** ▸ **FILE AN APPEAL**

Performance Objective

Task: Compose, format, key, proofread, and print a letter of appeal, and attach to this document photocopies of information to substantiate reimbursement requested.

Conditions: Typewriter or computer, printer, letterhead paper, envelope, attachments, thesaurus, English dictionary, medical dictionary, and pen or pencil.

Standards: Time: _____ minutes

                  Accuracy: _____

                  (Note: The time element and accuracy criteria may be given by your instructor.)

Scenario. After retyping and resubmitting Mary T. Avery's insurance claim in Assignment 9–7, the insurance company sends an EOB/RA (health insurance claim number 123098) with a check in the amount of $300 to the College Clinic for payment of the claim. Dr. Cutler wishes an appeal to be made for an increase of the payment to an additional $100. Note: This patient's marital status is single and the insured's identification number is T45098.

Directions. Use the retyped claim to Assignment 9–7 for Mary T. Avery. Follow these basic step-by-step procedures.

1. Refer to the end of Chapter 4 in the *Handbook* and follow the procedure to compose, format, key, proofread, and print a letter.

2. Include the beneficiary's name, health insurance claim number, dates of service in question, and items or services in question with name, address, and signature of the provider.

3. Compose a letter with an introduction that stresses the medical practice's qualifications, the physician's commitment to complying with regulations and providing appropriate services, and the importance of the practice to the payer's panel of physicians or specialists.

4. Provide a detailed account of the necessity of the treatment given and its relationship to the patient's problems and chief complaint. You might cross reference the medical record and emphasize parts of it that the reviewer may have missed.

5. Explain the reason why the provider does not agree with the payment. Use a blank sheet labeling it "Explanation of Benefits" because you do not have this printed document to attach.

6. Abstract excerpts from the coding resource book if necessary.

7. Direct the correspondence to Mr. Donald Pearson, a claims adjuster at the American Insurance Company.

8. Type an envelope for the letter.

9. Retain copies of all data sent for the physician's files.

ALTAPOINT PRACTICE MANAGEMENT SOFTWARE ASSIGNMENTS

ASSIGNMENT **9–10** ▸ **ENTER PAYMENTS FROM AN EXPLANATION OF BENEFITS DOUCUMENT INTO THE PRACTICE MANAGEMENT SYSTEM**

Performance Objective

Task: Enter insurance payment data from an explanation of benefits document into the practice management system

Conditions: Explanation of benefits document (Figure 9-8) and computer

Standards: Time:_____minutes

                 Accuracy:_____

                 (Note: The time element and accuracy criteria may be given by your instructor.)

Directions. Before attempting the Practice Management software assignment, refer to Appendix C and follow the instructions provided to familiarize yourself with the software. Then refer to the Practice Management software on the CD that accompanies the *Workbook*.

1. For this assignment, follow the instructions for entering payments from an explanation of benefits (EOB) document and enter the payments received from Teri Simpson's insurance company listed on the EOB dated March 16.

2. To obtain a grade, either print a hard copy of the patient's financial account record or have your instructor view the data onscreen for approval.

Assignment 9-10

UNITED MUTUAL INSURANCE
787 East 3433 South
Building 554
Salt Lake City, Utah 84109

PROVIDER REMITTANCE
Explanation of Benefits

Creekside Clinic
1100 E. North Union Ave.
Suite 101
Midvale, Utah 84047

PAGE:	1 of 1
DATE:	03/16/2007
ID NUMBER:	SIMP000001

PROVIDER: JEFFREY LYNDON, M.D.

Patient: Teri Simpson   Claim: 781126

FROM DATE	THRU DATE	PROC CODE	UNITS	AMT. BILLED	AMT. ALLOWED	DED.	COPAY	PYMT	R
02/09	02/09	99212	1	$60.00	$60.00	.00	.00	$48.00	
02/09	02/09	90658	1	$25.00	$25.00	.00	.00	$20.00	
02/09	02/09	90471	1	$15.00	$15.00	.00	.00	$12.00	
Claim Total				$100.00	$100.00	.00	.00	$80.00	

PAYMENT SUMMARY		TOTAL ALL CLAIMS		EFT INFORMATION	
Total Amt. Pd.	$80.00	Amt. Charged	$100.00	Number	345678
Prior Credit Bal.	.00	Amt. Allowed	$100.00	Date	04/16/2007
Prior Credit App.	.00	Deductible	.00	Amount	$80.00
New Credit Bal.	.00	Coinsurance	.00		
Net Disbursed	$80.00	Other Reduction	.00		
		Amt. Approved	$80.00		

Figure 9–8

ASSIGNMENT 9-11 ▸ **ENTER PAYMENTS FROM AN EXPLANATION OF BENEFITS DOUCUMENT INTO THE PRACTICE MANAGEMENT SYSTEM**

Performance Objective

Task: Enter insurance payment data from an explanation of benefits document into the practice management system

Conditions: Explanation of benefits document (Figure 9-9) and computer

Standards: Time:_____minutes

                       Accuracy:_____

                       (Note: The time element and accuracy criteria may be given by your instructor.)

Directions. Before attempting the Practice Management software assignment, refer to Appendix C and follow the instructions provided to familiarize yourself with the software. Then refer to the Practice Management software on the CD that accompanies the *Workbook*.

1. For this assignment, follow the instructions for entering payments from an explanation of benefits (EOB) document and enter the payments received from Michael Lee's insurance company listed on the EOB dated April 16.

2. To obtain a grade, either print a hard copy of the patient's financial account record or have your instructor view the data onscreen for approval.

Assignment 9-11

UNITED MUTUAL INSURANCE
787 East 3433 South
Building 554
Salt Lake City, Utah 84109

PROVIDER REMITTANCE
Explanation of Benefits

Creekside Clinic
1100 E. North Union Ave.
Suite 101
Midvale, Utah 84047

PAGE: 1 of 1
DATE: 04/16/2007
ID NUMBER: SIMP000002

PROVIDER: JEFFREY LYNDON, M.D.

Patient: Michael Lee   Claim: 783008

FROM DATE	THRU DATE	PROC CODE	UNITS	AMT. BILLED	AMT. ALLOWED	DED.	COPAY	PYMT	R
03/14	03/14	99213	1	$75.00	$75.00	.00	.00	$60.00	
03/14	03/14	12002	1	$80.00	$80.00	.00	.00	$64.00	
03/14	03/14	90703	1	$25.00	$20.00	.00	.00	$20.00	
03/14	03/14	90471	1	$15.00	$15.00	.00	.00	$12.00	
Claim Total				$195.00	$195.00	.00	.00	$156.00	

PAYMENT SUMMARY		TOTAL ALL CLAIMS		EFT INFORMATION	
Total Amt. Pd.	$156.00	Amt. Charged	$195.00	Number	345678
Prior Credit Bal.	.00	Amt. Allowed	$195.00	Date	04/16/2007
Prior Credit App.	.00	Deductible	.00	Amount	$156.00
New Credit Bal.	.00	Coinsurance	.00		
Net Disbursed	$156.00	Other Reduction	.00		
		Amt. Approved	$156.00		

Figure 9–9

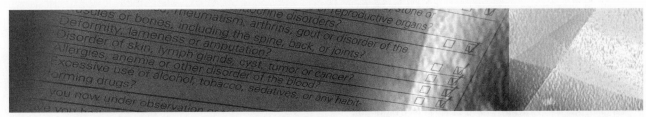

Office and Insurance Collection Strategies

KEY TERMS

Your instructor may wish to select some words pertinent to this chapter for a test. For definitions of the terms, further study, and/or reference, the words, phrases, and abbreviations may be found in the glossary at the end of the Handbook. *Key terms for this chapter follow.*

accounts receivable (A/R)

age analysis

AMA Code of Medical Ethics

automatic stay

balance

bankruptcy

bonding

cash flow

Code of Medical Ethics

collateral

collection ratio

credit

credit card

creditor

cycle billing

debit card

debt

debtor

discount

dun messages

embezzlement

estate administrator

estate executor

fee schedule

financial accounting record

garnishment

insurance balance billing

itemized statement

lien

manual billing

netback

no charge (NC)

nonexempt assets

professional courtesy

reimbursement

secured debt

skip

statute of limitations

unsecured debt

write-off

KEY ABBREVIATIONS

See how many abbreviations and acronyms you can translate and then use this as a handy reference list. Definitions for the key abbreviations are located near the back of the Handbook *in the glossary.*

A/R _____

ATM _____

CMS _____

COBRA _____

CPT _____

e-check _____

ERISA _____

FACT _____

FCBA _____

FCRA _____

FCT _____

FDCPA _____

FEHBA _____

HMO _____

N/A _____

NC _____

NSF _____

TILA _____

W2 _____

PERFORMANCE OBJECTIVES

The student will be able to:

- Define and spell the key terms and key abbreviations for this chapter, given the information from the *Handbook* glossary, within a reasonable time period and with enough accuracy to obtain a satisfactory evaluation.
- After reading the chapter, answer the fill-in-the-blanks, mix and match, multiple choice, and true/false review questions with enough accuracy to obtain a satisfactory evaluation.
- Select an appropriate dun message for a patient's bill, given a patient's ledger/statement, within a reasonable time period and with enough accuracy to obtain a satisfactory evaluation.
- Post a courtesy adjustment, given a patient's ledger/statement, within a reasonable period of time and with enough accuracy to obtain a satisfactory evaluation.
- Post a patient's charges and payment to the patient's financial accounting record, using the Mock Fee Schedule in Appendix A in this *Workbook*, within a reasonable time period and with enough accuracy to obtain a satisfactory evaluation.
- Compose a collection letter for a delinquent account, given letterhead stationery, within a reasonable time period and with enough accuracy to obtain a satisfactory evaluation.
- Complete a credit card voucher, given a patient's ledger/statement, within a reasonable time period and with enough accuracy to obtain a satisfactory evaluation.
- Complete a financial agreement, given a patient's ledger/statement, within a reasonable time period and with enough accuracy to obtain a satisfactory evaluation.

ALTAPOINT PRACTICE MANAGEMENT SOFTWARE OBJECTIVES

The student will be able to:

- Post payments to the financial accounting records of two patients and print hard copies within a reasonable time period and with enough accuracy to obtain a satisfactory evaluation.

STUDY OUTLINE

Cash Flow Cycle
  Accounts Receivable
  Patient Education
  Patient Registration Form
Fees
  Fee Schedule
  Fee Adjustments
  Communicating Fees
  Collecting Fees
Credit Arrangements
  Payment Options
Credit and Collection Laws
  Statute of Limitations
  Equal Credit Opportunity Act
  Fair Credit Reporting Act
  Fair Credit Billing Act
  Truth in Lending Act
  Truth in Lending Consumer Credit Cost Disclosure
  Fair Debt Collection Practices Act

The Collection Process
  Office Collection Techniques
  Insurance Collection
  Collection Agencies
  Credit Bureaus
  Credit Counseling
  Small Claims Court
  Tracing a Skip
  Special Collection Issues
Procedure: Seven-Step Billing and Collection Guidelines
Procedure: Telephone Collection Plan
Procedure: Create a Financial Agreement with a Patient
Procedure: File a Claim in Small Claims Court
Procedure: File an Estate Claim

 ASSIGNMENT **10–1** ▸ **REVIEW QUESTIONS**

Part I Fill in the Blank

Review the objectives, key terms, chapter information, glossary definitions of key terms, and figures before completing the following review questions.

1. Third-party payers are composed of

    a. _____

    b. _____

    c. _____

    d. _____

2. The unpaid balance due from patients for professional services rendered is known as a/an

    _____.

3. An important document that provides demographic and identifying data for

    each patient and assists in billing and collection is called a/an _____

    _____.

4. A term preferable to "write-off" when used in a medical practice is _____.

5. To verify a check, ask the patient for a/an _____

   and _____

6. The procedure of systematically arranging the accounts receivable, by age, from the

   date of service is called _____.

7. Write the formula for calculating the office accounts receivable (A/R) ratio.

   _____

   _____

   _____

8. What is the collection rate if a total of $40,300 was collected for the month and the

   total of the accounts receivable is $50,670? _____.

9. Are physicians' patient accounts single-entry accounts, open-book accounts, or

   written contract accounts? _____.

10. A court order attaching a debtor's property or wages to pay off a debt is known as _____.

11. An individual who owes on an account and moves, leaving no forwarding address, is

    called a/an _____.

12. Translate these credit and collection abbreviations.

NSF	_____	T	_____
WCO	_____	SK	_____
PIF	_____	FN	_____
NLE	_____	UE	_____

13. A straight petition in bankruptcy or absolute bankruptcy is also known as a/an_____.

14. A wage earner's bankruptcy is sometimes referred to as a/an _____.

15. State three bonding methods.

a. _____

b. _____

c. _____

16. A system of billing accounts at spaced intervals during the month on the basis of a breakdown of accounts by alphabet, account number, insurance type, or date of

service is known as _____.

Part II Mix and Match

17. Match the credit and collection terms in the right column with the descriptions, and fill in the blank with the appropriate letter.

_____	Reductions of the normal fee based on a specific amount of money or a percentage of the charge	a. debtor
_____	Phrase to remind a patient about a delinquent account	b. itemized statement
_____	Item that permits bank customers to withdraw cash at any hour from an automated teller machine	c. fee schedule
_____	Individual owing money	d. discounts
_____	Claim on the property of another as security for a debt	e. financial account record (ledger)
_____	Individual record indicating charges, payments, adjustments, and balances owed for services rendered	f. creditor
_____	Detailed summary of all transactions of a creditor's account	g. dun message
_____	Person to whom money is owed	h. debit card
_____	Listing of accepted charges or established allowances for specific medical procedures	i. lien

18. Match the following federal acts with their descriptions and fill in the blank with the appropriate letter.

_____	Law stating that a person has 60 days to complain about an error from the date that a statement is mailed	a. Equal Credit Opportunity Act
_____	Consumer protection act that applies to anyone who charges interest or agrees on payment of a bill in more than four installments, excluding a downpayment	b. Fair Credit Reporting Act
_____	Regulates collection practices of third-party debt collectors and attorneys who collect debts for others	c. Fair Credit Billing Act
_____	Federal law prohibiting discrimination in all areas of granting credit	d. Truth in Lending Act
_____	Regulates agencies that issue or use credit reports on consumers	e. Fair Debt Collection Practices Act

Part III Multiple Choice

Choose the best answer.

19. Signing another person's name on a check to obtain money or pay off a debt without permission is called

    a. embezzle

    b. steal

    c. garnish

    d. forgery

20. When sending monthly statements to patients for balances due, the postal service can forward mail if the addressed envelopes contain the statement

    a. "Please Forward"

    b. "Forwarding Service Requested"

    c. "Forwarding and Return Receipt Requested"

    d. "Send Forward"

21. When accepting a credit card as payment on an account, the proper guideline(s) to follow is/are to:

    a. ask for photo identification

    b. accept a card only from the person whose name is on the card

    c. get approval from the credit card company

    d. all of the above

22. A service offered by a nonprofit agency assisting people in paying off their debts is known as

    a. credit counseling

    b. debt solutions

    c. grant-in-aid under the Hill-Burton Act

    d. small claims court

23. Insurance payment checks should be stamped in the endorsement area on the back "For Deposit Only," which is called a/an

    a. conditional endorsement

    b. qualified endorsement

    c. special endorsement

    d. restrictive endorsement

Part IV True/False

Write "T" or "F" in the blank to indicate whether you think the statement is true or false.

_____   24. Insurance companies and the federal government do not recommend waiving copayments to patients.

_____   25. Regulation Z of the Truth in Lending Consumer Credit Cost Disclosure law applies if the patient is making three payments.

_____   26. Most state collection laws allow telephone calls to the debtor between 8 AM and 9 PM.

_____   27. When a patient has declared bankruptcy, it is permissible to continue to send monthly statements for a balance due.

_____   28. A collection agency must follow all the laws stated in the Fair Debt Collection Practices Act.

ASSIGNMENT **10-2** ▸ **SELECT A DUN MESSAGE**

Performance Objective

Task: Select an appropriate dun message and insert it on a patient's financial accounting record (ledger card).

Conditions: Use the patient's financial accounting record (Figure 10–1) and a typewriter.

Standards: Time: _____ minutes

                         Accuracy: _____

                         (Note: The time element and accuracy criteria may be given by your instructor.)

Directions. Read the scenario and refer to the patient's financial accounting record (Figure 10–1). Select appropriate dun messages for each month the patient has been billed. You may wish to refer to Figure 10–3 in the *Handbook*.

Scenario. Carrie Jones was on vacation in June and July and did not pay on her account. It is August (current year).

June 1, 20XX dun message   _____

July 1, 20XX dun message   _____

August 1, 20XX dun message   _____

After the instructor has returned your work to you, either make the necessary corrections and place your work in a three-ring notebook for future reference or, if you received a high score, place it in your portfolio for reference when applying for a job.

Acct   No. 10-2

STATEMENT
Financial Account
COLLEGE CLINIC
4567 Broad Avenue
Woodland Hills, XY 12345-0001
Tel. 555-486-9002
Fax No. 555-487-8976

Carrie Jones
15543 Dean Street
Woodland Hills, XY 12345

Phone No. (H)   (555) 439-8800   (W)   (555) 550-8706   Birthdate   05-14-72

Primary Insurance Co.   Prudential Insurance Company   Policy/Group No.   450998

	REFERENCE	DESCRIPTION	CHARGES	CREDITS PYMNTS.	ADJ.	BALANCE	
			BALANCE FORWARD ⟶			20	00
4-16--xx	99215	C hx/exam HC DM DX 582				154	99
4-17--xx		Prudential billed (4-16-xx)				154	99
5-27--xx		Rec'd insurance ck #435		30	00	124	99
6-1-xx		Billed pt				124	99
7-1-xx		Billed pt				124	99
8-1-xx		Billed pt				124	99

PLEASE PAY LAST AMOUNT IN BALANCE COLUMN

THIS IS A COPY OF YOUR FINANCIAL ACCOUNT AS IT APPEARS ON OUR RECORDS

Figure 10–1

ASSIGNMENT 10–3 ▸ MANUALLY POST A COURTESY ADJUSTMENT

Performance Objective

Task: Post a courtesy adjustment to a patient's financial accounting record (ledger card).

Conditions: Use the patient's financial accounting record (Figure 10–2) and a pen.

Standards: Time: _____ minutes

                  Accuracy: _____

                  (Note: The time element and accuracy criteria may be given by your instructor.)

Directions. Read the case scenario and refer to the patient's financial accounting record (Figure 10–2). You may wish to refer to Figure 10–3 in the *Handbook*. Post a courtesy adjustment to her financial accounting record.

Scenario. Maria Smith recently lost her job and is raising two children as a single parent. It is September 1 (current year). A discussion with Dr. Gerald Practon leads to a decision to write off the balance on the account.

After the instructor has returned your work to you, either make the necessary corrections and place your work in a three-ring notebook for future reference or, if you received a high score, place it in your portfolio for reference when applying for a job.

Acct No. 10-3

STATEMENT
Financial Account
COLLEGE CLINIC
4567 Broad Avenue
Woodland Hills, XY 12345-0001
Tel. 555-486-9002
Fax No. 555-487-8976

Ms. Maria Smith
3737 Unser Road
Woodland Hills, XY 12345

Phone No. (H) (555) 430-8877   (W)   (555) 908-1233   Birthdate 06-11-80

Primary Insurance Co.   Metropolitan Insurance Company   Policy/Group No.   4320870

	REFERENCE	DESCRIPTION	CHARGES		CREDITS PYMNTS.	ADJ.	BALANCE	
			BALANCE FORWARD ⟶				20	00
5-19-xx	99214	OV DX 582	61	51			81	51
5-20-xx		Metropolitan billed (5-19-xx)					81	51
6-20-xx		Rec'd ins ck #6778			25	00	56	51
7-1-xx		Pt billed					56	51
8-1-xx		Pt billed					56	51

PLEASE PAY LAST AMOUNT IN BALANCE COLUMN

THIS IS A COPY OF YOUR FINANCIAL ACCOUNT AS IT APPEARS ON OUR RECORDS

Figure 10–2

ASSIGNMENT **10-4** ▸ **MANUALLY POST A PATIENT'S CHARGES AND PAYMENT**

Performance Objective

Task: Post a payment to a patient's financial accounting record (ledger card).

Conditions: Use the patient's financial accounting record (Figure 10–3), the Mock Fee Schedule in Appendix A in this *Workbook*, and a pen.

Standards: Time: _____ minutes

                  Accuracy: _____

                  (Note: The time element and accuracy criteria may be given by your instructor.)

Directions. Read the case scenario, refer to the patient's financial accounting record (Figure 10–3), and refer to the Mock Fee Schedule in Appendix A in this *Workbook*. You may wish to refer to Figure 10–3 in the *Handbook*. Post the charges for the services rendered and payment to the patient's financial accounting record.

Scenario. On October 12 (current year), new patient Kenneth Brown came in for a Level III office visit and electrocardiogram (ECG). He has no insurance and paid $50 on his account with check number 3421.

    After the instructor has returned your work to you, either make the necessary corrections and place your work in a three-ring notebook for future reference or, if you received a high score, place it in your portfolio for reference when applying for a job.

Acct No. ___10-4___

STATEMENT
Financial Account
COLLEGE CLINIC
4567 Broad Avenue
Woodland Hills, XY 12345-0001
Tel. 555-486-9002
Fax No. 555-487-8976

Mr. Kenneth Brown
8896 Aster Drive
Woodland Hills, XY 12345

Phone No. (H) ___(555) 760-5211___   (W) ___(555) 987-3355___   Birthdate ___01-15-82___

Primary Insurance Co. ___none___   Policy/Group No. _____

REFERENCE	DESCRIPTION	CHARGES	CREDITS PYMNTS.	ADJ.	BALANCE
		BALANCE FORWARD ⟶			

PLEASE PAY LAST AMOUNT IN BALANCE COLUMN ⤒

THIS IS A COPY OF YOUR FINANCIAL ACCOUNT AS IT APPEARS ON OUR RECORDS

Figure 10–3

ASSIGNMENT **10–5** ▸ **COMPOSE A COLLECTION LETTER**

Performance Objective

Task: Key a letter for the physician's signature and post the entry on the patient's financial
                     accounting record (ledger card).

Conditions: Use the patient's financial accounting record (Figure 10–4), one sheet of letterhead
                     (Figure 10–5), a number 10 envelope, and a pen.

Standards: Time: _____ minutes

                     Accuracy: _____

                     (Note: The time element and accuracy criteria may be given by your instructor.)

Directions. Read the case scenario, refer to the patient's financial accounting record (Figure 10–4), and compose a
collection letter, using your signature and requesting payment. Type this letter on letterhead stationery in full block
format (paragraphs to left margin). Include a paragraph stating that a copy of the delinquent statement is enclosed.
You may wish to refer to Figure 10–16 in the *Handbook*. Post an entry on the patient's financial accounting record.

Scenario. It is December 1 (current year), and you have sent Mr. Ron Kelsey two statements with no response.
You tried to reach him by telephone without success and have decided to send him a collection letter (Figure 10–5).
    After the instructor has returned your work to you, either make the necessary corrections and place your work in
a three-ring notebook for future reference or, if you received a high score, place it in your portfolio for reference
when applying for a job.

Acct No. 10-5

STATEMENT
Financial Account
COLLEGE CLINIC
4567 Broad Avenue
Woodland Hills, XY 12345-0001
Tel. 555-486-9002
Fax No. 555-487-8976

Mr. Ron Kelsey
6321 Ocean Street
Woodland Hills, XY 12345

Phone No. (H) (555) 540-9800   (W) (555) 890-7766   Birthdate 03-25-75

Primary Insurance Co. XYZ Insurance Company   Policy/Group No. 8503Y

	REFERENCE	DESCRIPTION	CHARGES	CREDITS PYMNTS.	ADJ.	BALANCE	
				BALANCE FORWARD →			
07-09-xx	99283	ER new pt EPF hx/exam MC DM	66 23			66	23
07-10-xx		XYZ Insurance billed (3-9-xx)				66	23
09-20-xx		EOB rec'd pt has not met deductible				66	23
10-01-xx		Billed pt				66	23
11-01-xx		Billed pt				66	23

PLEASE PAY LAST AMOUNT IN BALANCE COLUMN ⬆

THIS IS A COPY OF YOUR FINANCIAL ACCOUNT AS IT APPEARS ON OUR RECORDS

Figure 10–4

COLLEGE CLINIC
4567 Broad Avenue
Woodland Hills, XY 12345-0001
Tel. (555) 486-9002
FAX (555) 487-8976

Figure 10–5

ASSIGNMENT 10–6 ▸ COMPLETE A CREDIT CARD VOUCHER

Performance Objective

Task: Complete a credit card voucher and post an entry on the patient's ledger.

Conditions: Use the patient's ledger card (Figure 10–6), a credit card voucher (Figure 10–7), and a pen.

Standards: Time: _____ minutes

                       Accuracy: _____

                       (Note: The time element and accuracy criteria may be give by your instructor.)

Directions. Read the case scenario and refer to the patient's ledger/statement (Figure 10–6). Fill in the credit card voucher (Figure 10–7) and post an appropriate entry on the ledger/statement. You may wish to refer to Figure 10–13 in the *Handbook*.

Scenario. It is November 6 (current year), and you receive a telephone call at the College Clinic. It is Kevin Long, who has an unpaid balance, and it is up to you to discuss this delinquency with Mr. Long and come to an agreement on how the account can be paid. After discussion, Mr. Long decides to pay the total balance due by MasterCard credit card, giving you his authorization and account number: 5676 1342 5437 XXX0 (expiration date, December 31, 20xx). His name is listed on the card as Kevin O. Long. You call the bank, and the authorization number given is 534889.

After the instructor has returned your work to you, either make the necessary corrections and place your work in a three-ring notebook for future reference or, if you received a high score, place it in your portfolio for reference when applying for a job.

Acct No. __10-6__

STATEMENT
Financial Account
COLLEGE CLINIC
4567 Broad Avenue
Woodland Hills, XY 12345-0001
Tel. 555-486-9002
Fax No. 555-487-8976

Mr. Kevin O. Long
2443 Davis Street
Woodland Hills, XY 12345

Phone No. (H) __(555) 244-5600__   (W) __(555) 970-4466__   Birthdate __08-15-76__

Primary Insurance Co. __Blue Cross__   Policy/Group No. __130-XX-0987__

	REFERENCE	DESCRIPTION	CHARGES		CREDITS		BALANCE	
					PYMNTS.	ADJ.		
		BALANCE FORWARD ➡						
09-08-xx	99205	OV Level V DX 582	132	28			132	28
09-09-xx		Blue Cross billed (9-8-xx)					132	28
10-12-xx		BC EOB rec'd pt has not met deductible					132	28
10-23-xx		Not covered by insurance. Balance due					132	28

PLEASE PAY LAST AMOUNT IN BALANCE COLUMN ⬆

THIS IS A COPY OF YOUR FINANCIAL ACCOUNT AS IT APPEARS ON OUR RECORDS

Figure 10–6

BANKCARD SALES SLIP 3PT.

MOORE® SPEEDISET® MOORESCAN® PATENTED 205 PRINTED IN USA
FORM 50983C (12-08) P689

DO NOT WRITE _____ ABOVE THIS LINE

A555A

EXPIRATION
DATE
CHECKED

SIGN HERE

X _____

The issuer of the card identified on this item is authorized to pay the amount shown as TOTAL upon proper presentation. I promise to pay such TOTAL (together with any other charges due thereon) subject to and in accordance with the agreement governing the use of such card.

↑ PLEASE DO NOT WRITE ABOVE THIS LINE ↑

QTY.	CLASS	DESCRIPTION	PRICE	AMOUNT

DATE	AUTHORIZATION	SUB TOTAL
	REG./DEPT. CLERK	TAX

TIPS / MISC.

VISA MasterCard 5882352   TOTAL

CUSTOMER: RETAIN THIS COPY FOR YOUR RECORDS

SALES SLIP
CUSTOMER COPY

Figure 10–7

A S S I G N M E N T **10–7** ► **C O M P L E T E   A   F I N A N C I A L   A G R E E M E N T**

___

Performance Objective

Task: Complete a financial agreement and post an entry on the patient's ledger.

Conditions: Use the patient's ledger card (Figure 10–8), a financial statement form (Figure 10–9), and a pen.

Standards: Time: _____ minutes

                       Accuracy: _____

                       (Note: The time element and accuracy criteria may be given by your instructor.)

Scenario. Mr. Joseph Small has a large balance due. Create a payment plan for this case. You have discussed the installment plan concerning the amount of the total debt, the downpayment, amount and date of each installment, and the date of final payment. On June 1 (current year), Mr. Small is paying $500 cash as a downpayment, and the balance is to be divided into five equal payments, due on the first of each month. There will be no monthly finance charge. Mr. Small's daytime telephone number is 555-760-5502. He is a patient of Dr. Brady Coccidioides.

Directions. Read the case scenario. Complete a financial agreement (Figure 10–9) by subtracting the downpayment from the total debt. Refer to the patient's ledger/statement (Figure 10–8) and post an appropriate entry to the ledger/statement using a pen. You may wish to refer to Figure 10–5 in the *Handbook*. Review the completed financial agreement with the patient (role played by another student). Ask the patient (role played by another student) to sign the financial agreement. Make a photocopy of the form for the patient to retain. File the original financial agreement in the patient's financial files in the office.

After the instructor has returned your work to you, either make the necessary corrections and place your work in a three-ring notebook for future reference or, if you received a high score, place it in your portfolio for reference when applying for a job.

Acct No. 10-7

STATEMENT
Financial Account
COLLEGE CLINIC
4567 Broad Avenue
Woodland Hills, XY 12345-0001
Tel. 555-486-9002
Fax No. 555-487-8976

Mr. Joseph Small
655 Sherry Street
Woodland Hills, XY 12345

Phone No. (H) (555) 320-8801   (W) (555) 760-5502   Birthdate 11-04-77

Primary Insurance Co.   Blue Shield   Policy/Group No. 870-XX-4398

	REFERENCE	DESCRIPTION	CHARGES		CREDITS PYMNTS.	ADJ.	BALANCE	
		BALANCE FORWARD ➤					20	00
04-19-xx	99215	OV Level	96	97			116	97
04-30-xx	99218	Adm hosp	74	22			191	19
04-30-xx	32440	Pneumonectomy, total	1972	10			2163	29
05-20-xx		Blue Shield billed (1-19 to 30-xx)					2163	29
05-15-xx		BS EOB Pt deductible $2000 rec'd ck #544			163	29	2000	00

PLEASE PAY LAST AMOUNT IN BALANCE COLUMN ⬆

THIS IS A COPY OF YOUR FINANCIAL ACCOUNT AS IT APPEARS ON OUR RECORDS

Figure 10–8

FINANCIAL AGREEMENT

For PROFESSIONAL SERVICES rendered or to be rendered to:

Patient _____ Daytime Phone _____

Parent if patient is a minor _____

1. Cash price for services . . . . $ _____
2. Cash down payment . . . . $ _____
3. Charges covered by insurance service plan . . . . $ _____
4. Unpaid balance of cash price. . . . . $ _____
5. Amount financed (the amount of credit provided to you) . . . . $ _____
6. FINANCE CHARGE (the dollar amount the credit will cost you) . . . . . $ _____
7. ANNUAL PERCENTAGE RATE
   (the cost of credit as a yearly rate) . . . . _____ %
8. Total of payments (5 + 6 above-the amount you will have
   paid when you have made all scheduled payments). . . . . $ _____
9. Total sales price (1 + 6 above-sum of cash price, financing
   charge and any other amounts financed by the creditor, not part of
   the finance charge) . . . . $ _____

You have the right at any time to pay the unpaid balance due under this agreement without penalty. You have the right at this time to receive an itemization of the amount financed.

☐ I want an itemization   ☐ I do not want an itemization

Total of payments (#8 above) is payable to Dr. _____

in _____ monthly installments of $ _____ each and _____ installments of

$ _____ each. The first installment being payable on _____ 20 _____

and subsequent installments on the same day of each consecutive month until paid in full.

NOTICE TO PATIENT

Do not sign this agreement if it contains any blank spaces. You are entitled to an exact copy of any agreement you sign. You have the right at any time to pay the unpaid balance due under this agreement.

The patient (parent or guardian) agrees to be and is fully responsible for total payment of services performed in this office including any amounts not covered by health insurance or prepayment program the responsible party may have. See your contract documents for any additional information about nonpayment, default, any required prepayment in full before the scheduled date and prepayment refunds and penalties.

Signature of patient or one parent if patient is a minor:

X _____

Doctor's Signature _____

Form 1826 • 1982

SCHEDULE OF PAYMENT

No.	Date Due	Amount of Installment	Date Paid	Amount Paid	Balance Owed
		Total Amount			
D.P.					
1					
2					
3					
4					
5					
6					
7					
8					
9					
10					
11					
12					
13					
14					
15					
16					
17					
18					
19					
20					
21					
22					
23					

Figure 10–9

ALTAPOINT PRACTICE MANAGEMENT SOFTWARE ASSIGNMENTS

ASSIGNMENT **10–8** ▸ **ENTER PAYMENTS FROM OTHER SOURCES INTO THE PRACTICE MANAGEMENT SYSTEM**

Performance Objective

Task: Enter payment received from a patient into the practice management system.

Conditions: Check from patient and computer.

Standards: Time: _____ minutes

                               Accuracy: _____

                               (Note: The time element and accuracy criteria may be given by your instructor.)

Directions. Before attempting the Practice Management software assignment, refer to Appendix C and follow the instructions provided to familiarize yourself with the software. Then refer to the Practice Management software on the CD that accompanies the *Workbook*.

1. For this assignment, follow the instructions for entering payment from other sources. Post the $100 payment (Check #1456) received in the mail from Jane R. Maywood as payment in full for her May 10 office visit. Post it to the full balance rather than the individual item.

2. To obtain a grade, either print a hard copy of the patient's financial account record or have your instructor view the data onscreen for approval.

ASSIGNMENT **10-9 ▸ ENTER PAYMENTS FROM OTHER SOURCES INTO THE PRACTICE MANAGEMENT SYSTEM**

Performance Objective

Task: Enter payment received from a patient into the practice management system.

Conditions: Check from patient and computer.

Standards: Time: _____ minutes

                    Accuracy: _____

                    (Note: The time element and accuracy criteria may be given by your instructor.)

Directions: Before attempting the Practice Management software assignment, refer to Appendix C and follow the instructions provided to familiarize yourself with the software. Then refer to the Practice Management software on the CD that accompanies the *Workbook*.

1. For this assignment, follow the instructions for entering payments from other sources. Post the $190 Visa payment telephoned in by Glen Waxman on August 15 as payment in full for his July 30 office visit. Post it to the full balance rather than the individual item.

2. To obtain a grade, either print a hard copy of the patient's financial account record or have your instructor view the data onscreen for approval.

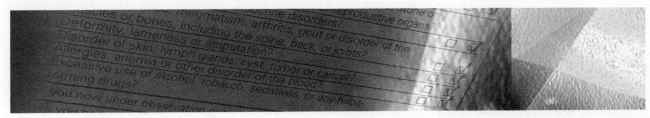

The Blue Plans, Private Insurance, and Managed Care Plans

KEY TERMS

Your instructor may wish to select some words pertinent to this chapter for a test. For definitions of the terms, further study, and/or reference, the words, phrases, and abbreviations may be found in the glossary at the end of the Handbook. *Key terms for this chapter follow.*

ancillary services

buffing

capitation

carve outs

churning

claims-review type of foundation

closed panel program

comprehensive type of foundation

copayment (copay)

deductible

direct referral

disenrollment

exclusive provider organization (EPO)

fee-for-service

formal referral

foundation for medical care (FMC)

gatekeeper

health maintenance organization (HMO)

in-area

independent (or individual) practice association (IPA)

managed care organizations (MCOs)

participating physician

per capita

physician provider group (PPG)

point-of-service (POS) plan

preferred provider organization (PPO)

prepaid group practice model

primary care physician (PCP)

self-referral

service area

staff model

stop loss

tertiary care

turfing

utilization review (UR)

verbal referral

withhold

KEY ABBREVIATIONS

See how many abbreviations and acronyms you can translate and then use this as a handy reference list. Definitions for the key abbreviations are located near the back of the Handbook *in the glossary.*

COBRA _____

copay _____

EBP _____

EPO _____

ERISA _____

FMS _____

HEDIS_____

HMO _____

IPA _____

MCO _____

NCQA _____

PCP _____

PHP _____

POS _____

PPG _____

PPO _____

QIO _____

QISMC _____

UR _____

PERFORMANCE OBJECTIVES

The student will be able to:

■ Define and spell the key terms and key abbreviations for this chapter, given the information from the *Handbook* glossary, within a reasonable time period and with enough accuracy to obtain a satisfactory evaluation.

■ After reading the chapter, answer the fill-in-the-blank, multiple choice, and true/false review questions with enough accuracy to obtain a satisfactory evaluation.

■ Complete treatment authorization forms of managed care plans, given completed new patient information forms, within a reasonable time period and with enough accuracy to obtain a satisfactory evaluation.

ALTAPOINT PRACTICE MANAGEMENT SOFTWARE OBJECTIVES

The student will be able to:

■ Enter transactions from an encounter form (superbill) and transmit an insurance claim electronically to the patient's insurance company within a reasonable time period and with enough accuracy to obtain a satisfactory evaluation.

STUDY OUTLINE

Private Insurance
Blue Cross and Blue Shield Plans

Managed Care
Prepaid Group Practice Health Plans
Benefits
Health Care Reform

Managed Care Systems
Health Maintenance Organizations
Exclusive Provider Organizations
Foundations for Medical Care
Independent Practice Associations

Preferred Provider Organizations
Physician Provider Groups
Point-of-Service Plans
Triple-Option Health Plans

Medical Review
Quality Improvement Organization
Utilization Review of Management

Management of Plans
Contracts
Preauthorization of Prior Approval
Diagnostic Tests

ASSIGNMENT **11-4 ▸ OBTAIN AUTHORIZATION FOR DIAGNOSTIC ARTHROSCOPY FOR A MANAGED CARE PLAN**

Performance Objective

Task: Complete a treatment authorization form to obtain permission for diagnostic arthroscopy with debridement for a patient from a managed care plan.

Conditions: Use a treatment authorization form (Figure 11–4) and a typewriter.

Standards: Time: _____ minutes

                 Accuracy: _____

                 (Note: The time element and accuracy criteria may be given by your instructor.)

Directions: Complete the treatment authorization form for this patient (Figure 11–4), date it August 12 of the current year, and submit it to the managed care plan. Refer to Figure 11–1 in the *Handbook* for visual guidance.

Scenario. Daniel Chan has been referred by his primary care physician, Dr. Gerald Practon, to an orthopedic surgeon, Dr. Raymond Skeleton. Both physicians are members of his managed care plan, Metropolitan Life. The patient comes into Dr. Skeleton's office complaining of pain, swelling, and crepitus of the right knee. The patient is having difficulty walking but indicates no recent injury to the knee.

   Mr. Chan lives at 226 West Olive Avenue, Woodland Hills, XY, 12340-0329, and his telephone number is 555-540-6700. His plan identification number is FTW90876, effective February 1, 20xx, and he was born February 23, 1971.

   After taking a history, completing a physical examination, and taking and reviewing radiographs, Dr. Skeleton suspects the patient has a tear of the medial meniscus and may require debridement of articular cartilage. This procedure will be performed on an outpatient basis at College Hospital. Authorization must be obtained for the surgical arthroscopy with debridement of articular cartilage. Dr. Practon's Metropolitan Life provider number is ML C01402X and Dr. Skeleton's Metropolitan Life provider number is ML C4561X.

   After the instructor has returned your work to you, either make the necessary corrections and place your work in a three-ring notebook for future reference or, if you received a high score, place it in your portfolio for reference when applying for a job.

College Clinic
4567 Board Avenue
Woodland Hills, XY 12345-0001
Telephone No. (555) 487-8976
Fax No. (555) 487-8976

MANAGED CARE PLAN AUTHORIZATION REQUEST

❏ Health Net   ❏ Met Life
❏ Pacificare   ❏ Travelers
❏ Secure Horizons   ❏ Pru Care
❏ Other

Member/Group No.

TO BE COMPLETED BY PRIMARY CARE PHYSICIAN OR OUTSIDE PROVIDER

Patient Name_____ Date_____

❏ Male ❏ Female Birthdate_____ Home Telephone Number_____

Address _____

Primary Care Physician_____ NPI_____

Referring Physician_____ NPI_____

Referred to _____ NPI_____

Address _____ Telephone No._____

Diagnosis Code_____ Diagnosis _____

Diagnosis Code_____ Diagnosis _____

Treatment Plan _____

Authorization requested for: ❏ Consult only   ❏ Treatment only   ❏ Consult/Treatment

❏ Consult/Procedure/Surgery   ❏ Diagnostic Tests

Procedure Code: _____ Description: _____

Procedure Code: _____ Description: _____

Place of service ❏ Office ❏ Outpatient ❏ Inpatient ❏ Other   Number of visits: _____

Facility: _____ Length of stay:_____

Physician's signature: _____

TO BE COMPLETED BY PRIMARY CARE PHYSICIAN

PCP Recommendations: _____ PCP Initials: _____

Date eligibility checked:_____

TO BE COMPLETED BY UTILIZATION MANAGEMENT

Authorized: _____ Auth. No:_____ Not Authorized _____

Deferred: _____ Modified: _____

Effective Date: _____ Expiration Date: _____ No. of visits: _____

Figure 11–4

ASSIGNMENT **11–5 ▸ OBTAIN AUTHORIZATION FOR CONSULTATION FROM A MANAGED CARE PLAN**

Performance Objective

Task: Complete a treatment authorization form to obtain permission for consultation for a patient from a managed care plan.

Conditions: Use a treatment authorization form (Figure 11–5) and a typewriter.

Standards: Time: _____ minutes

Accuracy: _____

(Note: The time element and accuracy criteria may be given by your instructor.)

Directions. Complete the treatment authorization form for this patient (Figure11–5), date it September 3 of the current year, and submit it to the managed care plan. Refer to Figure 11–1 in the *Handbook* for visual guidance.

Scenario. Frederico Fellini, with a history of getting up four times during the night with a slow urinary stream, was seen by his primary care physician, Dr. Gerald Practon. An intravenous pyelogram yielded negative results except for distention of the urinary bladder. Physical examination of the prostate showed an enlargement. The preliminary diagnosis is benign prostatic hypertrophy (BPH).

The patient will be referred to Dr. Douglas Lee, a urologist, for consultation (Level 4) and cystoscopy. Transurethral resection of the prostate is possible at a future date. Dr. Lee's address is 4300 Cyber Street, Woodland Hills, XY, 12345, and his office telephone number is 555-675-3322.

Dr. Practon's managed care contract is with PruCare, identification number PC C01402X, of which this patient is a member.

Mr. Fellini lives at 476 Miner Street, Woodland Hills, XY, 12345, and his telephone number is 555-679-0098. His PruCare plan identification number is VRG87655, effective January 1, 20xx. His birthdate is May 24, 1944.

After the instructor has returned your work to you, either make the necessary corrections and place your work in a three-ring notebook for future reference or, if you received a high score, place it in your portfolio for reference when applying for a job.

College Clinic
4567 Board Avenue
Woodland Hills, XY 12345-0001
Telephone No. (555) 487-8976
Fax No. (555) 487-8976

MANAGED CARE PLAN AUTHORIZATION REQUEST

❑ Health Net   ❑ Met Life
❑ Pacificare   ❑ Travelers
❑ Secure Horizons   ❑ Pru Care
❑ Other

Member/Group No.

**TO BE COMPLETED BY PRIMARY CARE
PHYSICIAN OR OUTSIDE PROVIDER**

Patient Name_____ Date_____
❑ Male ❑ Female Birthdate_____ Home Telephone Number_____
Address _____
Primary Care Physician_____ NPI_____
Referring Physician_____ NPI_____
Referred to_____ NPI_____
Address _____ Telephone No._____
Diagnosis Code_____ Diagnosis_____
Diagnosis Code_____ Diagnosis_____
Treatment Plan _____
Authorization requested for: ❑ Consult only   ❑ Treatment only ❑ Consult/Treatment
                             ❑ Consult/Procedure/Surgery   ❑ Diagnostic Tests
Procedure Code: _____ Description: _____
Procedure Code: _____ Description: _____
Place of service ❑ Office ❑ Outpatient ❑ Inpatient ❑ Other   Number of visits:_____
Facility: _____ Length of stay:_____
Physician's signature: _____

TO BE COMPLETED BY PRIMARY CARE PHYSICIAN

PCP Recommendations: _____ PCP Initials: _____
Date eligibility checked:_____

TO BE COMPLETED BY UTILIZATION MANAGEMENT
Authorized: _____ Auth. No:_____ Not Authorized _____
Deferred: _____ Modified: _____
Effective Date: _____ Expiration Date: _____ No. of visits: _____

Figure 11–5

ASSIGNMENT **11-6** ▸ **OBTAIN AUTHORIZATION FOR DIAGNOSTIC BODY SCAN FROM A MANAGED CARE PLAN**

Performance Objective

Task: Complete a treatment authorization form to obtain permission for diagnostic complete body bone scan and mammogram for a patient covered by a managed care plan.

Conditions: Use a treatment authorization form (Figure 11–6) and a typewriter.

Standards: Time: _____ minutes

                    Accuracy: _____

                    (Note: The time element and accuracy criteria may be given by your instructor.)

Directions. Complete the treatment authorization form for this patient (Figure 11–6), date it October 23 of the current year, and submit it to the managed care plan. Refer to Figure 11–1 in the *Handbook* for visual guidance.

Scenario. A patient, Debbie Dye, sees her primary care physician, Dr. Gerald Practon, for complaint of midback pain. She underwent a lumpectomy 2 years ago for a malignant neoplasm of the lower left breast; thus she has a history of breast cancer. She has been referred by Dr. Practon (PacifiCare identification number PC C01402X) to Dr. Donald Patos, an oncologist, for a complete workup. He finds that her complaint of midback pain warrants the need to refer her to XYZ Radiology for bilateral diagnostic mammography and a complete body bone scan.

Dr. Patos' address is 4466 East Canter Drive, Woodland Hills, XY, 12345, and his office telephone number is 555-980-5566. Dr. Patos' PacifiCare identification number is PC 5673X.

Ms. Dye lives at 6700 Flora Road, Woodland Hills, XY, 12345, and her telephone number is 555-433-6755. Her PacifiCare plan identification number is SR45380, effective January 1, 20xx. Her birth date is August 6, 1952.

XYZ Radiology's address is 4767 Broad Avenue, Woodland Hills, XY, 12345-0001, and the office telephone number is 555-486-9162.

After the instructor has returned your work to you, either make the necessary corrections and place your work in a three-ring notebook for future reference or, if you received a high score, place it in your portfolio for reference when applying for a job.

College Clinic
4567 Board Avenue
Woodland Hills, XY 12345-0001
Telephone No. (555) 487-8976
Fax No. (555) 487-8976

MANAGED CARE PLAN AUTHORIZATION REQUEST

❑ Health Net   ❑ Met Life
❑ Pacificare   ❑ Travelers
❑ Secure Horizons   ❑ Pru Care
❑ Other

Member/Group No.

TO BE COMPLETED BY PRIMARY CARE PHYSICIAN OR OUTSIDE PROVIDER

Patient Name_____ Date_____

❑ Male ❑ Female Birthdate_____ Home Telephone Number_____

Address _____

Primary Care Physician_____ NPI_____

Referring Physician_____ NPI_____

Referred to_____ NPI_____

Address _____ Telephone No._____

Diagnosis Code_____ Diagnosis_____

Diagnosis Code_____ Diagnosis_____

Treatment Plan _____

Authorization requested for: ❑ Consult only   ❑ Treatment only   ❑ Consult/Treatment
                               ❑ Consult/Procedure/Surgery   ❑ Diagnostic Tests

Procedure Code: _____ Description: _____

Procedure Code: _____ Description: _____

Place of service ❑ Office ❑ Outpatient ❑ Inpatient ❑ Other   Number of visits:_____

Facility: _____ Length of stay:_____

Physician's signature: _____

TO BE COMPLETED BY PRIMARY CARE PHYSICIAN

PCP Recommendations: _____ PCP Initials: _____

Date eligibility checked:_____

TO BE COMPLETED BY UTILIZATION MANAGEMENT

Authorized: _____ Auth. No:_____ Not Authorized _____

Deferred: _____ Modified: _____

Effective Date: _____ Expiration Date: _____ No. of visits: _____

Figure 11–6

ALTAPOINT PRACTICE MANAGEMENT SOFTWARE ASSIGNMENTS

ASSIGNMENT **11-7** ▸ **ENTER TRANSACTIONS FROM AN ENCOUNTER FORM (SUPERBILL) INTO THE PRACTICE MANAGEMENT SYSTEM AND TRANSMIT AN INSURANCE CLAIM ELECTRONICALLY**

Performance Objective

Task: Enter transactions from Denise Watson's encounter form (superbill) into the practice management system and transmit an insurance claim electronically.

Conditions: Patient's electronic data, encounter form (superbill) (Figure 11-7) and computer.

Standards: Time: _____ minutes

                 Accuracy: _____

                 (Note: The time element and accuracy criteria may be given by your instructor.)

Directions. Before attempting the Practice Management software assignment, refer to Appendix C and follow the instructions provided to familiarize yourself with the software. Then refer to the Practice Management software on the CD that accompanies the *Workbook*.

1. For this assignment, follow the instructions for entering transactions from an encounter form (superbill) and enter the charges for Denise Watson's office visit on June 15. If codes used in this assignment do not already appear in the system, refer to Assignment 5-13 in *Workbook* Chapter 5.

2. After the information has been entered, transmit the insurance claim to Ms. Watson's insurance company by following the instructions for transmitting a claim electronically.

3. Print a hard copy of the insurance claim to hand in to your instructor to receive a score.

4. A Performance Evaluation Checklist may be reproduced form the "Instruction Guide to the *Workbook*" chapter if your instructor wishes you to submit it to assist with scoring and comments.

   After the instructor has returned your work to you, either make the necessary corrections and place your work in a three-ring notebook for future reference or, if you received a high score, place it in your portfolio for reference when applying for a job.

Assignment 11-8

College Clinic

4567 Broad Avenue
Woodlands Hills, XY
12345-0001
Tel (555) 486-9002
Fax (555) 487-8976

Doctors No. _____

☐ PRIVATE   ☐ MANAGED CARE   ☐ MEDICAID   ☐ MEDICARE   ☐ TRICARE   ☐ W/C

ACCOUNT #	PATIENT'S LAST NAME	FIRST	INITIAL	TODAY'S DATE
	Watson	*Denise*	*L.*	*6/15/2007*

ASSIGNMENT: I hereby assign payment directly to College Clinic of the surgical and/or medical benefits, if any, otherwise payable to me for his/her services as described below.
SIGNED (Patient, or Parent, if Minor)   DATE:

	DESCRIPTION	CPT-4/MD	FEE		DESCRIPTION	CPT-4/MD	FEE		DESCRIPTION	CPT-4/MD	FEE
	OFFICE VISIT-NEW PATIENT				**WELL BABY EXAM**				**LABORATORY**		
	Level 1	99201			Intial	99381			Glucose Blood	82951	
✓	Level 2	99202	*65.00*		Periodic	99391			Hematocrit	85013	
	Level 3	99203			**OFFICE PROCEDURES**				Occult Blood	82270	
	Level 4	99204			Anscopy	46600			Urine Dip	81000	
	Level 5	99205			ECG 24-hr	93000			**X-RAY**		
	OFFICE VISIT-ESTAB, PATIENT				Fracture Rpr Foot	28470			Foot - 2 View	73620	
	Level 1	99211		✓	I & D	10060	*82.00*		Forearm - 2 View	73090	
	Level 2	99212			Suture Repair	12002			Nasal Bone - 3	70160	
	Level 3	99213							Spine LS - 2 view	72100	
	Level 4	99214			**INJECTIONS/VACCINATIONS**						
	Level 5	99215			DPT	90701			**MISCELLANEOUS**		
	OFFICE CONSULT-NP/EST				Influenza Vac	90658			Handling of Spec	99000	
	Level 3	99243			OPU-Poliovirus	90712			Supply	99070	
	Level 4	99244			Tetanus	90703			Venipuncture	36415	
	Level 5	99245			Immun Admin	90471					

COMMENTS:

Physician:

RETURN APPOINTMENT

_____ Week(s)   _____ Month(s)

DIAGNOSIS: DESCRIPTION   CODE
Primary: *Furuncle/Back* _____   *680.2*
Secondary: _____   _____
_____   _____
_____   _____

REC'D BY:
☐ BANK CARD
☐ CASH
☐ CHECK
  # _____

PREVIOUS BALANCE	⊖
TODAY'S FEE	*147.00*
AMOUNT REC'D/CO-PAY	
BALANCE	*147.00*

Figure 11–7

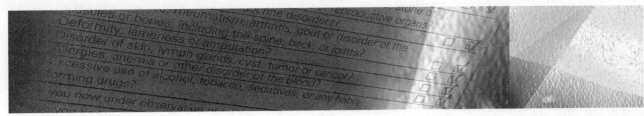

Medicare

KEY TERMS

Your instructor may wish to select some words pertinent to this chapter for a test. For definitions of the terms, further study, and/or reference, the words, phrases, and abbreviations may be found in the glossary at the end of the Handbook. *Key terms for this chapter follow.*

advance beneficiary notice (ABN)

approved charges

assignment

benefit period

Centers for Medicare and Medicaid Services (CMS)

Correct Coding Initiative (CCI)

crossover claim

diagnostic cost groups (DCGs)

disabled

end-stage renal disease (ESRD)

fiscal intermediary (FI)

formulary

hospice

hospital insurance

intermediate care facilities (ICFs)

limiting charge

medical necessity

Medicare

Medicare administrative contractor (MAC)

Medicare Part A

Medicare Part B

Medicare Part C

Medicare Part D

Medicare/Medicaid (Medi-Medi)

Medicare Secondary Payer (MSP)

Medicare Summary Notice (MSN)

Medigap (MG)

national alphanumeric codes

nonparticipating physician (nonpar)

nursing facility (NF)

participating physician (par)

Physician Quality Reporting Initiative (PQRI)

premium

prospective payment system (PPS)

Quality Improvement Organization (QIO)

qui tam action

reasonable fee

relative value unit (RVU)

remittance advice (RA)

resource-based relative value scale (RBRVS)

respite care

Supplemental Security Income (SSI)

supplementary medical insurance (SMI)

volume performance standard (VPS)

whistleblowers

KEY ABBREVIATIONS

See how many abbreviations and acronyms you can translate and then use this as a handy reference list. Definitions for the key abbreviations are located near the back of the Handbook *in the glossary.*

ABN _____

CAP _____

CLIA _____

CMS _____

CCI _____

COBRA _____

DC _____

DCGs _____

DDS _____

DEFRA _____

DME _____

DO _____

DPM _____

EGHP _____

EOB _____

ERA _____

ESRD _____

FI _____

GPCI _____

HCPCS _____

HMO _____

ICFs _____

ICU _____

LCD _____

LGHP _____

LMRP _____

MAAC _____

MAC _____

MCO _____

MD _____

Medi-Medi _____

MG _____

MMA _____

MSA _____

MSN _____

MSP _____

NCDs _____

NEMB _____

NF _____

nonpar physician _____

NPI _____

OASDI _____

OBRA _____

OCNA _____

OIG _____

OR _____

par physician _____

PAYRID _____

PFFS plan _____

PIN _____

POS plan _____

PPO _____

PQRI _____

PRO _____

PPS _____

PSO _____

QIO _____

RA _____

RBRVS _____

RFBS _____

RVU _____

SOF _____

SMI _____

SSI _____

TEFRA _____

UPIN _____

VA _____

VPS _____

PERFORMANCE OBJECTIVES

The student will be able to:

- Define and spell the key terms and key abbreviations for this chapter, given the information from the *Handbook* glossary, within a reasonable time period and with enough accuracy to obtain a satisfactory evaluation.
- After reading the chapter answer the fill-in-the-blanks, multiple choice, and true/false review questions, with enough accuracy to obtain a satisfactory evaluation.
- Fill in the correct meaning of each abbreviation, given a list of common medical abbreviations and symbols that appear in chart notes, within a reasonable time period and with enough accuracy to obtain a satisfactory evaluation.
- Complete each CMS-1500 (08-05) Health Insurance Claim Form for billing, given the patients' medical chart notes, ledger cards, and blank insurance claim forms, within a reasonable

time period and with enough accuracy to obtain a satisfactory evaluation.

- Post payments, adjustments, and balances on the patients' ledger cards, using the Medicare Mock Fee Schedule in Appendix A in this *Workbook*, within a reasonable time period and with enough accuracy to obtain a satisfactory evaluation.
- Compute mathematical calculations, given Medicare problem situations, within a reasonable time period and with enough accuracy to obtain a satisfactory evaluation.
- Using the *Current Procedural Terminology* (CPT) code book or the Mock Fee Schedule in Appendix A in this *Workbook* and the Healthcare Common Procedure Coding System (HCPCS) list of codes in Appendix B in this *Workbook*, select the HCPCS and/or procedural code numbers, given a series of medical services, procedures, or supplies, within a reasonable time period and with enough accuracy to obtain a satisfactory evaluation.

ALTAPOINT PRACTICE MANAGEMENT SOFTWARE OBJECTIVES

The student should be able to:

- Enter transactions from encounter forms (superbills) into the practice management system and transmit and print insurance claims

electronically to the insurance company within a reasonable time period and with enough accuracy to obtain a satisfactory evaluation.

STUDY OUTLINE

Background
Policies and Regulations
 Eligibility Requirements
 Health Insurance Card
 Enrollment Status
 Benefits and Nonbenefits
Additional Insurance Programs
 Medicare/Medicaid
 Medicare/Medigap
 Medicare Secondary Payer
 Automobile or Liability Insurance Coverage
Medicare Managed Care Plans
 Health Maintenance Organizations
 Carrier Dealing Prepayment Organization
Utilization and Quality Control
 Quality Improvement Organizations
 Federal False Claims Amendment Act
Medicare Billing Compliance Issues
 Clinical Laboratory Improvement Amendment

Payment Fundamentals
 Provider
 Prior Authorization
 Waiver of Liability Provision
 Elective Surgery Estimate
 Prepayment Screens
 Correct Coding Initiative
Medicare Reimbursement
 Chronology of Payment
 Reasonable Fee
 Resource-Based Relative Value Scale
 Healthcare Common Procedure Coding System (HCPCS)
Claim Submission
 Local Coverage Determination
 Medicare Administrative Contractors and Fiscal Agents
 Provider Identification Numbers
 Patient's Signature Authorization
 Time Limit

Paper Claims
Electronic Claims
Medicare/Medicaid Claims
Medicare/Medigap Claims
Medicare/Employer Supplemental Insurance
  Claims
Medicare/Supplemental and MSP Claims
Deceased Patients Claims
Physician Substitute Coverage
After Claim Submission
Remittance Advice
Medicare Summary Notice

**Beneficiary Representative/Representative
Payee**
Posting Payments
Review and Redetermination Process
**Procedure: Determine Whether Medicare is
Primary or Secondary and Determine**
Additional Benefits
**Procedure: Complete an Advance Beneficiary
Notice (ABN) Form**

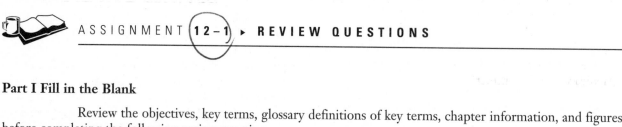

A S S I G N M E N T **12–1** ▸ **R E V I E W Q U E S T I O N S**

Part I Fill in the Blank

Review the objectives, key terms, glossary definitions of key terms, chapter information, and figures before completing the following review questions.

1. An individual becomes eligible for Medicare Parts A and B at age ___65___.

2. Medicare Part A is ___Hospital___ coverage, and Medicare Part B is ___Medical___ coverage.

3. Name an eligibility requirement that would allow aliens to receive Medicare benefits.

the applicant must have lived in the US as a permanent resident for 5 consecutive yrs.

4. Funding for the Medicare Part A program is obtained from

Special contributions from employees + self employed persons & employer matching contrabutions

and funding for the Medicare Part B program is obtained equally from

those who sign up for it & uncle Sam.

5. Define a Medicare Part A hospital benefit period. It begins the day a patient enters a hospital + ends when the patient hasn't been a bed patient in any hospital or nursing facility for 60 consecutive days

6. A program designed to provide pain relief, symptom management, and supportive services to terminally ill individuals and their families is known as

hospice

7. Short-term inpatient medical care for terminally ill individuals to give temporary

    relief to the caregiver is known as *respite care*

8. The frequency of Pap tests for Medicare patients is 1 every 24 months low risk, 1 every 12 months high risk

    and that for mammograms is 1 every 12 months.

9. Some third-party payers offer policies that fall under guidelines issued by the federal
    government and may cover prescription costs, Medicare deductibles, and copayments;

    these secondary or supplemental policies are known as *Secondary*
    insurance policies.

10. Name two types of health maintenance organization (HMO) plans that may have
    Medicare Part B contracts.

    p445
    a. HMO risk Plans
    b. HMO Cost Plans

11. The federal laws establishing standards of quality control and safety measures in

    clinical laboratories are known as *Clinical Laboratory Improvement Amendment (CLIA)*

12. Acceptance of assignment by a participating physician means that he or she agrees to

    accept payment from Medicare after the $ 131 ~~Medicare~~
    annual deductible has been met.

13. Philip Lenz is seen by Dr. Doe, who schedules an operative procedure in 1 month.

    This type of surgery is known as *elective surgery*,
    because it does not have to be performed immediately.

14. A Medicare insurance claim form showed an alphanumeric code, J0540, for an injection

    of 600,000 U of penicillin G. This number is referred to as a/an *modifier*

15. Organizations or claims processors under contract to the federal government that handle
    insurance claims and payments for hospitals under Medicare Part A are known as

    fiscal intermediary The National Blue Cross Association
    and those that process claims for physicians and other suppliers of services under

    Medicare Part B are called *Medicare administrative Contractors*.

16. A Centers for Medicare and Medicaid Services (CMS)–assigned provider

    identification number is known as a/an _National Provider identifier_ .

    Physicians who supply durable medical equipment must have a/an _Supplier_
    number.

17. If circumstances make it impossible to obtain a signature each time a paper claim is
    submitted or an electronic claim is transmitted, the Medicare patient's signature may

    be obtained either _Medicare patients signature on file_
    or _a form in the medical office_ , thus indicating the signature is on file.

18. The time limit for sending in a Medicare insurance claim is

    1 fiscal yr after the fiscal yr services were rendered

19. Mrs. Davis, a Medicare/Medicaid (Medi-Medi) patient, has a cholecystectomy. In
    completing the insurance claim form, the assignment portion is left blank in error.
    What will happen in this case?

    the claim will get rejected

    _____

20. If an individual is 65 years of age and is a Medicare beneficiary but is working and has
    a group insurance policy, where is the insurance claim form sent initially?

    to their group insurance

21. If a Medicare beneficiary is injured in an automobile accident, the physician submits
    the claim form to

    Medicare .

Part II Multiple Choice

Choose the best answer.

22. Medicare prescription drug benefits for individuals who purchase the insurance are available under

    a. Medicare part A

    b. Medicare part B

    c. Medicare part C

    (d.) Medicare part D

23. Medicare secondary payer (MSP) cases may involve

    a. Medicare-aged workers under group health plans of more than 20 covered employees

    b. Medicare-aged or disabled individuals who also receive benefits under the Department of Veterans Affairs and Medicare

    c. Medicare patient who is involved in an automobile accident

    (d.) All of the above

24. If a Medicare patient is to receive a medical service that may be denied payment either entirely or partially, the provider should

    a. Transmit a claim for adjudication to receive an official notice of denial

    (b.) Have the patient sign an Advance Beneficiary Notice

    c. Have the patient make a partial payment

    d. Ask the patient for payment

25. A decision by a Medicare administrative contractor (MAC) whether to cover (pay) a particular medical service on a contractor-wide basis in accordance with whether it is reasonable and necessary is known as a/an

    (a.) Local Coverage Determination

    b. Correct Coding Initiative edit

    c. Prepayment screen

    d. Redetermination process

26. According to regulations, a Medicare patient must be billed for a copayment

    a. at least once before a balance is adjusted off as uncollectable

    b. at least two times before a balance is adjusted off as uncollectable

    (c.) at least three times before a balance is adjusted off as uncollectable

    d. no more than four times before a balance is adjusted off as uncollectible

Part III True/False

Write "T" or "F" in the blank to indicate whether you think the statement is true or false.

_____T_____ 27. All patients who have a Medicare health insurance card have Part A hospital and Part B medical coverage.

_____T_____ 28. Prescription drug plans refer to the drugs in their formularies by tier numbers.

_____F_____ 29. Nonparticipating physicians may decide on a case-by-case basis whether to accept assignment when providing medical services to Medicare patients.

_____T_____ 30. Medicare's Correct Coding Initiative was implemented by the Centers for Medicare and Medicaid Services to eliminate unbundling of CPT codes.

_____T_____ 31. A Medicare/Medigap claim is not called a crossover claim.

ASSIGNMENT 12–2 ▸ CALCULATE MATHEMATICAL PROBLEMS

Performance Objective

Task: Calculate and insert the correct amounts for seven Medicare scenarios.

Conditions: Use a pen or pencil, the description of problem, and, for Problem 7, Figures 12–1 and 12–2.

Standards: Time: _____ minutes

Accuracy: _____

(Note: The time element and accuracy criteria may be given by your instructor.)

Directions. Submitting insurance claims, particularly Medicare claims, involves a bit of arithmetic. Several problems are given here so that you will gain experience with situations encountered daily in your work. The Medicare deductible is always subtracted from the allowed amount first before mathematic computations continue.

Problem 1. Mr. Doolittle has Medicare Part B coverage. He was well during the entire past year. On January 1, Mr. Doolittle is rushed to the hospital, where Dr. Input performs an emergency gastric resection. Medicare is billed for $450, and the doctor agrees to accept assignment. The patient has not paid any deductible. Complete the following statements by putting in the correct amounts.

Original Bill _____

   a. Medicare allows $400. Medicare payment: _____

   b. Patient owes Dr. Input: _____

   c. Dr. Input's courtesy adjustment: _____

   Mathematical computations:

Problem 2. Mrs. James has Medicare Part B coverage. She met her deductible when she was ill in March of this year. On November 1, Dr. Caesar performs a bilateral salpingo-oophorectomy, for which he bills her $300 and agrees to accept a Medicare assignment.

Original Bill _____

   a. Medicare allows $275. Medicare payment: _____

   b. Patient owes Dr. Caesar: _____

   c. Dr. Caesar's courtesy adjustment: _____

Mathematical computations for surgeon:

The assistant surgeon charged Mrs. James $60 (the Medicare limiting charge) and does not accept assignment. After receiving her check from Medicare, Mrs. James sends the surgeon his $60. Medicare has allowed $55 for the fee.

a. How much of the money was from Mrs. James' private funds? $_____.

b. How much did Medicare pay? $_____.

Mathematical computations for assistant surgeon:

Problem 3. You work for Dr. Coccidioides. He does not accept assignment. He is treating Mr. Robinson for allergies. Mr. Robinson has Medicare Part A. You send in a bill to Medicare for the $135 that Mr. Robinson

owes you. What portion of the bill will Medicare pay? _____

Problem 4. In June, Mr. Fay has an illness that incurs $89 in medical bills. He asks you to bill Medicare, and the physician does not accept assignment. He has paid the deductible at another physician's office.

a. If Medicare allows the entire amount of your fees, the Medicare check to the patient is

$_____ (which comes to you).

b. The patient's part of the bill to you is $_____.

Mathematical computations:

Problem 5. Mr. Iba, a Medicare patient with a Medigap insurance policy, is seen for an office visit and the fee is $80. The Medicare-approved amount is $54.44. The patient has met his deductible for the year.

a. The Medicare payment check is $ _____.

b. After the claim is submitted to the Medigap insurance, the Medigap payment check is

$_____.

Note: Chapter 12 in the *Handbook* gives details on Medigap coverage guidelines.

c. To zero out the balance, the Medicare courtesy adjustment is $ _____.

Mathematical computations:

Problem 6. Mrs. Smith, a Medicare patient, had surgery, and the participating physician's fee is $1250. This patient is working part-time, and her employer group health plan (primary insurance) allowed $1100, applied $500 to the deductible, and paid 80% of $600.

a. Amount paid by this plan: $ _____.

b. The spouse's employer group health plan (secondary insurance) is billed for the balance, which is

$ _____, and this program also has a $500 deductible. This plan pays 100% of the fee billed, minus the deductible.

c. The spouse's employer group plan makes a payment of $ _____.

You send copies of remittance advice from the two group health plans and submit a claim to Medicare (the third insurance) for $1250. The balance at this point is $ _____.

Mathematical computations:

Problem 7. Beverly James has Medicare Part B coverage. She has $242 in medical bills and has met $100 of the $131 (2007 deductible). Dr. Practon agrees to accept assignment.

Original Bill   _____

a. Medicare allows $200. Medicare payment: _____

b. Beverly James owes Dr. Practon: _____

c. Dr. Practon's courtesy adjustment: _____

Mathematical computations:

Problem 8. Oliver Mills has Medicare Part B coverage. He fell at home and suffered a sprain and Dr. Skeleton treated him. His medical bill totaled $370 and he has met $60 of the $131 (2007 deductible). Dr. Skeleton agrees to accept assignment.

Original Bill   _____

   a. Medicare allows $280. Medicare payment: _____

   b. Oliver Mills owes Dr. Skeleton: _____

   c. Dr. Skeleton's courtesy adjustment: _____

   Mathematical computations:

Problem 9. Maria Sanchez has Medicare Part B coverage. She has $565 in medical bills at Dr. Cardi's office and met $45 of the $131 (2007 deductible) at another physician's office. Dr. Cardi agrees to accept assignment.

Original Bill   _____

   a. Medicare allows $480. Medicare payment: _____

   b. Maria Sanchez owes Dr. Cardi: _____

   c. Dr. Cardi's courtesy adjustment: _____

   Mathematical computations:

Problem 10. In the late 1980s, Medicare's Resource-Based Relative Value System (RBRVS) became the way payment was determined each year. However, since the early 1990s, annual fee schedules have been supplied by local fiscal intermediaries, and so the RBRVS has become more useful in determining practice cost to convert patients to capitation in negotiations of managed care contracts. Because physicians may request determination of fees for certain procedures to discover actual cost and what compensation ratios should be, it is important to know how Medicare fees are determined. Each year the *Federal Register* publishes geographic practice cost indices by Medicare carrier and locality as well as relative value units and related information. This assignment will give you some mathematical practice in using figures for annual conversion factors to determine fees for given procedures in various regions of the United States. Refer to Figures 12–1 and 12–2, which are pages of the *Federal Register*.

a. HCPCS Code 47600: Removal of gallbladder. The medical practice is located in Phoenix, Arizona.

	Work	*Overhead*	*Malpractice*
RVUs	_____	_____	_____
GPCI	× _____	× _____	× _____

+ _____ + _____ + _____ = Total adjusted RVUs _____

2007 Conversion factor $37.8975 × Total adjusted RVUs _____ = allowed

amount $ _____.

b. HCPCS Code 47715: Excision of bile duct cyst. The medical practice is located in Arkansas.

	Work	*Overhead*	*Malpractice*
RVUs	_____	_____	_____
GPCI	× _____	× _____	× _____

+ _____ + _____ + _____ = Total adjusted RVUs _____

2007 Conversion factor $37.8975 × Total adjusted RVUs _____ = allowed

amount $ _____.

c. HCPCS Code 48146: Pancreatectomy. The medical practice is located in Fresno, California.

	Work	*Overhead*	*Malpractice*
RVUs	_____	_____	_____
GPCI	× _____	× _____	× _____

+ _____ + _____ + _____ = Total adjusted RVUs _____

2007 Conversion factor $37.8975 × Total adjusted RVUs _____ = allowed

amount $ _____.

ADDENDUM D.---GEOGRAPHIC PRACTICE COST INDICES BY MEDICARE CARRIER AND LOCALITY

Carrier number	Locality number	Locality name	Work	Practice expense	Mal-practice	
510	5	Birmingham, AL	0.981	0.913	0.824	
510	4	Mobile, AL	0.964	0.911	0.824	
510	2	North Central AL	0.970	0.867	0.824	
510	1	Northwest AL	0.985	0.869	0.824	
510	6	Rest of AL	0.975	0.851	0.824	
510	3	Southeast AL	0.972	0.869	0.824	
1020	1	Alaska	1.106	1.255	1.042	
1030	5	Flagstaff (city), AZ	0.983	0.911	1.255	
1030	1	Phoenix, AZ	1.003	1.016	1.255	
1030	7	Prescott (city), AZ	0.983	0.911	1.255	
1030	99	Rest of Arizona	0.987	0.943	1.255	
1030	2	Tucson (city), AZ	0.987	0.989	1.255	
1030	8	Yuma (city), AZ	0.983	0.911	1.255	
520	13	Arkansas	0.960	0.856	0.302	
2050	26	Anaheim-Santa Ana, CA	1.046	1.220	1.370	
542	14	Bakersfield, CA	1.028	1.050	1.370	
542	11	Fresno/Madera, CA	1.006	1.009	1.370	
542	13	Kings/Tulare, CA	0.999	1.001	1.370	
2050	18	Los Angeles, CA (1st of 8)	1.060	1.196	1.370	
2050	19	Los Angeles, CA (2nd of 8)	1.060	1.196	1.370	

Figure 12–1

ADDENDUM B.—RELATIVE VALUE UNITS (RVUs) AND RELATED INFORMATION

HCPCS[1]	MOD	Status	Description	Work RVUs	Practice expense RVUs[2]	Mal-practice RVUs	Total	Global period	Up-date
47399	....	C	Liver surgery procedure	0.00	0.00	0.00	0.00	YYY	S
47400	....	A	Incision of liver duct	19.11	8.62	1.38	29.11	090	S
47420	....	A	Incision of bile duct	15.48	9.59	2.01	27.08	090	S
47425	....	A	Incision of bile duct	14.95	11.84	2.48	29.27	090	S
47440	....	A	Incision of bile duct	18.51	10.61	2.23	31.35	090	S
47460	....	A	Incision of bile duct sphincter	14.57	15.71	1.84	32.12	090	N
47480	....	A	Incision of gallbladder	8.14	7.68	1.61	17.43	090	S
47490	....	A	Incision of gallbladder	6.11	3.61	0.38	10.10	090	N
47500	....	A	Injection for liver x-rays	1.98	1.53	0.14	3.65	000	N
47505	....	A	Injection for liver x-rays	0.77	1.34	0.14	2.25	000	N
47510	....	A	Insert catheter, bile duct	7.47	2.90	0.25	10.62	090	N
47511	....	A	Insert bile duct drain	10.02	2.90	0.25	13.17	090	N
47525	....	A	Change bile duct catheter	5.47	1.61	0.16	7.24	010	N
47530	....	A	Revise, reinsert bile tube	5.47	1.53	0.19	7.19	090	N
47550	....	A	Bile duct endoscopy	3.05	1.58	0.35	4.98	000	S
47552	....	A	Biliary endoscopy, thru skin	6.11	1.38	0.21	7.70	000	S
47553	....	A	Biliary endoscopy, thru skin	6.42	3.84	0.63	10.89	000	N
47554	....	A	Biliary endoscopy, thru skin	9.16	3.97	0.68	13.81	000	N
47555	....	A	Biliary endoscopy, thru skin	7.64	2.66	0.30	10.60	000	N
47556	....	A	Biliary endoscopy, thru skin	8.66	2.66	0.30	11.62	000	N
47600	....	A	Removal of gallbladder	10.80	7.61	1.60	20.01	090	S
47605	....	A	Removal of gallbladder	11.66	8.23	1.77	21.66	090	S
47610	....	A	Removal of gallbladder	14.01	9.47	2.02	25.50	090	S
47612	....	A	Removal of gallbladder	14.91	14.39	3.08	32.38	090	S
47620	....	A	Removal of gallbladder	15.97	11.35	2.39	29.71	090	S
47630	....	A	Removal of bile duct stone	8.40	3.79	0.40	12.59	090	N
47700	....	A	Exploration of bile ducts	13.90	7.71	1.60	23.21	090	S
47701	....	A	Bile duct revision	26.87	8.30	1.92	37.09	090	S
47710	....	A	Excision of bile duct tumor	18.64	12.19	2.49	33.32	090	S
47715	....	A	Excision of bile duct cyst	14.66	8.31	1.73	24.70	090	S
47716	....	A	Fusion of bile duct cyst	12.67	6.63	1.55	20.85	090	S
47720	....	A	Fuse gallbladder and bowel	12.03	9.26	1.95	23.34	090	S
47721	....	A	Fuse upper gi structures	14.57	11.55	2.50	28.62	090	S
47740	....	A	Fuse gallbladder and bowel	14.08	10.32	2.16	26.56	090	S
47760	....	A	Fuse bile ducts and bowel	20.15	11.74	2.56	34.45	090	S
47765	....	A	Fuse liver ducts and bowel	19.25	14.77	3.00	37.02	090	S
47780	....	A	Fuse bile ducts and bowel	20.63	13.22	2.76	36.61	090	S
47800	....	A	Reconstruction of bile ducts	17.91	13.37	2.46	33.74	090	S
47801	....	A	Placement, bile duct support	11.41	5.54	0.82	17.77	090	S
47802	....	A	Fuse liver duct and intestine	16.19	10.38	1.77	28.34	090	S
47999	....	C	Bile tract surgery procedure	0.00	0.00	0.00	0.00	YYY	S
48000	....	A	Drainage of abdomen	13.25	7.13	1.42	21.80	090	S
48001	....	A	Placement of drain, pancreas	15.71	8.22	1.91	25.84	090	S
48005	....	A	Resect/debride pancreas	17.77	9.29	2.16	29.22	090	S
48020	....	A	Removal of pancreatic stone	13.12	6.86	1.59	21.57	090	S
48100	....	A	Biopsy of pancreas	10.30	4.26	0.80	15.36	090	S
48102	....	A	Needle biopsy, pancreas	4.48	2.44	0.25	7.17	010	N
48120	....	A	Removal of pancreas lesion	12.93	9.83	2.09	24.85	090	S
48140	....	A	Partial removal of pancreas	18.47	13.44	2.86	34.77	090	S
48145	....	A	Partial removal of pancreas	19.30	15.88	3.20	38.38	090	S
48146	....	A	Pancreatectomy	21.97	16.67	1.94	40.58	090	S
48148	....	A	Removal of pancreatic duct	14.57	8.32	1.70	24.59	090	S
48150	....	A	Partial removal of pancreas	34.55	22.79	4.80	62.14	090	S
48151	....	D	Partial removal of pancreas	0.00	0.00	0.00	0.00	090	0
48152	....	A	Pancreatectomy	31.33	22.79	4.80	58.92	090	S
48153	....	A	Pancreatectomy	34.55	22.79	4.80	62.14	090	S
48154	....	A	Pancreatectomy	31.33	22.79	4.80	58.92	090	S
48155	....	A	Removal of pancreas	19.65	20.63	4.31	44.59	090	S
48160	....	N	Pancreas removal, transplant	0.00	0.00	0.00	0.00	XXX	0
48180	....	A	Fuse pancreas and bowel	21.11	12.74	2.66	36.51	090	S
48400	....	A	Injection, intraoperative	1.97	1.04	0.24	3.25	ZZZ	S
48500	....	A	Surgery of pancreas cyst	12.17	8.62	1.68	22.47	090	S
48510	....	A	Drain pancreatic pseudocyst	11.34	7.62	1.46	20.42	090	S
48520	....	A	Fuse pancreas cyst and bowel	13.11	11.43	2.46	27.00	090	S
48540	....	A	Fuse pancreas cyst and bowel	15.95	12.80	2.68	31.43	090	S
48545	....	A	Pancreatorrhaphy	14.81	7.75	1.81	24.37	090	S
48547	....	A	Duodenal exclusion	21.42	11.20	2.61	35.23	090	S

[1] All numeric CPT HCPCS Copyright 1993 American Medical Association.
[2] *Indicates reduction of Practice Expense RVUs as a result of OBRA 1993.

Figure 12–2

ASSIGNMENT 12–3 ▸ LOCATE HCPCS ALPHANUMERIC CODES

Performance Objective

Task: Insert the correct HCPCS codes for problems presented.

Conditions: Use a pen or pencil, the CPT code book, and Appendix B in this *Workbook*.

Standards: Time: _____ minutes

                 Accuracy: _____

                 (Note: The time element and accuracy criteria may be given by your instructor.)

Directions. As you have learned from the *Handbook*, it is necessary to use three levels of codes (CPT, HCPCS, and regional codes) when submitting Medicare claims. Refer to Appendix B in this *Workbook* to complete this HCPCS coding exercise for Medicare claims.

1. Cellular therapy   _____

2. Injection amygdalin, laetrile, vitamin B_{17} _____

3. Lidocaine (Xylocaine) injection for local anesthetic   _____

4. Splint, wrist   _____

5. Crutches   _____

6. Cervical head harness   _____

7. 1 ml gamma globulin   _____

8. Injection, vitamin B_{12} _____

9. Contraceptives (unclassified drugs)   _____

10. Surgical tray   _____

11. Penicillin, procaine, aqueous, injection   _____

   Now get some practice in selecting HCPCS modifiers. For this part of the assignment, in addition to referring to Appendix B in this *Workbook*, you will need to refer to your CPT code book or Appendix A in this *Workbook* to complete these Medicare problems.

12. Second surgical opinion by a professional review organization,
    detailed history and examination, low-complexity decision making   _____

13. Chiropractic manipulation of spine, one region, acute treatment   _____

14. Office visit by a locum tenens physician of established patient,
    problem-focused history and examination with straightforward
    decision making   _____

15. Strapping of thumb of left hand   _____

ASSIGNMENT **12–4** ▸ **LOCATE HCPCS PREVENTIVE CARE
EXAMINATION CODES**

HCPCS Preventive Care Examination Codes

Since 2005, a Medicare beneficiary is allowed a one-time "Welcome to Medicare" physical examination within the first 6 months that he or she is on Part B (see *Handbook* Table 12–1).

G0344 Initial preventive physical examination; face-to-face visit, services limited to new beneficiary during the first 6 months of Medicare Part B enrollment.

G0366 Electrocardiogram (ECG), routine ECG with at least 12 leads; performed as a component of the initial preventive physical examination with interpretation and report. (bundled into payment for another service that is not specified).

G0367 Electrocardiogram, tracing only, without interpretation and report, performed as a component of the initial preventive physical examination.

G0368 Electrocardiogram, interpretation and report only, performed as a component of the initial preventative physical examination. (paid under physician fee schedule).

Directions. Read the scenarios and refer to the HCPCS Preventive Care Examination codes to assist you in selecting the correct code.

1. Within 6 months after enrollment in Medicare Part B, Mary Sanchez is seen in Dr. Cardi's office for a physical examination and then he sends her over to the College Hospital for the ECG with interpretation.

   Hospital HCPCS Code _____

   Provider who interprets ECG HCPCS Code _____

   Physician's HCPCS Code _____

2. Dr. Donald Smith, a hospital-based clinic physician, does a physical examination and an ECG tracing with report and interpretation on David Bloch within 6 months of his enrollment in Medicare Part B.

   Hospital HCPCS Codes _____ and _____

   Physician's HCPCS Code _____

3. Dr. Gerald Practon performs both the physical examination and the ECG tracing with report and interpretation in his office on Anna Scofield within 6 months of her enrollment in Medicare Part B.

   Physician's HCPCS Codes _____ and _____

Insurance Claim Assignments

Assignments presented in this section are to give you hands-on experience in completing a variety of Medicare insurance cases by using the CMS-1500 (08-05) claim form. Periodically, newsletters are issued by Medicare fiscal intermediaries relaying new federal policies and guidelines. This may change block requirements on the claim form, codes (procedural and diagnostic) that are covered in the Medicare program, or mean lower reimbursement or denial of reimbursement for a particular code number. Cases shown do not reflect payment policies for a particular procedure or service; this depends on federal guidelines and local medical review policies (LMRPs) at the time of claim submission.

The cases presented in this section are:

Assignment 12–5   Medicare

Assignment 12–6   Medicare/Medicaid (Medi-Medi)

Assignment 12–7   Medicare Secondary Payer (MSP) [advanced]

Assignment 12–8   Medicare/Medigap

Assignment 12–9   Medicare Railroad, Retiree with Advance Beneficiary Notice [advanced]

Assignment 12–10   Medicare/Medicaid (Medi-Medi)

Additional cases presented on the CD-ROM (Student Software Challenge) are:

Computer Case 8   Medicare

Computer Case 9   Medicare/Medigap

Computer Case 10   Medicare/Medicaid

ASSIGNMENT **12–5 ▸ COMPLETE A CLAIM FORM FOR A MEDICARE CASE**

Performance Objective

Task: Complete a CMS-1500 (08-05) claim form for a Medicare case, post transactions to the financial accounting record, and define patient record abbreviations.

Conditions: Use the patient's medical record (Figure 12–3) and financial statement (Figure 12–4), one health insurance claim form (print from CD or Evolve website), a typewriter or computer, procedural and diagnostic code books, and Appendices A and B in this *Workbook*.

Standards: Claim Productivity Measurement

Time: _____ minutes

Accuracy: _____

(Note: The time element and accuracy criteria may be given by your instructor.)

Directions

1. Complete the CMS-1500 (08-05) claim form, using Office for Civil Rights (OCR) guidelines for a Medicare case. If your instructor wants you to direct it to your local fiscal intermediary, obtain the name and address by going to the Evolve website listed in Internet Resources at the end of Chapter 12 in the *Handbook*. Refer to Elsa M. Mooney's patient record for information. Refer to Appendix A in this *Workbook* to locate the fees to be recorded on the claim and posted to the financial statement. Date the claim December 21. Dr. Cardi is a participating physician who is accepting assignment, and Mrs. Mooney has already met her deductible for the year owing to previous medical expenses with another physician. Use the participating provider Medicare fee.

2. Refer to Chapter 7 (Figure 7–8) of the *Handbook* for instructions on how to complete this claim form and a Medicare template.

3. Use your CPT code book or Appendix A in this *Workbook* to determine the correct five-digit code number and modifiers for each professional service rendered. Use your HCPCS Level II code book or refer to Appendix B in this *Workbook* for HCPCS procedure codes and modifiers.

4. Record all transactions on the financial accounting record and indicate when you have billed Medicare.

5. On January 12, Medicare sent check No. 115620 and paid 80% of the allowed amount for services rendered on December 15, 20xx. Post this amount to the patient's financial account and indicate the balance due from the patient.

6. A Performance Evaluation Checklist may be reproduced from the "Instruction Guide to the Workbook" chapter if your instructor wishes you to submit it to assist with scoring and comments.

After the instructor has returned your work to you, either make the necessary corrections and place your work in a three-ring notebook for future reference or, if you received a high score, place it in your portfolio for reference when applying for a job.

Abbreviations pertinent to this record:

Pt	_____	LC	_____
N	_____	MDM	_____
EKG	_____	adv	_____
STAT	_____	rtn	_____
CPK	_____	ofc	_____
Dx	_____	echo	_____
ASCVD	_____	RTO	_____

Additional Coding and Fee Calculations

1. Refer to Mrs. Mooney's medical record, abstract information, and code procedures that would be billed by outside providers.

Site	Description of Service	Code
a. College Hospital Laboratory	_____	_____
b. College Hospital Physiology	_____	_____
c. College Hospital Physiology	_____	_____
d. College Hospital Radiology	_____	_____

2. Refer to the Mock Fee Schedule shown in Appendix A in this *Workbook* and complete the following questions:

A. If Dr. Cardi is not participating in the Medicare program, what is the maximum (limiting charge) he can bill for the professional services rendered?

Office visit $ _____   ECG $ _____

B. In the case of a nonparticipating physician, how much will Medicare pay for these services? Note: Use the nonparticipating fees as the allowed amount.

Office visit $ _____   ECG $ _____

C. How much is the patient's responsibility for these services?

Office visit $ _____   ECG $ _____

D. How much will the courtesy adjustment be on the patient's financial record?

Office visit $ _____   ECG $ _____

3. Locate a financial accounting record (ledger).

   Note: Refer to the step-by-step procedures at the end of Chapter 3 in the *Handbook* and graphic examples Figures 3–16 and 10–3.

4. Insert the patient's name and address, including ZIP code in the box.

5. Enter the patient's personal data.

6. Ledger lines: Insert date of service (DOS), reference (CPT code number, check number, or dates of service for posting adjustments or when insurance was billed), description of the transaction, charge amounts, payments, adjustments, and running current balance. The posting date is the actual date the transaction is recorded. If the DOS differs from the posting date, list the DOS in the reference or description column.

   Note: A good bookkeeping practice is to take a red pen and draw a line across the financial accounting record (ledger) from left to right to indicate the last entry billed to the insurance company.

PATIENT RECORD NO. 12-5

Mooney	Elsa	M.	02-06-30	F	555-452-4968
LAST NAME	FIRST NAME	MIDDLE NAME	BIRTH DATE	SEX	HOME PHONE

5750 Canyon Road   Woodland Hills   XY   12345
ADDRESS   CITY   STATE   ZIP CODE

555-806-3244   Mooney@wb.net
CELL PHONE   PAGER NO.   FAX NO.   E-MAIL ADDRESS

321-XX-2653   R9865549
PATIENT'S SOC. SEC. NO.   DRIVER'S LICENSE

retired secretary
PATIENT'S OCCUPATION   NAME OF COMPANY

ADDRESS OF EMPLOYER   PHONE

husband deceased
SPOUSE OR PARENT   OCCUPATION

EMPLOYER   ADDRESS   PHONE

Medicare   self
NAME OF INSURANCE   INSURED OR SUBSCRIBER

321-XX-2653A
POLICY/CERTIFICATE NO.   GROUP NO.

REFERRED BY: George Gentle, MD, 1000 N. Main Street, Woodland Hills, XY 12345   NPI# 40213102XX

DATE	PROGRESS NOTES
12-15-xx	New pt referred by Dr. Gentle comes in complaining of chest pain and shortness of
	breath; a detailed history was taken. A detailed examination was essentially N. EKG done
	to rule out myocardial infarction; normal sinus rhythm, no abnormalities noted. Pt sent to
	College Hospital for STAT cardiac enzymes (CPK), 2D echocardiogram
	(transthoracic/real-time with Doppler), and complete chest x-ray.
	Working Dx: angina—ASCVD (LC MDM). Pt adv to rtn to ofc this afternoon for test results.
	PC/llf *Perry Cardi, MD*

Figure 12–3

STATEMENT
Financial Account
COLLEGE CLINIC
4567 Broad Avenue
Woodland Hills, XY 12345-0001
Tel. 555-486-9002
Fax No. 555-487-8976

Acct No. _12-5_

[handwritten: Copy over to Elsa's Form in Ch 12 in Handouts]

Mrs. Elsa M. Mooney
5750 Canyon Road
Woodland Hills, XY 12345-0001

Phone No. (H) _(555) 452-4968_ (W) _____

Birthdate _02-06-30_

Primary Insurance Co. _Medicare_

Policy/Group No. _321-XX-2653A_

REFERENCE		DESCRIPTION	CHARGES	CREDITS		BALANCE
				PYMNTS.	ADJ.	
			BALANCE FORWARD ➤			70 92
12-15-xx	99203	Init OV, D hx/exam, LC decision making	70.92 ~~30 43~~ 33.25 ~~03 25~~		30 43 282	~~30 25~~ 30 43
12-15-xx	9 3000	EKG with interpret & report	34 26			34 26
2-1-xx init OV		Init OV, D hx/exam, LC decision making Medicare payment account adjustment		64 92 30 43	600 282	600 282 —
2-1-xx EKG		EKG with interpret & report Medicare payment account adjustment		31 36	290	290 —

PLEASE PAY LAST AMOUNT IN BALANCE COLUMN ⬆

THIS IS A COPY OF YOUR FINANCIAL ACCOUNT AS IT APPEARS ON OUR RECORDS

Figure 12–4

ASSIGNMENT **12–6** ▸ COMPLETE A CLAIM FORM FOR A
                    MEDICARE/MEDICAID CASE

Performance Objective

Task: Complete a CMS-1500 (08-05) claim form for a Medicare/Medicaid case, post transactions
                     to the financial accounting record, and define patient record abbreviations.

Conditions: Use the patient's medical record (Figure 12–5) and financial statement (Figure 12–6),
                     one health insurance claim form (print from CD or Evolve website), a typewriter or
                     computer, procedural and diagnostic code books, and appendices A and B in this *Workbook*.

Standards: Claim Productivity Measurement

                     Time: _____ minutes

                     Accuracy: _____

                     (Note: The time element and accuracy criteria may be given by your instructor.)

Directions

1. Complete the CMS-1500 (08-05) claim form, using OCR guidelines for a Medicare/Medicaid case. If your
   instructor wants you to direct it to your local Medicare fiscal intermediary, obtain the name and address by
   going to the Evolve website listed in Internet Resources at the end of Chapter 12 in the *Handbook*. Refer to
   Mrs. Helen P. Nolan's patient record for information. Refer to Appendix A in this *Workbook* to locate the fees
   to be recorded on the claim and posted to the financial statement. Date the claim May 31.

2. Refer to Chapter 7 and Figure 7–9 of the *Handbook* for instructions on how to complete the CMS-1500
   (08-05) claim form.

3. Use your CPT code book or Appendix A in this *Workbook* to determine the correct five-digit code number and
   modifiers for each professional service rendered. Use your HCPCS Level II code book or refer to Appendix B in
   this *Workbook* for HCPCS procedure codes and modifiers.

4. Record all transactions on the financial record and indicate the proper information when you have billed
   Medicare/Medicaid. On July 1, you receive a check (number 107621) from Medicare for $600, and on July 15
   you receive a voucher (number 3571) from Medicaid for $200. Record these payments on the account, and show
   a courtesy adjustment to zero the account.

5. A Performance Evaluation Checklist may be reproduced from the "Instruction Guide to the *Workbook*" chapter
   if your instructor wishes you to submit it to assist with scoring and comments.

   After the instructor has returned your work to you, either make the necessary corrections and place your work in
   a three-ring notebook for future reference or, if you received a high score, place it in your portfolio for reference
   when applying for a job.

Abbreviations pertinent to this record:

Pt	_____	phys	_____
hx	_____	prep	_____
BP	_____	hosp	_____
ext	_____	EPF	_____
Dx	_____	exam	_____
int	_____	MC	_____
adv	_____	MDM	_____
pre-op	_____	slt	_____
adm	_____	PF	_____
UA	_____	SF	_____
auto	_____	RTO	_____
FBS	_____	wk	_____
micro	_____	OV	_____
CXR	_____	p.r.n.	_____

Additional Coding and Fee Calculations

1. Refer to Mrs. Nolan's medical record, abstract information, and code procedures that would be billed by outside providers.

Site	*Description of Service*	*Code*
a. College Hospital Laboratory	_____	_____
b. College Hospital Laboratory	_____	_____
c. College Hospital Laboratory	_____	_____
d. College Hospital Radiology	_____	_____

2. Calculate Dr. Cutler's assistant surgeon fee, which is 18.5% of the primary surgeon's fee:

   Hemorrhoidectomy with fistulectomy: $ _____

3. Locate a financial accounting record (ledger).

   Note: Refer to the step-by-step procedures at the end of Chapter 3 in the *Handbook* and graphic examples Figures 3–16 and 10–3.

4. Insert the patient's name and address, including ZIP code in the box.

5. Enter the patient's personal data.

6. Ledger lines: Insert date of service (DOS), reference (CPT code number, check number, or dates of service for posting adjustments or when insurance was billed), description of the transaction, charge amounts, payments, adjustments, and running current balance. The posting date is the actual date the transaction is recorded. If the DOS differs from the posting date, list the DOS in the reference or description column.

Note: A good bookkeeping practice is to take a red pen and draw a line across the financial accounting record (ledger) from left to right to indicate the last entry billed to the insurance company.

PATIENT RECORD NO. 12-6

Nolan	Helen	P.	05-10-37	F	555-660-9878
LAST NAME	FIRST NAME	MIDDLE NAME	BIRTH DATE	SEX	HOME PHONE

2588 Cedar Street	Woodland Hills	XY	12345
ADDRESS	CITY	STATE	ZIP CODE

		555-660-9878		Nolan@wb.net
CELL PHONE	PAGER NO.	FAX NO.		E-MAIL ADDRESS

732-XX-1573	J4022876
PATIENT'S SOC. SEC. NO.	DRIVER'S LICENSE

homemaker	
PATIENT'S OCCUPATION	NAME OF COMPANY

ADDRESS OF EMPLOYER	PHONE

James J. Nolan	retired journalist	07-22-36
SPOUSE OR PARENT	OCCUPATION	BIRTH DATE

EMPLOYER	ADDRESS	PHONE

Medicare/Medicaid	
NAME OF INSURANCE	INSURED OR SUBSCRIBER

732-XX-1573B	19-60-2358490-1-XX
MEDICARE NO.	MEDICAID NO.

REFERRED BY: James B. Jeffers, MD, 100 S. Broadway, Woodland Hills, XY 12345   NPI# 12345069XX

DATE	PROGRESS NOTES
5-1-xx	New pt comes in complaining of constipation, rectal bleeding, and rectal pain. Detailed
	hx taken, BP 120/80. A detailed exam revealed ext hemorrhoids. Diagnostic proctoscopy
	done to further evaluate the hemorrhoids and control bleeding using bipolar cautery.
	Dx: int & ext bleeding hemorrhoids and anorectal fistula. Adv hospitalization for removal
	of hemorrhoids and fistula repair.
	RR/llf *Rex Rumsey, MD*
5-8-xx	Pre-op testing done prior to adm to College Hospital (UA auto/with micro., hemogram
	auto, FBS quantitative, CXR single frontal view). Admit, phys exam & prep of hospital
	records. Hemorrhoidectomy with fistulectomy performed (authorization no. 7699220012).
	Dr. Clarence Cutler assisted.
	RR/llf *Rex Rumsey, MD*
5-9-xx	Hosp visit (EPF hx/exam MC MDM). Pt comfortable, slt pain.
	RR/llf *Rex Rumsey, MD*
5-10-xx	Hosp visit (PF hx/exam SF MDM). No pain.
	RR/llf *Rex Rumsey, MD*
5-11-xx	Discharged pt to home. RTO in 1 wk.
	RR/llf *Rex Rumsey, MD*
5-17-xx	OV (PF hx/exam SF MDM). Pt doing well, surgical site healed. Return p.r.n.
	RR/llf *Rex Rumsey, MD*

Figure 12–5

STATEMENT
Financial Account
COLLEGE CLINIC
4567 Broad Avenue
Woodland Hills, XY 12345-0001
Tel. 555-486-9002
Fax No. 555-487-8976

Acct. No. 12-6

Helen P. Nolan
2588 Cedar Street
Woodland Hills, XY 12345

Phone No. (H)   (555) 660-9878   (W) _____   Birthdate   05-10-37

Primary Insurance Co.   Medicare/Medicaid   Policy/Group No. 732-XX-1573B

| | REFERENCE | DESCRIPTION | CHARGES | CREDITS | | BALANCE |
				PYMNTS.	ADJ.	
20XX			BALANCE FORWARD ➡			
05-01-xx		NP OV				
05-01-xx		Proctoscopy				
05-08-xx		Hemorrhoidectomy with fistulectomy				
05-09-xx		HV				
05-10-xx		HV				
05-11-xx		Discharge				
05-17-xx		OV				

PLEASE PAY LAST AMOUNT IN BALANCE COLUMN ⬆

THIS IS A COPY OF YOUR FINANCIAL ACCOUNT AS IT APPEARS ON OUR RECORDS

Figure 12–6

ASSIGNMENT 12–7 ▸ COMPLETE A CLAIM FORM FOR A MEDICARE/SECONDARY PAYER CASE

Performance Objective

Task: Complete a CMS-1500 (08-05) claim form, for an MSP case, post transactions to the financial accounting record, and define patient record abbreviations.

Conditions: Use the patient's medical record (Figure 12–7) and financial statement (Figure 12–8), one health insurance claim form (print from CD or Evolve website), a typewriter or computer, procedural and diagnostic code books, and appendices A and B in this *Workbook*.

Standards: Claim Productivity Measurement

Time: _____ minutes

Accuracy: _____

(Note: The time element and accuracy criteria may be given by your instructor.)

Directions

1. Complete the CMS-1500 (08-05) claim form, using OCR guidelines for an MSP case, and direct it to the primary insurance carrier. This assignment requires two claim forms, so make a photocopy of the CMS-1500 (08-05) claim form for the second claim. Refer to Peter F. Donlon's patient record for information. Refer to Appendix A in this *Workbook* to locate the fees to be recorded on the claim and posted to the financial statement. Date the claim May 14. Dr. Antrum is not accepting assignment in this case. For a nonparticipating physician, use the limiting charge column of the mock fee schedule. This should also be considered the allowed amount.

2. See Chapter 7 (Figure 7–10) of the *Handbook* for help in completing these forms.

3. Use your CPT code book or Appendix A in this *Workbook* to determine the correct five-digit code number and modifiers for each professional service rendered. Refer to your HCPCS Level II code book or Appendix B in this *Workbook* for HCPCS procedure codes and modifiers.

4. Record all transactions on the financial record and indicate when you have billed the primary insurance carrier.

5. On June 5, Coastal Health Insurance Company paid $800 (check number 45632) on this claim. Post this payment to the patient's financial account and indicate the balance that will be billed to Medicare the following day. Note: The explanation of benefits from Coastal Health would be sent to Medicare with a completed CMS-1500 (08-05) claim form.

6. A Performance Evaluation Checklist may be reproduced from the "Instruction Guide to the *Workbook*" chapter if your instructor wishes you to submit it to assist with scoring and comments.

After the instructor has returned your work to you, either make the necessary corrections and place your work in a three-ring notebook for future reference or, if you received a high score, place it in your portfolio for reference when applying for a job.

Abbreviations pertinent to this record:

ER	_____	&	_____
p.m.	_____	adm	_____
EPF	_____	MC	_____
hx	_____	imp	_____
exam	_____	PF	_____
LC	_____	SF	_____
MDM	_____	hosp	_____
est	_____	RTO	_____
pts	_____	OV	_____
cm	_____	surg	_____
consult	_____	sched	_____
c̄	_____	ofc	_____
D	_____	post-op	_____
C	_____	wk	_____
M	_____		
MRI	_____		
px	_____		

Additional Coding and Fee Calculations

1. Refer to Mr. Donlon's medical record, abstract information, and code procedures that would be billed by outside providers.

Site	Description of Service	Code
a. Emergency room (ER) physician	_____	_____
b. ER consult	_____	_____
c. College Hospital Radiology	_____	_____
d. College Hospital Radiology	_____	_____

2. Use your diagnostic code book and code the symptoms that the patient presented with in the ER

     Symptom   *Code*

 a. _____   _____

 b. _____   _____

 c. _____   _____

3. On the septoplasty surgery (May 10, 20xx), assume that Coastal Health Insurance Company paid $459.74.

 a. What would the Medicare payment be? _____

 b. What would the patient responsibility be? _____

 c. What would the courtesy adjustment be? _____

4. Locate a financial accounting record (ledger).

 Note: Refer to the step-by-step procedures at the end of Chapter 3 in the *Handbook* and graphic examples Figures 3–16 and 10–3.

5. Insert the patient's name and address, including ZIP code in the box.

6. Enter the patient's personal data.

7. Ledger lines: Insert date of service (DOS), reference (CPT code number, check number, or dates of service for posting adjustments or when insurance was billed), description of the transaction, charge amounts, payments, adjustments, and running current balance. The posting date is the actual date the transaction is recorded. If the DOS differs from the posting date, list the DOS in the reference or description column.

 Note: A good bookkeeping practice is to take a red pen and draw a line across the financial accounting record (ledger) from left to right to indicate the last entry billed to the insurance company.

PATIENT RECORD NO. 12-7

Donlon	Peter	F	08-09-38	M	555-762-3580
LAST NAME	FIRST NAME	MIDDLE NAME	BIRTH DATE	SEX	HOME PHONE

1840 East Chevy Chase Drive	Woodland Hills	XY	12345
ADDRESS	CITY	STATE	ZIP CODE

CELL PHONE	PAGER NO.	FAX NO.	E-MAIL ADDRESS

987-XX-4321	Y2100968
PATIENT'S SOC. SEC. NO.	DRIVER'S LICENSE

chef	Harbor Town Eatery
PATIENT'S OCCUPATION	NAME OF COMPANY

1116 Harbor Way, Woodland Hills, XY 12345	555-762-0050
ADDRESS OF EMPLOYER	PHONE

wife deceased	
SPOUSE OR PARENT	OCCUPATION

Coastal Health Insurance Co., 10 N. Main Street, Woodland Hills, XY 12345	555-369-4401
NAME OF PRIMARY INSURANCE ADDRESS	PHONE

NAME OF INSURANCE	INSURED OR SUBSCRIBER

34276	45A
POLICY/CERTIFICATE NO.	GROUP NO.
Medicare	987-XX-4321A
NAME OF SECONDARY INSURANCE	MEDICARE NO.

REFERRED BY:

DATE	PROGRESS NOTES
5-1-xx	Called to ER on Sunday, 11 p.m. ER physician, Dr. Rene Whitney (NPI # 77 536222XX) performed an EPF hx/exam
	with LC MDM on one of my est pts who was injured at home while walking across lawn pushing garbage can;
	tripped and hit his head on curb. Pt complains of acute headache, nausea, and nasal pain caused by impact and skin
	laceration. Sutured a 2.0 cm simple laceration of nose. Pt vomited twice in ER. Requested ER consult c̄ neurologist,
	Dr. Parkinson (C hx/exam M MDM), who ordered MRI of brain (without contrast) and complete skull series. I performed
	a C hx and px & adm pt to College Hospital; MDM MC. Imp: Concussion without skull fracture, no loss of
	consciousness; nasal laceration; deviated septum which may need reconstruction. Disability from work from 5-1 to 5-17
	CA/llf *Concha Antrum, MD*
5-2-xx	Hospital visit (PF hx/exam LC MDM).
	CA/llf *Concha Antrum, MD*
5-3-xx	Hospital visit (PF hx/exam SF MDM).
	CA/llf *Concha Antrum, MD*
5-4-xx	Discharge from hospital. See hosp records for daily notes. RTO in 2 day for suture removal.
	CA/llf *Concha Antrum, MD*
5-6-xx	OV. Sutures removed; wound healed. Discussed deviated septum and recommended septoplasty. Surg sched for
	5/10/xx at College Hospital.
	CA/llf *Concha Antrum, MD*
5-10-xx	Adm to College Hospital (D hx/exam LC MDM). Performed septoplasty. Pt doing well; moved to recovery room.
	CA/llf *Concha Antrum, MD*
5-11-xx	Pt doing well, no hemorrhage, discharged home.
	CA/llf *Concha Antrum, MD*
5-12-xx	Pt comes into ofc with postop anterior nasal hemorrhage. Cauterized rt side. RTO in 1 wk.
	CA/llf *Concha Antrum, MD*

Figure 12–7

STATEMENT
Financial Account
COLLEGE CLINIC
4567 Broad Avenue
Woodland Hills, XY 12345-0001
Tel. 555-486-9002
Fax No. 555-487-8976

Acct. No. __12-7__

Peter F. Donlon
1840 East Chevy Chase Drive
Woodland Hills, XY 12345

Phone No. (H) ___(555) 762-3580___   (W) ___(555)762-0050___

Birthdate ___08-09-38___

Insurance Co. ___Coastal Health Insurance Co./Medicare___

Policy/Group No. ___34276 Grp. 45A___
Medicare No. ___987-XX-4321A___

	REFERENCE	DESCRIPTION	CHARGES	CREDITS PYMNTS.	ADJ.	BALANCE
20XX			BALANCE FORWARD →			
05-01-xx		Initial hospital care				
05-01-xx		Skin repair				
05-02-xx		HV				
05-03-xx		HV				
05-04-xx		Discharge				
05-06-xx		Suture removal				
05-10-xx		Admit-Septoplasty				
05-11-xx		Discharge				
05-12-xx		Postop OV				

PLEASE PAY LAST AMOUNT IN BALANCE COLUMN ⬆

THIS IS A COPY OF YOUR FINANCIAL ACCOUNT AS IT APPEARS ON OUR RECORDS

Figure 12–8

ASSIGNMENT 12-8 ▸ COMPLETE A CLAIM FOR A MEDICARE/MEDIGAP CASE

Performance Objective

Task: Complete a CMS-1500 (08-05) claim form for a Medicare/Medigap case, post transactions to the financial accounting record, and define patient record abbreviations.

Conditions: Use the patient's medical record (Figure 12–9) and financial statement (Figure 12–10), one health insurance claim form (print from CD or Evolve website), a typewriter or computer, procedural and diagnostic code books, and appendices A and B in this *Workbook*.

Standards: Claim Productivity Measurement

Time: _____ minutes

Accuracy: _____

(Note: The time element and accuracy criteria may be given by your instructor.)

Directions

1. Complete the CMS-1500 (08-05) claim form, using Medicare/Medigap OCR guidelines. If your instructor wants you to direct it to your local fiscal intermediary, obtain the name and address by going to the Evolve website listed in Internet Resources at the end of Chapter 12 in the *Handbook*. This case involves a patient who has a Medigap supplemental policy that is secondary payer. Refer to Jeremiah W. Diffenderffer's patient record and financial statement for information. See Medicare participating provider fees in Appendix A in this *Workbook* to locate the fees to be recorded on the claim and posted to the financial statement. Date the claim June 13. Dr. Coccidioides is accepting assignment in this case. Mr. Diffenderffer has met his deductible for the year, owing to previous care by Dr. Coccidioides.

2. Refer to Chapter 7 and Figure 7–10 of the *Handbook* for instructions on how to complete the CMS-1500 (08-05) claim form.

3. Use your CPT code book or Appendix A in this *Workbook* to determine the correct five-digit code number and modifiers for each professional service rendered. Refer to your HCPCS Level II code book or Appendix B in this *Workbook* for HCPCS procedure codes and modifiers.

4. Record all transactions on the financial record, and indicate the proper information when you have billed Medicare and Medigap.

5. On August 3, Medicare check number 654821 was received in the amount of $270.05, paying 80% of the allowable amount for all services except the medication charge, of which they allowed $10. Post this payment to the patient's financial account, and calculate and post the courtesy adjustment. On August 15, United American Insurance Company check number 3254 was received in the amount of $67.51, paying 20% of the allowable amount for all services, including the $10 allowed amount determined by Medicare for the medication. Post this payment to the patient's financial statement, and indicate the balance due from the patient.

6. A Performance Evaluation Checklist may be reproduced from the "Instruction Guide to the *Workbook*" chapter if your instructor wishes to submit it to assist with scoring and comments.

After the instructor has returned your work to you, either make the necessary corrections and place your work in a three-ring notebook for future reference or, if you received a high score, place it in your portfolio for reference when applying for a job.

Abbreviations pertinent to this record:

Est	_____	hx	_____
oft	_____	exam	_____
p.m.	_____	HC	_____
SOB	_____	MDM	_____
adv	_____	imp	_____
AP	_____	RTO	_____
lat	_____	wk	_____
tech	_____	c/o	_____
CXR	_____	HCN	_____
ABG	_____	PF	_____
PFT	_____	SF	_____
a.m.	_____	IV	_____
RTO	_____	ml	_____
CPX	_____	appt	_____
C	_____		

Additional Coding

1. Refer to Mr. Diffenderffer's medical record, abstract information, and code procedures that would be billed by outside providers.

Site	Description of Service	Code
a. College Hospital Laboratory	_____	_____
b. College Hospital Respiratory Department	_____	_____

2. Locate a financial accounting record (ledger).

   Note: Refer to the step-by-step procedures at the end of Chapter 3 in the *Handbook* and graphic examples Figures 3–16 and 10–3.

3. Insert the patient's name and address, including ZIP code in the box.

4. Enter the patient's personal data.

5. Ledger lines: Insert date of service (DOS), reference (CPT code number, check number, or dates of service for posting adjustments or when insurance was billed), description of the transaction, charge amounts, payments, adjustments, and running current balance. The posting date is the actual date the transaction is recorded. If the DOS differs from the posting date, list the DOS in the reference or description column.

Note: A good bookkeeping practice is to take a red pen and draw a line across the financial accounting record (ledger) from left to right to indicate the last entry billed to the insurance company.

PATIENT RECORD NO. 12-8

Diffenderffer	Jeremiah	W	08-24-31	M	555-471 9930
LAST NAME	FIRST NAME	MIDDLE NAME	BIRTH DATE	SEX	HOME PHONE

120 Elm Street	Woodland Hills	XY	12345	
ADDRESS	CITY	STATE	ZIP CODE	

555-218-0087		555-471-9930		Diffenderffer@wb.net
CELL PHONE	PAGER NO.	FAX NO.		E-MAIL ADDRESS

731-XX-7401	none
PATIENT'S SOC. SEC. NO.	DRIVER'S LICENSE

retired painter	
PATIENT'S OCCUPATION	NAME OF COMPANY

ADDRESS OF EMPLOYER	PHONE

deceased	
SPOUSE OR PARENT	OCCUPATION

Medicare	731-XX-7401T
NAME OF INSURANCE	MEDICARE NO

United American Insurance Company, P.O. Box 810, Dallas, TX 75221	555-328-2841
NAME OF OTHER INSURANCE	ADDRESS	PHONE

007559715	UNITXY003
POLICY/CERTIFICATE NO.	PAYERID NO.

REFERRED BY: John M. Diffenderffer (brother)

DATE	PROGRESS NOTES
6-1-xx	Est pt telephoned ofc this p.m. stating he has been involved in a long painting project in
	his home and when he breathed paint fumes in his kitchen today he experienced
	SOB & coughing. Dr. Coccidioides is out of the ofc this p.m. and was paged. Physician
	adv pt to come into ofc for AP & lat chest x-ray and bilateral bronchogram this afternoon.
	Chest x-ray and bronchogram taken by x-ray tech.
	RH/llf *Rene Holmes, CMA*
6-2-xx	CXR and bronchogram showed pulmonary emphysema. Adv pt by phone to have ABG for
	direct O_2 saturation and PFT (spirometry) at College Hospital this a.m. and RTO for CPX
	this afternoon.
	BC/llf *Brady Coccidioides, MD*
6-2-xx	Pt returns for C hx/exam HC MDM. Imp: emphysema, bronchitis and pneumonitis due to
	inhalation of fumes and vapors. Adv no more painting; bed rest. RTO 1 wk.
	BC/llf *Brady Coccidioides, MD*
6-5-xx	Pt calls as ofc is closing c/o difficulty breathing; he has been ambulating and climbing
	stairs. HCN PF hx/exam SF MDM. Administered Coramine (nikethamide) medication IV
	(unclassified drug, 1.5 ml two ampules @ 12.50 each). Imp: recurrent bronchitis and pneumonitis,
	exertional dyspnea. Adv complete bed rest. RTO for appt on 6-9-xx.
	BC/llf *Brady Coccidioides, MD*

Figure 12–9

STATEMENT
Financial Account
COLLEGE CLINIC
4567 Broad Avenue
Woodland Hills, XY 12345-0001
Tel. 555-486-9002
Fax No. 555-487-8976

Acct. No. 12-8

Jeremiah W. Diffenderffer
120 Elm Street
Woodland Hills, XY 12345

Phone No. (H)   (555) 471-9930   (W) _____

Birthdate   08-24-31

Insurance Co.   Medicare/United American Insurance Co.

Policy/Group No.   007559715
Medicare No.   731-XX-7401T

| | REFERENCE | DESCRIPTION | CHARGES | CREDITS | | BALANCE | |
				PYMNTS.	ADJ.		
20XX			BALANCE FORWARD ➔			20	00
06-01-xx		Chest x-ray					
06-01-xx		Bronchogram					
06-02-xx		OV					
06-05-xx		HC					
06-05-xx		IV administration					
06-05-xx		Medication					

PLEASE PAY LAST AMOUNT IN BALANCE COLUMN

THIS IS A COPY OF YOUR FINANCIAL ACCOUNT AS IT APPEARS ON OUR RECORDS

Figure 12–10

ASSIGNMENT 12–9 ▸ COMPLETE A CLAIM FORM FOR A MEDICARE CASE
WITH AN ADVANCE BENEFICIARY NOTICE

Performance Objective

Task: Complete a CMS-1500 (08-05) claim form for a Medicare case and an advance beneficiary
                     notice, post transactions to the financial accounting record, and define patient record
                     abbreviations.

Conditions: Use the patient's record (Figure 12–11) and financial statement (Figure 12–12), an advance
                     beneficiary notice form (Figure 12–13), two health insurance claim forms (print from CD or
                     Evolve website), a typewriter or computer, procedural and diagnostic code books, and
                     appendices A and B in this *Workbook*.

Standards: Claim Productivity Measurement

                     Time: _____ minutes

                     Accuracy: _____

                     (Note: The time element and accuracy criteria may be given by your instructor.)

Directions

1. Complete a CMS-1500 (08-05) claim form for a Medicare case, using OCR guidelines. If your instructor wants
   you to direct it to your local Medicare Railroad fiscal intermediary, obtain the name and address by going to the
   Evolve website listed in Internet Resources at the end of Chapter 12 in the *Handbook*. This assignment requires
   two claim forms, so make a photocopy for the second claim. Refer to Raymond D. Fay's patient record for
   information. Refer to Appendix A in this *Workbook* to locate the fees to be recorded on the claim and posted
   to the financial statement. Date the claim December 31. Dr. Antrum is a participating physician and is
   accepting assignment in this case.

2. Refer to Figure 7–8 in the *Handbook* for instructions on how to complete the CMS-1500 (08-05) claim form.

3. The nystagmus service is disallowed by Medicare, and an advance beneficiary notice needs to be completed.
   Refer to Figure 12–10 in the *Handbook* for a completed example of this form. Note: When a noncovered service
   is provided, a fee will not be listed in the Medicare fee schedule; therefore, list the regular (mock) fee.

4. Use your CPT code book or Appendix A in this *Workbook* to determine the correct five-digit code number and
   modifiers for each professional service rendered. Use your HCPCS Level II code book or refer to Appendix B in
   this *Workbook* for HCPCS procedure codes and modifiers. The patient has met $71 of the $131 deductible.

5. Record all transactions on the financial accounting record, and indicate the proper information when you have
   billed Medicare.

6. A Performance Evaluation Checklist may be reproduced from the "Instruction Guide to the *Workbook*" chapter
   if your instructor wishes you to submit it to assist with scoring and comments.

   After the instructor has returned your work to you, either make the necessary corrections and place your work in
a three-ring notebook for future reference or, if you received a high score, place it in your portfolio for reference
when applying for a job.

Abbreviations pertinent to this record:

Pt	_____	RTO	_____
D	_____	rtn	_____
hx	_____	OV	_____
exam	_____	appt(s)	_____
retn	_____	wk	_____
R/O	_____	inj.	_____
LC	_____	Dx	_____
MDM	_____	PF	_____
N	_____	SF	_____
X	_____	sx	_____
incl	_____	disc	_____

Additional Fee Calculations

1. Medicare sent payment on this claim, allowing 80% of the amount after the partial deductible was met, which was subtracted from the amount of this claim. Medicare denied payment on code 92531 as a noncovered service.

   a. What is the amount of the Medicare check?   _____

   b. What is the amount of the patient responsibility?   _____

   c. Is there a courtesy adjustment?   _____

2. Locate a financial accounting record (ledger).

   Note: Refer to the step-by-step procedures at the end of Chapter 3 in the *Handbook* and graphic examples Figures 3–16 and 10–3.

3. Insert the patient's name and address, including ZIP code in the box.

4. Enter the patient's personal data.

5. Ledger lines: Insert date of service (DOS), reference (CPT code number, check number, or dates of service for posting adjustments or when insurance was billed), description of the transaction, charge amounts, payments, adjustments, and running current balance. The posting date is the actual date the transaction is recorded. If the DOS differs from the posting date, list the DOS in the reference or description column.

   Note: A good bookkeeping practice is to take a red pen and draw a line across the financial accounting record (ledger) from left to right to indicate the last entry billed to the insurance company.

PATIENT RECORD NO. 12-9

Fay	Raymond		02-03-32	M	555-788-9090
LAST NAME	FIRST NAME	MIDDLE NAME	BIRTH DATE	SEX	HOME PHONE

33 North Pencil Avenue	Woodland Hills	XY	12345	
ADDRESS	CITY	STATE	ZIP CODE	

	555-250-4890	555-788-9090		fay@wb.net
CELL PHONE	PAGER NO.	FAX NO.		E-MAIL ADDRESS

887-66-1235	R8966543
PATIENT'S SOC. SEC. NO.	DRIVER'S LICENSE

retired railroad engineer	
PATIENT'S OCCUPATION	NAME OF COMPANY

ADDRESS OF EMPLOYER	PHONE

Marilyn B. Fay	homemaker
SPOUSE OR PARENT	OCCUPATION

EMPLOYER	ADDRESS	PHONE

Medicare Railroad	self
NAME OF INSURANCE	INSURED OR SUB SCRIBER

A 887-XX-1235A
MEDICARE NO.

REFERRED BY: George Gentle, MD, 1000 N. Main St., Woodland Hills, XY 12345   NPI# 402131102XX

DATE	PROGRESS NOTES
10-31-xx	New pt presents, a D hx was taken. Pt complains of skin rash and dizziness for 3 days.
	A detailed exam reveals rash on chest and arms. Retn in 4 days for tests to R/O eye/ear
	causes for dizziness and food allergies (LC MDM).
	CA/llf *Concha Antrum, MD*
11-4-xx	Comprehensive audiometric threshold evaluation (with speech)—N. 10 intradermal
	allergy tests; delayed reaction. Bilateral mastoid X (complete)—N. Spontaneous nystagmus
	test, incl. gaze—N. RTO in 3 days for skin test results.
	CA/llf *Concha Antrum, MD*
11-7-xx	Rtn OV for allergy skin test results—positive for 3 substances. Pt to purchase allergen
	extract and make sequential appts next wk for daily immunotherapy inj. Dx: food allergies.
	CA/llf *Concha Antrum, MD*
11-14-xx thru	Immunotherapy; 3 inj. per/day
11-18-xx	CA/llf *Concha Antrum, MD*
11-21-xx thru	Immunotherapy; 3 inj. per/day
11-25-xx	CA/llf *Concha Antrum, MD*
11-28-xx thru	Immunotherapy; 3 inj. per/day
12-2-xx	CA/llf *Concha Antrum, MD*
12-5-xx thru	Immunotherapy; 3 inj. per/day
12-8-xx	CA/llf *Concha Antrum, MD*
12-9-xx	OV (PF hx/exam SF MDM) Pt. sx improved. Received final inj and evaluated for disch.
	CA/llf *Concha Antrum, MD*

Figure 12–11

Acct No. 12-9

STATEMENT
Financial Account
COLLEGE CLINIC
4567 Broad Avenue
Woodland Hills, XY 12345-0001
Tel. 555-486-9002
Fax No. 555-487-8976

Raymond Fay
33 North Pencil Avenue
Woodland Hills, XY 12345

Phone No. (H) _____(555) 788-9090_____ (W) _____ Birthdate 02-03-32 _____

Primary Insurance Co. ___Medicare Railroad_____ Policy/Group No. A 887-XX 1235A ____

Secondary Insurance Co. _____N/A_____ Policy/Group No. _____

| DATE | REF-ERENCE | DESCRIPTION | CHARGES | CREDITS | | BALANCE |
				PYMNTS.	ADJ.	
20xx				BALANCE FORWARD →		
10-31-xx		OV				
11-4-xx		Audiometry evaluation				
11-4-xx		Intradermal allergy tests				
11-4-xx		Bilateral mastoid x-rays				
11-4-xx		Spontaneous nystagmus test				
11-7-xx		Allergy test results				
11-14 to 11-18-xx		Immunotherapy inj. (3/day X 5)				
11-21 to 11-25-xx		Immunotherapy inj. (3/day X 5)				
11-28 to 12-2-xx		Immunotherapy inj. (3/day X 5)				
12-5 to 12-9-xx		Immunotherapy inj. (3/day X 5)				
12-9-xx		OV				

PLEASE PAY LAST AMOUNT IN BALANCE COLUMN ⇧

THIS IS A COPY OF YOUR FINANCIAL ACCOUNT AS IT APPEARS ON OUR RECORDS

Figure 12–12

College Clinic
4567 Broad Avenue
Woodland Hills, XY 12345-0001

Patient's Name: _____   Medicare # (HICN): _____

ADVANCE BENEFICIARY NOTICE (ABN)

NOTE: You need to make a choice about receiving these health care items or services.

We expect that Medicare will not pay for the item(s) or service(s) that are described below. Medicare does not pay for all of your health care costs. Medicare only pays for covered items and services when Medicare rules are met. The fact that Medicare may not pay for a particular item or service does not mean that you should not receive it. There may be a good reason your doctor recommended it. Right now, in your case, **Medicare probably will not pay for –**

Items or Services:	init OV, D hx/exam LC decision making EKG ~~with interpret & report~~
Because:	new pt referred by Dr Gentle came in with complaints of chest pain + shortness of breath

The purpose of this form is to help you make an informed choice about whether or not you want to receive these items or services, knowing that you might have to pay for them yourself. Before you make a decision about your options, you should **read this entire notice carefully.**
• Ask us to explain, if you don't understand why Medicare probably won't pay.
• Ask us how much these items or services will cost you **(Estimated cost: $ _105.18_**), in case you have to pay for them yourself or through other insurance.

PLEASE CHOOSE ONE OPTION. CHECK ONE BOX. SIGN & DATE YOUR CHOICE.

☑ **Option 1. YES. I want to receive these items or services.**

I understand that Medicare will not decide whether to pay unless I receive these items or services. Please submit my claim to Medicare. I understand that you may bill me for items or services and that I may have to pay the bill while Medicare is making its decision. If Medicare does pay, you will refund to me any payments I made to you that are due to me. If Medicare denies payment, I agree to be personally and fully responsible for payment. That is, I will pay personally, either out of pocket or through any other insurance that I have. I understand I can appeal Medicare's decision.

☐ **Option 2. NO. I have decided not to receive these items or services.**

I will not receive these items or services. I understand that you will not be able to submit a claim to Medicare and that I will not be able to appeal your opinion that Medicare won't pay.

_12-15- xx_ _____   _Elsa Mooney_ _____
Date   **Signature of patient or person acting on patient's behalf**

NOTE: Your health information will be kept confidential. Any information that we collect about you on this form will be kept confidential in our offices. If a claim is submitted to Medicare, your health information on this form may be shared with Medicare. Your health information which Medicare sees will be kept confidential by Medicare.

OMB Approval No. 0938-0566   Form No. CMS-R-131-G   (June 2002)

Figure 12–13

ASSIGNMENT 12–10 ▸ COMPLETE A CLAIM FORM FOR A
MEDICARE/MEDICAID CASE

Performance Objective

Task: Complete a CMS-1500 (08-05) claim form for a Medicare/Medicaid case, post transactions to
                     the financial accounting record, and define patient record abbreviations.

Conditions: Use the patient's medical record (Figure 12–14) and financial statement (Figure 12–15), one
                     health insurance claim form (print from CD or Evolve website), a typewriter or computer,
                     procedural and diagnostic code books, and appendices A and B in this *Workbook.*

Standards: Claim Productivity Measurement

                     Time: _____ minutes

                     Accuracy: _____

                     (Note: The time element and accuracy criteria may be given by your instructor.)

Directions

1. Complete the CMS-1500 (08-05) claim form, using OCR guidelines for a Medicare/Medicaid case. If your
   instructor wants you to direct it to your local Medicare fiscal intermediary, obtain the name and address by
   going to the Evolve website listed in Internet Resources at the end of Chapter 12 in the *Handbook.* Refer to
   Mr. Harris Fremont's patient record for information. Refer to Appendix A in this *Workbook* to locate the fees
   to be recorded on the claim and posted to the financial statement. Date the claim October 31.

2. Refer to Chapter 7 and Figure 7–9 of the *Handbook* for instructions on how to complete the CMS-1500 (08-05)
   claim form.

3. Use your CPT code book or Appendix A in this *Workbook* to determine the correct five-digit code number and
   modifiers for each professional service rendered. Use your HCPCS Level II code book or refer to Appendix B
   in this *Workbook* for HCPCS procedure codes and modifiers.

4. Record all transactions on the financial account and indicate the proper information when you have billed
   Medicare/Medicaid.

5. On December 12, Medicare paid $125 (check number 281362) on this claim. Post this payment to the patient's
   financial account. On December 29, you receive a voucher number 7234 from Medicaid for $45. Post this
   payment to the patient's financial account and show the courtesy adjustment.

6. A Performance Evaluation Checklist may be reproduced from the "Instruction Guide to the *Workbook*" chapter
   if your instructor wishes you to submit it to assist with scoring and comments.

   After the instructor has returned your work to you, either make the necessary corrections and place your work in
a three-ring notebook for future reference or, if you received a high score, place it in your portfolio for reference
when applying for a job.

Abbreviations pertinent to this record:

NP	_____	pt	_____
c/o	_____	lab	_____
hx	_____	CBC	_____
R	_____	auto	_____
L	_____	diff	_____
N	_____	ESR	_____
Rx	_____	R/O	_____
adv	_____	PF	_____
rtn	_____	SF	_____
LC	_____	prn	_____
MDM	_____	imp	_____

Additional Coding

1. Refer to Mr. Fremont's medical record, abstract information, and code procedures that would be billed by outside providers.

Site	Description of Service	Code
a. ABC Laboratory	_____	_____
b. ABC Laboratory	_____	_____
c. ABC Laboratory	_____	_____
d. ABC Laboratory	_____	_____

2. Use your diagnostic code book and code the symptoms of which the patient complained.

Symptom	Code
a. _____	_____
b. _____	_____

3. Locate a financial accounting record (ledger).

Note: Refer to the step-by-step procedures at the end of Chapter 3 in the *Handbook* and graphic examples Figures 3–16 and 10–3.

4. Insert the patient's name and address, including ZIP code in the box.

5. Enter the patient's personal data.

6. Ledger lines: Insert date of service (DOS), reference (CPT code number, check number, or dates of service for posting adjustments or when insurance was billed), description of the transaction, charge amounts, payments, adjustments, and running current balance. The posting date is the actual date the transaction is recorded. If the DOS differs from the posting date, list the DOS in the reference or description column.

   Note: A good bookkeeping practice is to take a red pen and draw a line across the financial accounting record (ledger) from left to right to indicate the last entry billed to the insurance company.

PATIENT RECORD NO. 12-10

Fremont	Harris		07-10-23	M	555-899-0109
LAST NAME	FIRST NAME	MIDDLE NAME	BIRTH DATE	SEX	HOME PHONE

735 North Center Street	Woodland Hills,	XY	12345	
ADDRESS	CITY	STATE	ZIP CODE	

CELL PHONE	PAGER NO.	FAX NO.		E-MAIL ADDRESS

454-XX-9569	none	
PATIENT'S SOC. SEC. NO.	DRIVER'S LICENSE	

retired baseball coach	
PATIENT'S OCCUPATION	NAME OF COMPANY

ADDRESS OF EMPLOYER	PHONE

Emily B. Fremont	homemaker
SPOUSE OR PARENT	OCCUPATION

EMPLOYER	ADDRESS	PHONE

Medicare/Medicaid	
NAME OF INSURANCE	INSURED OR SUBSCRIBER

454-XX-9569A	56-10-0020205-0-XX
MEDICARE NO.	MEDICAID NO.

REFERRED BY: Raymond Skeleton, MD

DATE	PROGRESS NOTES
10-2-xx	NP referred by Dr. Skeleton. He comes in c/o discomfort around toes of both feet and
	has difficulty walking. Pt states he dropped shelf on feet about a month ago. A detailed
	hx reveals gout and mycotic nails. X-ray R and L feet (2 views) N. Detailed exam reveals
	bilateral mycotic nails & ingrown nail on great R toe. Rx: Electrically débride and trimmed
	overgrowth of all nails and adv to rtn if pain continues in great R toe (LC MDM). Gave pt
	order to have lab work done at ABC Laboratory (CBC w/auto diff., ESR (automated), uric acid level)
	R/O gout. Imp: Mycotic nails; difficulty walking.
	NP/llf *Nick Pedro, DPM*
10-18-xx	Pt returns c/o ingrown nail on R great toe (PF hx/exam SF MDM). Lab work done on
	10/2/xx showed no signs of gout. Performed wedge excision of skin/nail fold.
	Rtn prn. Imp: Ingrown nail – great R toe; toe pain.
	NP/llf *Nick Pedro, DPM*

Figure 12–14

Acct No. 12-10

STATEMENT
Financial Account
COLLEGE CLINIC
4567 Broad Avenue
Woodland Hills, XY 12345-0001
Tel. 555-486-9002
Fax No. 555-487-8976

Harris Fremont
735 North Center Street
Woodland Hills, XY 12345

Phone No. (H)____555-899-0109____(W)_____   Birthdate____7/10/23_____

Primary Insurance Co.__Medicare_____   Policy/Group No.__454XX9569A__

Secondary Insurance Co.__Medicaid_____   Policy/Group No.__561000202050XX__

DATE	REF-ERENCE	DESCRIPTION	CHARGES	CREDITS		BALANCE
				PYMNTS.	ADJ.	
20xx		BALANCE FORWARD ➡				
10-2-xx		NP OV				
10-2-xx		X-rays R/L feet				
10-2-xx		Débridement nails				
10-18-xx		OV				
10-18-xx		Wedge excision R. great toe				

PLEASE PAY LAST AMOUNT IN BALANCE COLUMN ⬆

THIS IS A COPY OF YOUR FINANCIAL ACCOUNT AS IT APPEARS ON OUR RECORDS

Figure 12–15

ALTAPOINT PRACTICE MANAGEMENT
SOFTWARE ASSIGNMENTS

ASSIGNMENT 12–11 ▸ ENTER TRANSACTIONS FROM AN ENCOUNTER
FORM (SUPERBILL) INTO THE PRACTICE
MANAGEMENT SYSTEM AND TRANSMIT AN
INSURANCE CLAIM ELECTRONICALLY

Performance Objective

Task: Enter transactions from Deborah Valle's encounter form (superbill) into the practice management system and transmit an insurance claim electronically.

Conditions: Patient's electronic data, encounter form (superbill) (Figure 12-16), and computer.

Standards: Time: _____ minutes

Accuracy: _____

(Note: The time element and accuracy criteria may be given by your instructor.)

Directions. Before attempting the Practice Management software assignment, refer to Appendix C and follow the instructions provided to familiarize yourself with the software. Then refer to the Practice Management software on the CD that accompanies the *Workbook*.

1. For this assignment, follow the instructions for entering transactions from an encounter form (superbill) and enter the charges for Deborah Valle's new patient office visit on August 12.

2. After the information has been entered, transmit the insurance claim to Ms. Valle's insurance company by following the instructions for transmitting a claim electronically.

3. Print a hard copy of the insurance claim to hand in to your instructor to receive a score.

4. A Performance Evaluation Checklist may be reproduced form the "Instruction Guide to the *Workbook*" chapter if your instructor wishes you to submit it to assist with scoring and comments.

After the instructor has returned your work to you, either make the necessary corrections and place your work in a three-ring notebook for future reference or, if you received a high score, place it in your portfolio for reference when applying for a job.

Assignment 12-11

College Clinic

4567 Broad Avenue
Woodlands Hills, XY
12345-0001
Tel (555) 486-9002
Fax (555) 487-8976

Doctors No. _____

☐ PRIVATE   ☐ MANAGED CARE   ☐ MEDICAID   ☐ MEDICARE   ☐ TRICARE   ☐ W/C

ACCOUNT #		TODAY'S DATE		
VALL000001		8/12/2007		

LAST NAME	FIRST NAME	MIDDLE INITIAL	DOB	SEX
Valle	Deborah	S.	9/16/1964	F

HOME PHONE	CELL PHONE PAGER	PATIENT EMAIL
(801) 555-8817		

ADDRESS	EMPLOYER NAME
2160 Maiden Lane Midvale, UT 84047	

SSN	DRIVER'S LICENSE	EMPLOYER ADDRESS
555-12-4321	B438716	

NAME OF SPOUSE OR PARENT	PATIENT OCCUPATION
Richard Valle	Housewife

NAME OF INSURANCE CO.	EMPLOYER PHONE
United Western Benefits	

ADDRESS OF INSURANCE CO.	POLICY NUMBER	GROUP NUMBER
151 S. Market St. Salt Lake City, UT 84131	A555-17-1718	AL-119

ASSIGNMENT: I hereby assign payment directly to College Clinic of the surgical and/or medical benefits, if any, otherwise payable to me for his/her services as described below.
SIGNED (Patient, or Parent, if Minor)   DATE:

DESCRIPTION	CPT-4/MD	FEE	DESCRIPTION	CPT-4/MD	FEE	DESCRIPTION	CPT-4/MD	FEE
OFFICE VISIT-NEW PATIENT			**WELL BABY EXAM**			**LABORATORY**		
✓ Level 1	99201	50.00	Intial	99381		Glucose Blood	82951	
Level 2	99202		Periodic	99391		Hematocrit	85013	
Level 3	99203		**OFFICE PROCEDURES**			Occult Blood	82270	
Level 4	99204		Anscopy	46600		Urine Dip	81000	
Level 5	99205		ECG 24-hr	93000		**X-RAY**		
OFFICE VISIT-ESTAB, PATIENT			Fracture Rpr Foot	28470		Foot - 2 View	73620	
Level 1	99211		I & D	10060		Forearm - 2 View	73090	
Level 2	99212		Suture Repair	12002		Nasal Bone - 3	70160	
Level 3	99213					✓ Spine LS - 2 view	72100	110.00
Level 4	99214		**INJECTIONS/VACCINATIONS**					
Level 5	99215		DPT	90701		**MISCELLANEOUS**		
OFFICE CONSULT-NP/EST			IM-Antibiotic	90788		Handling of Spec	99000	
Level 3	99243		Influenza Vac	90658		Supply	99070	
Level 4	99244		Tetanus	90703		Venipuncture	36415	
Level 5	99245		Immun Admin	90471				

COMMENTS:

Physician:

DIAGNOSIS:	DESCRIPTION	CODE	REC'D BY:		
Primary:	Lower back pain	724.2	☐ BANK CARD	PREVIOUS BALANCE	⊖
Secondary:			☐ CASH	TODAY'S FEE	160.00
			☐ CHECK	AMOUNT REC'D/CO-PAY	
			# _____	BALANCE	160.00

RETURN APPOINTMENT

_____ Week(s)   _____ Month(s)

Figure 12–16

ASSIGNMENT 12-12 ▸ ENTER TRANSACTIONS FROM AN ENCOUNTER FORM (SUPERBILL) INTO THE PRACTICE MANAGEMENT SYSTEM AND TRANSMIT AN INSURANCE CLAIM ELECTRONICALLY

Performance Objective

Task: Enter Transactions from Rahmed Taj's encounter form (superbill) into the practice management system and transmit an insurance claim electronically.

Conditions: Patient's electronic data, encounter form (superbill) (Figure 12-17), and computer.

Standards: Time: _____ minutes

Accuracy: _____

(Note: The time element and accuracy criteria may be given by your instructor.)

Directions. Before attempting the Practice Management software assignment, refer to Appendix C and follow the instructions provided to familiarize yourself with the software. Then refer to the Practice Management software on the CD that accompanies the *Workbook*.

1. For this assignment, follow the instructions for entering transactions from an encounter form (superbill) and enter the charges for Rahmed Taj's new patient office visit on August 22.

2. After the information has been entered, transmit the insurance claim to Rahmed Taj's insurance company by following the instructions for transmitting a claim electronically.

3. Print a hard copy of the insurance claim to hand in to your instructor to receive a score.

4. A Performance Evaluation Checklist may be reproduced form the "Instruction Guide to the *Workbook*" chapter if your instructor wishes you to submit it to assist with scoring and comments.

After the instructor has returned your work to you, either make the necessary corrections and place your work in a three-ring notebook for future reference or, if you received a high score, place it in your portfolio for reference when applying for a job.

Assignment 12-12

College Clinic

4567 Broad Avenue
Woodlands Hills, XY
12345-0001
Tel (555) 486-9002
Fax (555) 487-8976

Doctors No. _____

☒ PRIVATE   ☐ MANAGED CARE   ☐ MEDICAID   ☐ MEDICARE   ☐ TRICARE   ☐ W/C

ACCOUNT # TAJ0000001	TODAY'S DATE 8/22/2007		

LAST NAME Taj	FIRST NAME Rahmed	MIDDLE INITIAL	DOB 7/30/1975	SEX M

HOME PHONE (801) 555-4168	CELL PHONE PAGER	PATIENT EMAIL

ADDRESS 808 S. Rampart St. Midvale, UT 84046   EMPLOYER NAME Alta Data Systems

SSN 555-37-6512   DRIVER'S LICENSE B716803   EMPLOYER ADDRESS 1100 East South Union Ave Midvale, UT 84041

NAME OF SPOUSE OR PARENT   PATIENT OCCUPATION Computer Operator

NAME OF INSURANCE CO. United Western Benefits   EMPLOYER PHONE (801) 555-2313

ADDRESS OF INSURANCE CO. 151 S. Market St. Salt Lake City, UT 84131   POLICY NUMBER A555-77-1826   GROUP NUMBER AL-271

ASSIGNMENT: I hereby assign payment directly to College Clinic of the surgical and/or medical benefits, if any, otherwise payable to me for his/her services as described below.
SIGNED (Patient, or Parent, if Minor)   DATE:

DESCRIPTION	CPT-4/MD	FEE	DESCRIPTION	CPT-4/MD	FEE	DESCRIPTION	CPT-4/MD	FEE
OFFICE VISIT-NEW PATIENT			**WELL BABY EXAM**			**LABORATORY**		
Level 1	99201		Intial	99381		Glucose Blood	82951	
✓ Level 2	99202	65.00	Periodic	99391		Hematocrit	85013	
Level 3	99203		**OFFICE PROCEDURES**			Occult Blood	82270	
Level 4	99204		Anscopy	46600		Urine Dip	81000	
Level 5	99205		ECG 24-hr	93000		**X-RAY**		
OFFICE VISIT-ESTAB. PATIENT			Fracture Rpr Foot	28470		Foot - 2 View	73620	
Level 1	99211		I & D	10060		Forearm - 2 View	73090	
Level 2	99212		Suture Repair	12002		✓ Nasal Bone - 3	70160	85.00
Level 3	99213					Spine LS - 2 view	72100	
Level 4	99214		**INJECTIONS/VACCINATIONS**					
Level 5	99215		DPT	90701		**MISCELLANEOUS**		
OFFICE CONSULT-NP/EST			IM-Antibiotic	90788		Handling of Spec	99000	
Level 3	99243		Influenza Vac	90658		Supply	99070	
Level 4	99244		Tetanus	90703		Venipuncture	36415	
Level 5	99245		Immun Admin	90471				

COMMENTS:

Physician:

RETURN APPOINTMENT
____ Week(s)   ____ Month(s)

DIAGNOSIS: DESCRIPTION   CODE
Primary: Fractured Nasal Septum   802.0
Secondary: _____   ____
_____   ____
_____   ____

REC'D BY:
☐ BANK CARD
☐ CASH
☐ CHECK
   # _____

PREVIOUS BALANCE	⊖
TODAY'S FEE	150.00
AMOUNT REC'D/CO-PAY	
BALANCE	150.00

Figure 12–17

ASSIGNMENT **12-13** ▸ **ENTER TRANSACTIONS FROM AN ENCOUNTER FORM (SUPERBILL) INTO THE PRACTICE MANAGEMENT SYSTEM AND TRANSMIT AN INSURANCE CLAIM ELECTRONICALLY**

Performance Objective

Task: Enter transactions from Tadamori Mori's encounter form (superbill) into the practice management system and transmit an insurance claim electronically.

Conditions: Patient's electronic data, encounter form (superbill) (Figure 12-18), and computer.

Standards: Time: _____ minutes

                 Accuracy: _____

                 (Note: The time element and accuracy criteria may be given by your instructor.)

Directions. Before attempting the Practice Management software assignment, refer to Appendix C and follow the instructions provided to familiarize yourself with the software. Then refer to the Practice Management software on the CD that accompanies the *Workbook*.

1. For this assignment, follow the instructions for entering transactions from an encounter form (superbill) and enter the charges for Tadamori Mori's new patient office visit on June 1.

2. After the information has been entered, transmit the insurance claim to Tadamori Mori's insurance company by following the instructions for transmitting a claim electronically.

3. Print a hard copy of the insurance claim to hand in to your instructor to receive a score.

4. A Performance Evaluation Checklist may be reproduced from the "Instruction Guide to the *Workbook*" chapter if your instructor wishes you to submit it to assist with scoring and comments.

   After the instructor has returned your work to you, either make the necessary corrections and place your work in a three-ring notebook for future reference or, if you received a high score, place it in your portfolio for reference when applying for a job.

Assignment 12-13

College Clinic

4567 Broad Avenue
Woodlands Hills, XY
12345-0001
Tel (555) 486-9002
Fax (555) 487-8976

Doctors No. _____

☒ PRIVATE   ☐ MANAGED CARE   ☐ MEDICAID   ☐ MEDICARE   ☐ TRICARE   ☐ W/C

ACCOUNT #	TODAY'S DATE
MORI000001	6/01/2007

LAST NAME	FIRST NAME	MIDDLE INITIAL	DOB	SEX
Mori	Tadamori		6/20/1980	M

HOME PHONE	CELL PHONE PAGER	PATIENT EMAIL
(801) 555-9132		

ADDRESS	EMPLOYER NAME
920 N. Hill St. Midvale, UT 84047	Alta Data Systems

SSN	DRIVER'S LICENSE	EMPLOYER ADDRESS
555-17-XXXX	T386412	1100 East South Union Ave Midvale, UT 84047

NAME OF SPOUSE OR PARENT	PATIENT OCCUPATION
	Computer Operator

NAME OF INSURANCE CO.	EMPLOYER PHONE
United Western Benefits	(801) 555-2313

ADDRESS OF INSURANCE CO.	POLICY NUMBER	GROUP NUMBER
151 S. Market St. Salt Lake City, UT 84131	A555-66-6679	AL-119

ASSIGNMENT: I hereby assign payment directly to College Clinic of the surgical and/or medical benefits, if any, otherwise payable to me for his/her services as described below.
SIGNED (Patient, or Parent, if Minor)   DATE:

	DESCRIPTION	CPT-4/MD	FEE		DESCRIPTION	CPT-4/MD	FEE		DESCRIPTION	CPT-4/MD	FEE
	OFFICE VISIT-NEW PATIENT				**WELL BABY EXAM**				**LABORATORY**		
	Level 1	99201			Intial	99381			Glucose Blood	82951	
✓	Level 2	99202	65.00		Periodic	99391			Hematocrit	85013	
	Level 3	99203			**OFFICE PROCEDURES**				Occult Blood	82270	
	Level 4	99204			Anscopy	46600			Urine Dip	81000	
	Level 5	99205			ECG 24-hr	93000			**X-RAY**		
	OFFICE VISIT-ESTAB, PATIENT			✓	Fracture Rpr Foot	28470	150.00	✓	Foot - 2 View	73620	80.00
	Level 1	99211			I & D	10060			Forearm - 2 View	73090	
	Level 2	99212			Suture Repair	12002			Nasal Bone - 3	70160	
	Level 3	99213							Spine LS - 2 view	72100	
	Level 4	99214			**INJECTIONS/VACCINATIONS**						
	Level 5	99215			DPT	90701			**MISCELLANEOUS**		
	OFFICE CONSULT-NP/EST				IM-Antibiotic	90788			Handling of Spec	99000	
	Level 3	99243			Influenza Vac	90658		✓	Supply	99070	95.00
	Level 4	99244			Tetanus	90703			Venipuncture	36415	
	Level 5	99245			Immun Admin	90471					

COMMENTS:	RETURN APPOINTMENT
Physician:	____ Week(s) ____ Month(s)

DIAGNOSIS:	DESCRIPTION	CODE	REC'D BY:		
Primary:	Closed fracture metatarsus	825.25	☐ BANK CARD	PREVIOUS BALANCE	⊖
Secondary:			☐ CASH	TODAY'S FEE	390.00
			☐ CHECK	AMOUNT REC'D/CO-PAY	
			# _____	BALANCE	390.00

Figure 12–18

STUDENT SOFTWARE CHALLENGE

ASSIGNMENT **12–14 ▸ ASSIGNMENTS FOR MEDICARE CASES 8 THROUGH 10 ONSCREEN COMPLETION OF CMS-1500 (08-05) INSURANCE CLAIM FORMS**

Performance Objective

Task: Enter transactions from patients' onscreen encounter forms (superbills) and complete block-by-block onscreen health insurance claim forms.

Conditions: Onscreen encounter forms (superbills) and computer.

Standards: Time: _____ minutes

                 Accuracy: _____

                 (Note: The time element and accuracy criteria may be given by your instructor.)

Directions. Before attempting the assignments, refer to *Workbook* Appendix C and follow the instructions provided to familiarize yourself with the Student Software Challenge section of the software. Then insert the CD that accompanies the *Workbook* into the computer disk drive.

1. For these assignments, follow the instructions for entering data into the onscreen CMS-1500 (08-05) health insurance claim form, completing blocks 1 through 33 for cases 8 through 10.

2. Use your CPT code book or Appendix A in this *Workbook* to determine the correct five-digit code number and modifiers for each professional service rendered.

3. A Performance Evaluation Checklist may be reproduced from the "Instruction Guide to the *Workbook*" chapter if your instructor wishes you to submit it to assist with scoring and comments.

4. Print a hard copy of the completed health insurance claim form for each case.

5. After the instructor has returned your work to you, either make the necessary corrections and place your work in a three-ring notebook for future reference, or if you received a high score, place it in your portfolio for reference when applying for a job.

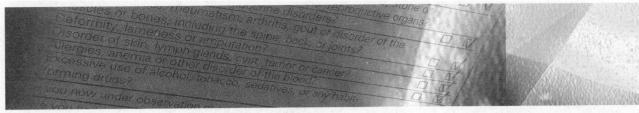

Medicaid and Other State Programs

KEY TERMS

Your instructor may wish to select some words pertinent to this chapter for a test. For definitions of the terms, further study, and/or reference, the words, phrases, and abbreviations may be found in the glossary at the end of the Handbook. *Key terms for this chapter follow.*

categorically needy

coinsurance copayment

covered services

Early and Periodic Screening, Diagnosis, and
  Treatment (EPSDT)

fiscal agent

Maternal and Child Health Program (MCHP)

Medicaid (MCD)

Medi-Cal

medically needy (MN)

prior approval

recipient

share of cost

State Children's Health Insurance Program (SCHIP)

Supplemental Security Income (SSI)

KEY ABBREVIATIONS

See how many abbreviations and acronyms you can translate and then use this as a handy reference list. Definitions for the key abbreviations are located near the back of the Handbook *in the glossary.*

CMS _____

DEFRA _____

EPSDT _____

FPL _____

HMO _____

MCD _____

MCHP _____

MCO _____

MQMB _____

MN _____

OBRA _____

OOY _____

POS _____

QI _____

QMB _____

RA _____

SCHIP _____

SLMB _____

SSI _____

TANF _____

TEFRA _____

PERFORMANCE OBJECTIVES

The student will be able to:

- Define and spell the key terms and key abbreviations for this chapter, given the information from the *Handbook* glossary, within a reasonable time period and with enough accuracy to obtain a satisfactory evaluation.
- After reading the chapter, answer the fill-in-the-blank, multiple choice, and true/false review questions with enough accuracy to obtain a satisfactory evaluation.
- Fill in the correct meaning of each abbreviation, given a list of common medical abbreviations and symbols that appear in chart notes, within a

reasonable time period and with enough accuracy to obtain a satisfactory evaluation.

- Given the patient's medical chart notes, ledger cards, and blank insurance claim forms, complete each CMS-1500 (08-05) Health Insurance Claim Form for billing within a reasonable time period and with enough accuracy to obtain a satisfactory evaluation.
- Correctly post payments, adjustments, and balances on the patient's ledger cards, using the Mock Fee Schedule in Appendix A in this *Workbook*, within a reasonable time period and with enough accuracy to obtain a satisfactory evaluation.

STUDY OUTLINE

History

Medicaid Programs
   Maternal and Child Health Program
   Low-Income Medicare Recipients

Medicaid Eligibility
   Verifying Eligibility
   Categorically Needy
   Medically Needy

**Maternal and Child Health Program
Eligibility**
   Accepting Medicaid Patients
   Identification Card
   Point-of-Service Machine
   Retroactive Eligibility

Medicaid Benefits
   Covered Services
   Disallowed Services

Medicaid Managed Care

Claim Procedure
   Copayment
   Prior Approval
   Time Limit
   Reciprocity
   Claim Form

After Claim Submission
   Remittance Advice
   Appeals

Medicaid Fraud Control

ASSIGNMENT **13-1** ▸ REVIEW QUESTIONS

Part I Fill in the Blank

   Review the objectives, key terms, glossary definitions of key terms, chapter information, and figures before completing the following review questions.

1. Medicaid is administered by ___the State___ with partial ___government___ funding.

2. Medicaid is not an insurance program. It is a/an ___medical care___ program.

3. In all other states, the program is known as Medicaid, but in California the program is

called ___Medi-Cal___

4. Because the federal government sets minimum requirements, states are free to enhance the Medicaid program. Name two ways in which Medicaid programs vary from state to state.

   a. _Maternal & child Health Program_

   b. ~~Low income Medicar~~ _State childrens Health_

5. SCHIP means _State Childrens Health Insurance Program_ and MCHP means _insurance program_

   Maternal & child Health Program and covers children of what age group?

   _0-21_

6. Name the three aid programs for low-income Medicare patients.

   a. _Medicaid Qualified Medicare Beneficiary Program_

   b. _Specified low-income Medicare Beneficiary Program_

   c. _Qualified Individuals Program_

7. Name two broad classifications of people eligible for Medicaid assistance.

   a. _Categorically Needy_

   b. _Medically Needy_

8. The name of the program for the prevention, early detection, and treatment of conditions of children receiving welfare is known as _Early ~~Prevention~~ & Periodic Screening, Diagnosis & treatment_.

   It is abbreviated as _EPSDT_.

9. Your Medicaid patient seen today needs long-term hemodialysis services. You telephone for authorization to get verbal approval. Four important items to obtain are:

   a. ~~Covered Services~~ ③ _any verbal # given by the field office_
   ④ _treatment authorization form indicating that the service was_
   b. ~~Point of Service plan~~ _already authorized must be sent in as follow-up to the phone call_
   ① _Date & time that authorization was given_
   ② _Name of the person who gave authorization_

10. The time limit for submitting a Medicaid claim varies from _2_ to
    _18_ from the date the service is rendered. In your state, the time limit is

    _12_

11. The insurance claim form for submitting Medicaid claims in all states is

    CMS 1500

12. Your Medicaid patient also has TRICARE. What billing procedure do you follow? Be exact in your steps for a dependent of an active military person.

    a. Bill tricare 1st

    b. Bill medicare 2nd

13. Five categories of adjudicated claims that may appear on a Medicaid remittance advice document are:

    a. adjustments

    b. approvals

    c. denials

    d. suspends

    e. audit/refund

14. Name three levels of Medicaid appeals.

    a. go 1st to regional fiscal Agent or Medicaid bureau

    b. 2nd Department of Social Welfare or Human Services

    c. 3rd Appellate Court that evaluate decisions by local & government agencies

Part II Multiple Choice

Choose the best answer.

15. When professional services are rendered, the Medicaid identification card or electronic verification must show eligibility for

    (a.) day of service

    b. year of service

    c. month of service

    d. week of service

16. When a Medicaid patient is injured in an automobile accident and the car has liability insurance, this involves a third-party payer so the insurance claim is sent to the

    a. patient

    (b.) automobile insurance carrier

    c. Medicaid fiscal agent

    d. none of the above

17. The only state without a Medicaid program that is similar to those existing in other states that has an alternative prepaid medical assistantance program is

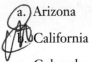

   a. Arizona

   b. California

   c. Colorado

   d. New Mexico

18. A patient's Medicaid eligibility may be verified by

   a. touch-tone telephone

   b. modem

   c. special Medicaid terminal equipment

   d. all of the above

19. When a Medicaid patient requires a piece of durable medical equipment, the physician must

   a. write a prescription

   b. obtain prior authorization, preferably written

   c. instruct the patient on how to use the equipment

   d. give name and address of where to purchase the equipment

20. Medicare beneficiaries who are disabled but have annual incomes below the federal poverty level may be eligible for

   a. Medicaid Qualified Medicare Beneficiary Program

   b. Qualifying Individuals Program

   c. Specified Low-Income Medicare Beneficiary Program

   d. all of the above

Part III True/False

Write "T" or "F" in the blank to indicate whether you think the statement is true or false.

   T 21. Cerebral palsy is a condition that qualifies a child for benefits under the Maternal and Child Health Program.

   T 22. There is only one type of copayment requirement in the Medicaid program.

   F 23. When filing a claim for a Medicaid managed care patient, transmit the claim to the managed care organization and not the Medicaid fiscal agent.

   F 24. Providers must enroll for participation in the Medicaid program with the fiscal agent for their region.

   F 25. A state agency that investigates complaints of mistreatment in long-term care facilities is the Medicaid Fraud Control Unit (MFCU).

A S S I G N M E N T **13–2** ▸ **CRITICAL THINKING**

Performance Objective

Task: After reading the scenario, answer questions, using critical thinking skills.

Conditions: Use a pen or pencil.

Standards: Time: _____ minutes

                 Accuracy: _____

                 (Note: The time element and accuracy criteria may be given by
                 your instructor.)

Directions. After reading the scenario, answer questions, using your critical thinking skills. Record your answers on the blank lines.

Scenario. Mrs. Ho suddenly experiences a pain in her right lower abdominal area and rushes to a local hospital for emergency care. Laboratory work verifies that she has a ruptured appendix, and immediate surgery is recommended. Is prior authorization required in a bonafide emergency situation like this?

_____

In referring to the instructions for completing a CMS-1500 (08-05) claim form for a Medicaid case, which two blocks on the CMS-1500 (08-05) claim form need to be completed for emergency services?

_____

ASSIGNMENT 13-3 ▸ COMPLETE A CLAIM FORM FOR A MEDICAID CASE

Performance Objective

Task: Complete a CMS-1500 (08-05) claim form, post transactions to the financial accounting record, and define patient record abbreviations.

Conditions: Use the patient's record (Figure 13–1) and financial statement (Figure 13–2), one health insurance claim form (print from CD or Evolve website), a typewriter or computer, procedural and diagnostic code books, and Appendices A and B in this *Workbook*.

Standards: Claim Productivity Measurement

Time: _____ minutes

Accuracy: _____

(Note: The time element and accuracy criteria may be given by your instructor.)

Directions

1. Using OCR guidelines, complete the Health Insurance Claim Form and direct it to Medicaid for Rose Clarkson by referring to her patient record. Date the claim September 6. Refer to Appendix A in this *Workbook* to locate the fees to record on the claim and post them to the financial statement. If your instructor wants you to insert the name and address of your Medicaid fiscal agent on the claim, obtain the address by going to the Evolve website listed in Internet Resources at the end of Chapter 13 in the *Handbook*.

2. Refer to Chapter 7 (Figure 7–7) in the *Handbook* for instructions on how to complete this claim form and a Medicaid template.

3. Use your *Current Procedural Terminology* (CPT) code book or Appendix A in this *Workbook* to determine the correct five-digit code number and modifiers for each professional service rendered. Use your Healthcare Common Procedure Coding System (HCPCS) Level II code book or refer to Appendix B in this *Workbook* for HCPCS procedure codes and modifiers.

4. Record all transactions on the financial account, and indicate the date when you have billed Medicaid.

5. Refer to Appendix A in this *Workbook* for the clinic and hospital provider numbers that are needed for completing Medicaid forms.

6. A Performance Evaluation Checklist may be reproduced from the "Instruction Guide to the Workbook" chapter if your instructor wishes you to submit it to assist with scoring and comments.

PATIENT RECORD NO. 13-3

Clarkson	Rose		03-09-44	F	555-487-2209
LAST NAME	FIRST NAME	MIDDLE NAME	BIRTH DATE	SEX	HOME PHONE

3408 Jackson Street	Hempstead	XY	11551-0300	
ADDRESS	CITY	STATE	ZIP CODE	

	555-340-2200			
CELL PHONE	PAGER NO.	FAX NO.		E-MAIL ADDRESS

030-XX-9543	R3207897
PATIENT'S SOC. SEC. NO.	DRIVER'S LICENSE

unemployed	
PATIENT'S OCCUPATION	NAME OF COMPANY

ADDRESS OF EMPLOYER	PHONE

SPOUSE OR PARENT	OCCUPATION

EMPLOYER	ADDRESS	PHONE

Medicaid	self
NAME OF INSURANCE	INSURED OR SUBSCRIBER

CC99756329346X	
MEDICAID NO.	GROUP NO.

REFERRED BY: James Jackson, MD, 100 North Main Street, Hempstead, XY 11551   NPI# 72011337XX

DATE	PROGRESS NOTES
9-4-xx	New pt presents complaining of cough & SOB. A detailed hx was taken which revealed
	mitral valve prolapse. A D exam was done indicating elevated cardiac and respiratory rates,
	diminished breath sounds, distended neck veins, and edema of both ankles. 12 lead ECG
	performed; normal sinus rhythm and elevated heart rate. Echocardiogram done
	(2D, complete with pulsed wave Doppler) to evaluate mitral valve, cardiac chamber size, and ventricular
	function; presence of mitral valve regurgitation. Single view chest x-ray indicated presence
	of fluid in lungs. Primary diagnosis: congestive heart disease and mitral valve prolapse
	(LC MDM). Pt given Rx for diuretic, digitalis, and vasodilator. Restrict fluid and sodium
	intake. Retn in 2 wks.
	PC/llf *Perry Cardi, MD*

Figure 13–1

Acct No.   13-3

STATEMENT
Financial Account
COLLEGE CLINIC
4567 Broad Avenue
Woodland Hills, XY 12345-0001
Tel. 555-486-9002
Fax No. 555-487-8976

Rose Clarkson
3408 Jackson Street
Hempstead, XY 11551-0300

Phone No. (H)_____(555) 487-2209_____ (W) _____   Birthdate_____3-9-44_____

Primary Insurance Co. _____Medicaid_____   Policy/Group No. ___C99756E____

Secondary Insurance Co. _____None_____   Policy/Group No. _____

| DATE | REFERENCE | DESCRIPTION | CHARGES | CREDITS | | BALANCE |
				PYMNTS.	ADJ.	
20xx			BALANCE FORWARD ➤			
9-4-xx		OV NP				
9-4-xx		12 lead ECG				
9-4-xx		Echocardiogram				
9-4-xx		Doppler echo, pulsed wave				
9-4-xx		Chest x-ray				

PLEASE PAY LAST AMOUNT IN BALANCE COLUMN ⬆

THIS IS A COPY OF YOUR FINANCIAL ACCOUNT AS IT APPEARS ON OUR RECORDS

Figure 13–2

After the instructor has returned your work to you, either make the necessary corrections and place your work in a three-ring notebook for future reference or, if you received a high score, place it in your portfolio for reference when applying for a job.

Abbreviations pertinent to this record:

Pt _____   LC _____

SOB _____   MDM _____

hx _____   Rx _____

D _____   retn _____

ECG _____   wks _____

1. Locate a financial accounting record (ledger).

   Note: Refer to the step-by-step procedures at the end of Chapter 3 in the *Handbook* and graphic examples Figures 3–16 and 10–3.

2. Insert the patient's name and address, including ZIP code in the box.

3. Enter the patient's personal data.

4. Ledger lines: Insert date of service (DOS), reference (CPT code number, check number, or dates of service for posting adjustments or when insurance was billed), description of the transaction, charge amounts, payments, adjustments, and running current balance. The posting date is the actual date the transaction is recorded. If the DOS differs from the posting date, list the DOS in the reference or description column.

   Note: A good bookkeeping practice is to take a red pen and draw a line across the financial accounting record (ledger) from left to right to indicate the last entry billed to the insurance company.

ASSIGNMENT **13–4** ▸ **COMPLETE A CLAIM FORM FOR A MEDICAID CASE**

Performance Objective

Task: Complete a CMS-1500 (08-05) claim form for a Medicaid case, post transactions to the financial accounting record, and define patient record abbreviations.

Conditions: Use the patient's record (Figure 13–3) and financial statement (Figure 13–4), one health insurance claim form (print from CD or Evolve website), a typewriter or computer, procedural and diagnostic code books, and appendices A and B in this *Workbook*.

Standards: Claim Productivity Measurement

Time: _____ minutes

Accuracy: _____

(Note: The time element and accuracy criteria may be given by your instructor.)

Directions

1. Using OCR guidelines, complete the Health Insurance Claim Form and direct it to Medicaid for Stephen M. Drake by referring to his patient record. Refer to Appendix A in this *Workbook* to locate the fees to record on the claim, and post them to the financial statement. On May 1, the fee for the injection of Bicillin is $10. As learned in Chapter 6, injectable drugs and medications may be billed separately for Medicaid patients. Date the claim May 26. If your instructor wants you to insert the name and address of your Medicaid fiscal agent on the claim, obtain it by going to the Evolve website listed in Internet Resources at the end of Chapter 13 in the *Handbook*. Do not list services not charged for (NC) on the claim form; however, do list postoperative follow-up visits during the global period on the financial statement. Locate the correct code number in the CPT Medicine section.

   Remember that the physician must always sign all forms on Medicaid cases; stamped signatures are not allowed.

2. Refer to Chapter 7 (Figure 7–7) in the *Handbook* for instructions on how to complete this claim form and a Medicaid template.

3. Use your CPT code book or Appendix A in this *Workbook* to determine the correct five-digit code number and modifiers for each professional service rendered. Use your HCPCS Level II code book or refer to Appendix B in this *Workbook* for HCPCS procedure codes and modifiers.

4. Record all transactions of the financial account and indicate the date when you have billed Medicaid.

5. Refer to Appendix A in this *Workbook* for the clinic and hospital provider numbers that are needed for completing Medicaid forms.

PATIENT RECORD NO. 13-4

Drake	Stephen	M	04-03-91	M	555-277-5831
LAST NAME	FIRST NAME	MIDDLE NAME	BIRTH DATE	SEX	HOME PHONE

2317 Charnwood Avenue	Woodland Hills	XY	12345	
ADDRESS	CITY	STATE	ZIP CODE	

CELL PHONE	PAGER NO.	FAX NO.	E-MAIL ADDRESS

566-XX-0081
PATIENT'S SOC. SEC. NO.   DRIVER'S LICENSE

full time student
PATIENT'S OCCUPATION   NAME OF COMPANY

ADDRESS OF EMPLOYER   PHONE

Mrs. Virginia B. Drake (mother)   none-family on welfare
SPOUSE OR PARENT   OCCUPATION

EMPLOYER   ADDRESS   PHONE

Medicaid
NAME OF INSURANCE   INSURED OR SUBSCRIBER

Child's identification number   19-37-1524033-16X
POLICY/CERTIFICATE NO.   GROUP NO.

REFERRED BY: James B. Jeffers, MD, 100 S. Broadway, Woodland Hills, XY 12345   Provider No. 12345069XX

DATE	PROGRESS NOTES
5-1-xx	NP comes in complaining of severe sore throat since April 4. A detailed hx was taken.
	Mother states Stephen has had many bouts of tonsillitis since age 4. He has missed
	school on three occasions this year due to throat infections. Did complete phys exam (D)
	which showed enlargement & inflam of tonsils. Temp 101.2. Strep culture done
	(screening) with a preliminary report; positive for strep. Administered penicillin G (Bicillin)
	1.2 million units IM and wrote Rx to start AB and continue x 10 d. Imp: Acute tonsillitis
	(LC MDM). RTO 1 week.
	GP/llf *Gerald Practon, MD*
5-8-xx	Pt returns; sore throat improved but still swollen. Tonsils are 4+ hypertrophic. Received
	medical records from past primary physician which indicated hx of 5 bouts of strep over
	last 3 yrs. Adv. tonsillectomy and adenoidectomy. Phoned for prior authorization 3 p.m.,
	Auth. No. 45042, given by Mrs. Jane Michaels. Pt to be admitted tomorrow for one day
	surgery (PF HX/PX SF MDM).
	GP/llf *Gerald Practon, MD*
5-9-xx	Admit to College Hospital. Tonsillectomy and adenoidectomy performed. Pt doing well,
	discharged 4:00 P.M. RTC 1 week.
	GP/llf *Gerald Practon, MD*
5-17-xx	PO visit. No complaints. Temp 98.1. Retn if necessary (PF HX/PX SF MDM).
	GP/llf *Gerald Practon, MD*

Figure 13–3

Acct No. 13-4

STATEMENT
Financial Account
COLLEGE CLINIC
4567 Broad Avenue
Woodland Hills, XY 12345-0001
Tel. 555-486-9002
Fax No. 555-487-8976

Stephen M. Drake
c/o Virginia B.Drake
2317 Charnwood Avenue
Woodland Hills, XY 12345

Phone No. (H) _____ (555) 277-5831 _____ (W) _____   Birthdate _____ 4-3-91 _____

Primary Insurance Co. _____ Medicaid _____   Policy/Group No. ___ 19-37-1524033-16X

Secondary Insurance Co. ___ N/A _____   Policy/Group No. _____

| DATE | REFERENCE | DESCRIPTION | CHARGES | CREDITS | | BALANCE |
				PYMNTS.	ADJ.	
20xx		BALANCE FORWARD ➜				
5-1-xx		NP OV				
5-1-xx		Strep culture				
5-1-xx		Injection AB				
5-1-xx		Bicillin				
5-8-xx		OV				
5-9-xx		T & A				
5-17-xx		PO OV				

PLEASE PAY LAST AMOUNT IN BALANCE COLUMN ⇨

THIS IS A COPY OF YOUR FINANCIAL ACCOUNT AS IT APPEARS ON OUR RECORDS

Figure 13–4

6. On July 1, Medicaid paid $200 on this claim. Post this payment (warrant number 766504) to the patient's financial account and adjust the balance, using the same line.

7. A Performance Evaluation Checklist may be reproduced from the "Instruction Guide to the *Workbook*" chapter if your instructor wishes you to submit it to assist with scoring and comments.

   After the instructor has returned your work to you, either make the necessary corrections and place your work in a three-ring notebook for future reference or, if you received a high score, place it in your portfolio for reference when applying for a job.

Abbreviations pertinent to this record:

NP	_____	imp	_____
hx	_____	LC	_____
phys	_____	MDM	_____
D	_____	RTO	_____
inflam	_____	yrs	_____
temp	_____	adv	_____
strep	_____	PF	_____
IM	_____	SF	_____
Rx	_____	RTC	_____
AB	_____	PO	_____
X	_____	retn	_____
d	_____		

Additional Coding

1. Using your diagnostic code book, code the symptoms that the patient presented with on May 1, 20xx.

   Symptom   *Code*

   a. _____ _____

   b. _____ _____

   c. _____ _____

2. Locate a financial accounting record (ledger).

Note: Refer to the step-by-step procedures at the end of Chapter 3 in the *Handbook* and graphic examples Figures 3–6 and 10–3.

3. Insert the patient's name and address, including ZIP code in the box.

4. Enter the patient's personal data.

5. Ledger lines: Insert date of service (DOS), reference (CPT code number, check number, or dates of service for posting adjustments or when insurance was billed), description of the transaction, charge amounts, payments, adjustments, and running current balance. The posting date is the actual date the transaction is recorded. If the DOS differs from the posting date, list the DOS in the reference or description column.

Note: A good bookkeeping practice is to take a red pen and draw a line across the financial accounting record (ledger) from left to right to indicate the last entry billed to the insurance company.

ASSIGNMENT **13–5** ▸ **COMPLETE A CLAIM FORM FOR A MEDICAID CASE**

Performance Objective

Task: Complete a CMS-1500 (08-05) claim form for a Medicaid case, post transactions to the financial accounting record, and define patient record abbreviations.

Conditions: Use the patient's record (Figure 13–5) and financial statement (Figure 13–6), one health insurance claim form (print from CD or Evolve website), a typewriter or computer, procedural and diagnostic code books, and appendices A and B in this *Workbook*.

Standards: Claim Productivity Measurement

Time: _____ minutes

Accuracy: _____

(Note: The time element and accuracy criteria may be given by your instructor.)

Directions

1. Using OCR guidelines, complete the Health Insurance Claim Form and direct it to Medicaid for Barry L. Brooke by referring to his patient record. Refer to Appendix A in this *Workbook* to locate the fees to record on the claim, and post them to the financial statement. The financial statement should be sent in care of (c/o) the patient's parents because he is a minor. Date the claim June 10. If your instructor wants you to insert the name and address of your Medicaid fiscal agent on the claim, obtain it by going to the Evolve website listed in Internet Resources at the end of Chapter 13 in the *Handbook*.

2. Refer to Chapter 7 (Figure 7–7) in the *Handbook* for instructions on how to complete this claim form and a Medicaid template.

3. Use your CPT code book or Appendix A in this *Workbook* to determine the diagnostic codes and the correct five-digit code number and modifiers for each professional service rendered. Use your HCPCS Level II code book or refer to Appendix B in this *Workbook* for HCPCS procedure codes and modifiers.

4. Record all transactions on the financial account and indicate the date when you have billed Medicaid.

5. Refer to Appendix A in this *Workbook* for the clinic and hospital provider numbers that are needed for completing Medicaid forms.

6. On July 1, Medicaid paid $75 (warrant number 329670) on this claim. Post this payment to the patient's financial statement and adjust the balance.

7. A Performance Evaluation Checklist may be reproduced from the "Instruction Guide to the *Workbook*" chapter if your instructor wishes you to submit it to assist with scoring and comments.

PATIENT RECORD NO. 13-5

Brooke	Barry	L		02-03-90	M	555-487-9770
LAST NAME	FIRST NAME	MIDDLE NAME		BIRTH DATE	SEX	HOME PHONE

3821 Ocean Drive	Woodland Hills	XY	12345
ADDRESS	CITY	STATE	ZIP CODE

			brooke@wb.net
CELL PHONE	PAGER NO.	FAX NO.	E-MAIL ADDRESS

776-XX-1931
PATIENT'S SOC. SEC. NO.   DRIVER'S LICENSE

child—full time student
PATIENT'S OCCUPATION   NAME OF COMPANY

ADDRESS OF EMPLOYER   PHONE

Robert D. Brooke (father)   none—family on welfare (father totally disabled)
SPOUSE OR PARENT   OCCUPATION

EMPLOYER   ADDRESS   PHONE

Medicaid   Barry
NAME OF INSURANCE   INSURED OR SUB SCRIBER

54-32-7681533-10X
MEDICAID NO.

REFERRED BY: Virginia B. Drake (friend)

DATE	PROGRESS NOTES
5-28-xx	Sunday evening, new pt seen in ER at College Hospital. Pt twisted L knee while playing
	baseball at Grove Park. X-rays (3 views of L knee) were ordered –N for fx. Imp: effusion
	and ligament strain lt knee. Tx: aspirated lt knee and removed 5 cc bloody fluid.
	Discussion is held with mother and son; bracing versus casting. Mother insists on a cast
	because she states he is noncompliant and thinks he will remove the brace and injure his
	leg further. Barry agrees to have cast. Applied long leg fiberglass walking cast. Pt to be
	seen in office in 2 wks (D HX/PX M MDM).
	RS/llf *Raymond Skeleton, MD*
6-10-xx	Pt returns c/o continued knee pain and wants cast removed. He is in tears and says he
	has been miserable. Mother agrees to have cast removed; leg examined. Fitted pt with
	orthotic device for his knee (straight-leg canvas immobilizer, longitudinal, prefabricated $85).
	Ordered MRI without contrast of L knee to be done at College Hospital Radiology. Pt given directions and
	precautions regarding ambulation with brace (EPF HX/PX LC MDM). RTO 2 wks.
	RS/llf *Raymond Skeleton, MD*

Figure 13–5

Acct No. 13-5

STATEMENT
Financial Account
COLLEGE CLINIC
4567 Broad Avenue
Woodland Hills, XY 12345-0001
Tel. 555-486-9002
Fax No. 555-487-8976

Barry L Brooke
c/o Robert D. Brooke
3821 Ocean Drive
Woodland Hills, XY 12345

Phone No. (H) _____ (555) 487-9770 _____ (W) _____   Birthdate _____ 2-3-90 _____

Primary Insurance Co. _____ Medicaid _____   Policy/Group No. _____ 5432768153310X _____

Secondary Insurance Co. _____   Policy/Group No. _____

| DATE | REFERENCE | DESCRIPTION | CHARGES | CREDITS | | BALANCE |
				PYMNTS.	ADJ.	
20xx		BALANCE FORWARD ➡				
5-28-xx		ER				
5-28-xx		Aspiration L knee				
5-28-xx		Cast application				
6-10-xx		OV				
6-10-xx		L Knee immobilizer				

PLEASE PAY LAST AMOUNT IN BALANCE COLUMN ⬆

THIS IS A COPY OF YOUR FINANCIAL ACCOUNT AS IT APPEARS ON OUR RECORDS

Figure 13–6

After the instructor has returned your work to you, either make the necessary corrections and place your work in a three-ring notebook for future reference or, if you received a high score, place it in your portfolio for reference when applying for a job.

Abbreviations pertinent to this record:

Pt	_____	lt	_____
ER	_____	tx	_____
L	_____	cc	_____
N	_____	MRI	_____
fx	_____	RTO	_____
imp	_____	wks	_____

Additional Coding

1. Refer to Barry Brooke's medical record, abstract information, and code procedures that would be billed by outside providers.

Site	*Description of Service*	*Code*
a. College Hospital Radiology	_____	_____
b. College Hospital Central Supply	_____	_____
c. College Hospital Radiology	_____	_____

2. Locate a financial accounting record (ledger).

   Note: Refer to the step-by-step procedures at the end of Chapter 3 in the *Handbook* and graphic examples Figures 3–16 and 10–3.

3. Insert the patient's name and address, including ZIP code in the box.

4. Enter the patient's personal data.

5. Ledger lines: Insert date of service (DOS), reference (CPT code number, check number, or dates of service for posting adjustments or when insurance was billed), description of the transaction, charge amounts, payments, adjustments, and running current balance. The posting date is the actual date the transaction is recorded. If the DOS differs from the posting date, list the DOS in the reference or description column.

   Note: A good bookkeeping practice is to take a red pen and draw a line across the financial accounting record (ledger) from left to right to indicate the last entry billed to the insurance company.

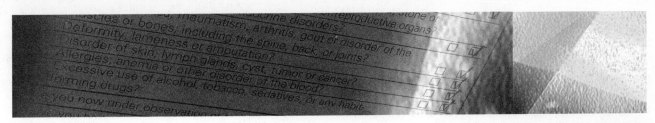

TRICARE and CHAMPVA

KEY TERMS

Your instructor may wish to select some words pertinent to this chapter for a test. For definitions of the terms, further study, and/or reference, the words, phrases, and abbreviations may be found in the glossary at the end of the Handbook. *Key terms for this chapter follow.*

active duty service member (ADSM)

allowable charge

authorized provider

beneficiary

catastrophic cap

catchment area

Civilian Health and Medical Program of the Department of Veterans Affairs (CHAMPVA)

cooperative care

coordination of benefits

cost-share

Defense Enrollment Eligibility Reporting System (DEERS)

emergency

fiscal intermediary (FI)

health benefits advisor (HBA)

Health Care Finder (HCF)

medically (or psychologically) necessary

military treatment facility (MTF)

nonparticipating provider (nonpar)

other health insurance (OHI)

participating provider (par)

partnership program

point-of-service (POS) option

preauthorization

primary care manager (PCM)

quality assurance program

service benefit program

service-connected injury

service retiree (military retiree)

sponsor

summary payment voucher

total, permanent, service-connected disability

TRICARE Extra

TRICARE for Life (TFL)

TRICARE Prime

TRICARE service center (TSC)

urgent care

veteran

KEY ABBREVIATIONS

See how many abbreviations and acronyms you can translate and then use this as a handy reference list. Definitions for the key abbreviations are located near the back of the Handbook *in the glossary.*

ADSM	_____	MD	_____
CHAMPVA	_____	MHS	_____
DDM	_____	MTF	_____
DDS	_____	NAS	_____
DEERS	_____	OHI	_____
DO	_____	par	_____
DPM	_____	PCM	_____
DSC	_____	POS	_____
FI	_____	RFMS	_____
FTM	_____	SHCP	_____
HAC	_____	TFL	_____
HBA	_____	TMA	_____
HCF	_____	TPR	_____
		TPRADFM	_____
		TSC	_____
		USFHP	_____
		VA	_____

PERFORMANCE OBJECTIVES

The student will be able to:

■ Define and spell the key terms and key abbreviations for this chapter, given the information from the *Handbook* glossary, within a reasonable time period and with enough accuracy to obtain a satisfactory evaluation.

■ After reading the chapter, answer the fill-in-the-blanks, multiple choice, and true/false review questions with enough accuracy to obtain a satisfactory evaluation.

■ Fill in the correct meaning of each abbreviation, given a list of common medical abbreviations and symbols that appear in chart notes, within a reasonable time period and with enough accuracy to obtain a satisfactory evaluation.

■ Given the patient's medical chart notes, ledger cards, and blank insurance claim forms, complete each CMS-1500 (08-05) Health Insurance Claim Form for billing within a reasonable time period and with enough accuracy to obtain a satisfactory evaluation.

■ Using the Mock Fee Schedule in Appendix A in this *Workbook*, correctly post payments, adjustments, and balances on the patients' ledger cards within a reasonable time period and with enough accuracy to obtain a satisfactory evaluation.

■ Compute mathematical calculations, given TRICARE problem situations, within a reasonable time period and with enough accuracy to obtain a satisfactory evaluation.

ALTAPOINT PRACTICE MANAGEMENT SOFTWARE OBJECTIVES

The student should be able to:

● Enter transactions from encounter form (superbills) and complete, print, and transmit electronic insurance claims to the insurance company using the practice management system, within a reasonable time period and with enough accuracy to obtain a satisfactory evaluation.

STUDY OUTLINE

History of TRICARE

TRICARE Programs
Eligibility
Nonavailability Statement

TRICARE Standard
Enrollment
Identification Card
Benefits
Fiscal Year
Authorized Providers of Health Care
Preauthorization
Payment

TRICARE Extra
Enrollment
Identification Card
Benefits
Network Provider
Preauthorization
Payments

TRICARE Prime
Enrollment
Identification Card
Benefits
Primary Care Manager
Preauthorization
Payments

TRICARE for Life
Enrollment
Identification Card
Benefits
Referral and Preauthorization
Payment

TRICARE Plus
Enrollment
Identification Card
Benefits
Payment

TRICARE Prime Remote Program
Enrollment
Identification Card
Benefits
Referral and Preauthorization
Payments

Supplemental Health Care Program
Enrollment
Identification Card
Benefits
Referral and Preauthorization
Payments

TRICARE Hospice Program

TRICARE and HMO Coverage

CHAMPVA Program
Eligibility
Enrollment
Identification Card
Benefits
Provider
Preauthorization

Medical Record Access
Privacy Act of 1974
Computer Matching and Privacy Protection Act of 1988

Claims Procedure
Fiscal Intermediary
TRICARE Standard and CHAMPVA
TRICARE Extra and TRICARE Prime
TRICARE Prime Remote and Supplemental Health Care Program
TRICARE for Life
TRICARE/CHAMPVA and Other Insurance
Medicaid and TRICARE/CHAMPVA
Medicare and TRICARE
Medicare and CHAMPVA
Dual or Double Coverage
Third-Party Liability
Workers' Compensation

After Claim Submission
TRICARE Summary Payment Voucher
CHAMPVA Explanation of Benefits Document
Quality Assurance
Claims Inquiries and Appeals

Procedure: Completing a CHAMPVA Claim Form

A S S I G N M E N T ► **REVIEW QUESTIONS**

Part I Fill in the Blank

Review the objectives, key terms, glossary definitions of key terms, chapter information, and figures before completing the following review questions.

1. CHAMPUS, the acronym for Civilian Health and Medical Program of the

   Uniformed Services, is now called ___TRICARE___ and was organized to control escalating medical costs and to standardize benefits for active-duty families and military retirees.

2. An active duty service member is known as a/an ___Sponsor___; once

   retired, this former member is called a/an ___Service retiree___.

3. An individual who qualifies for TRICARE is known as a/an ___beneficiary___.

4. A system for verifying an individual's TRICARE eligibility is called

   ___DEERS___.

5. Mrs. Hancock, a TRICARE beneficiary, lives 2 miles from a Uniformed Services Medical Treatment Facility but needs to be hospitalized for mental health care services at Orlando Medical Center, a civilian hospital. What type of authorization does she require?

   ___preauthorization saying it's Medically Necessary___

6. TRICARE Standard and CHAMPVA beneficiary identification cards are issued to ___all dependants 10yrs___

   and ___older___. Information must be obtained from ___front___

   and ___back___ of the card and placed on the health insurance claim form.

7. Programs that allow TRICARE Standard beneficiaries to receive treatment, services,

   or supplies from civilian providers are called ___Cooperative care___ and ___partnership program___.

8. For patients whose sponsor is a rank of E4 and below, the TRICARE Standard

   deductible for outpatient care is how much per patient? ___$50___

   Per family? ___$100___

9. For patients whose sponsor is a rank of E5 and above, the TRICARE Standard

   deductible for outpatient care is how much per patient? ___$150___

   Per family? ___$350___

10. For TRICARE Standard, dependents of active duty members pay what percentage for outpatient services after the deductible has been met? __20%__
What percentage does TRICARE pay? __80%__

11. For retired members or their dependents on TRICARE Standard, what is their deductible responsibility for outpatient services? Per person? __$150__
Per family? __$300__

12. For TRICARE Standard, retired members or their dependents pay what percentage for outpatient services after the deductible has been met? __25%__
What percentage does TRICARE pay? __75%__

13. A voluntary TRICARE health maintenance organization type of option is known as __TRICARE Prime__.

14. CHAMPVA is the acronym for __Civilan Health & Medical Program of the Veterans Administrator, now__ known as the __beneficiaries__.

15. Those individuals who serve in the United States Armed Forces, finish their service, and are honorably discharged are known as __Veterans__.

16. CHAMPVA is not an insurance program but is considered as a/an __service benefit__ program.

17. Which individuals are entitled to CHAMPVA medical benefits?
a. __Vet's spouse or unmarried child of w/ total disability, permanent in nature, resulting from a service connected__
b. __Vet's spouse or unmarried child - vet died as a result of a service connected disability or who @ the time of death had a total disability, permanent in nature injury__
c. __Vet, surviving spouse & children - vet died in the line of duty while in active service__

18. The public law establishing a person's right to review and contest inaccuracies in personal medical records is known as the __Privacy Act of 1974__.

19. An organization that contracts with the government to process TRICARE and CHAMPVA health insurance claims is known as a/an __Medicare HAC__.

20. The time limit for submitting a TRICARE Standard or CHAMPVA claim for outpatient service is __w/in 1 year from the date of service__;
for inpatient service, it is __1 year from the date of service__.

Part II Multiple Choice

Choose the best answer.

21. The TRICARE fiscal year

    a. begins January 1 and ends December 31

    b. begins April 1 and ends March 30

    c. begins June 1 and ends May 30

    d. begins October 1 and ends September 30

22. A health care professional who helps a patient who is under the TRICARE Standard program obtain preauthorization for care is called a/an

    a. primary care physician (PCP)

    b. health care finder (HCF)

    c. health benefits advisor (HBA)

    d. participating provider

23. TRICARE standard beneficiaries pay a certain amount each year for the cost-share and annual deductible, which is known as

    a. catastrophic cap

    b. limiting charge

    c. coinsurance

    d. payment limitation

24. To qualify for TRICARE for Life (TFL), a beneficiary must be

    a. a TRICARE beneficiary

    b. eligible for Medicare Part A

    c. enrolled in Medicare Part B

    d. all of the above

25. The time limit for filing a TRICARE Standard claim is

    a. the end of the calendar year after the fiscal year in which services were furnished

    b. within 1 year from the date a service is provided

    c. within 1 year from the month of service

    d. within 2 years from when service is provided

Part III True/False

Write "T" or "F" in the blank to indicate whether you think the statement is true or false.

___T___ 26. Medically necessary treatment needed for immediate illness or injury that would not result in further disability or death if not treated immediately is known as *urgent care*.

___T___ 27. TRICARE beneficiaries who use nonauthorized providers and receive medical services may be responsible for their entire bill.

___T___ 28. When an individual on TRICARE Prime shows you their identification card, it guarantees TRICARE eligibility.

___F___ 29. TRICARE Prime Remote (TPR) is a program designed for military retirees and their families.

___F___ 30. Beneficiaries of the CHAMPVA program have complete freedom of choice in selecting their civilian health care providers.

ASSIGNMENT **14–2** ▸ **CRITICAL THINKING**

Performance Objective

Task: After reading the scenarios, answer questions, using critical thinking skills.

Conditions: Use a pen or pencil.

Standards: Time: _____ minutes

                   Accuracy: _____

                   (Note: The time element and accuracy criteria may be given by your instructor.)

Directions. After reading the scenarios, answer questions, using your critical thinking skills. Record your answers on the blank lines.

1. If Bertha Evans is seen for an office visit and has other insurance besides TRICARE, and she is the dependent of an active military person, whom do you bill first?

   _____

2. If Jason Williams, a TRICARE beneficiary who became disabled at age 10 years and who is also receiving Medicare Part A benefits, is seen for a consultation, whom do you bill first?

   _____

3. If Tanner Vine, a CHAMPVA and Medicaid beneficiary, is seen on an emergency basis in the office, whom do you bill first?

   _____

ASSIGNMENT 14–3 ▸ CALCULATE MATHEMATICAL PROBLEMS

Performance Objective

Task: Calculate and insert the correct amounts for three TRICARE scenarios.

Conditions: Use a pen or pencil, the description of the problem, and calculation formulas.

Standards: Time: _____ minutes

                Accuracy: _____

                (Note: The time element and accuracy criteria may be given by your instructor.)

Directions. Calculate and insert the correct amounts for the following scenarios using these formulas.

Basic calculation formulas:

TRICARE
$	TRICARE allowed amount
– _____	Minus deductible
$	Balance on which pmt calculated
× ____ %	Multiply TRICARE plan %
$	TRICARE payment

PATIENT
$	Allowed amount after deductible
× ____ %	Multiply TRICARE plan %
$	
+ _____	Add any deductible amt owed
$	Amount patient pays

ADJUSTED AMOUNT
$	Billed amount
– _____	Minus allowable amount
$	Adjusted amount

Problem 1. On October 1, in consultation, Dr. Caesar sees the wife of a Navy man who is stationed at Port Hueneme. Dr. Caesar orders her to the hospital because of a suspected ectopic pregnancy. She undergoes a laparotomy and salpingectomy. Her husband is a rank of E4 and below. Here are her bills. Indicate what TRICARE Standard will pay.

Outpatient Services: *TRICARE Standard*

	Bill/Allowable	TRICARE payment	Patient Owes
Consultation	$75	$_____	$_____

Inpatient services:

Salpingectomy	$600
Assistant surgeon	$120
Anesthesiologist	$400

3-day stay (drugs, laboratory tests, operating room)	$2500	

| Total | $_____ | $_____ |

Mathematical computations:

Problem 2. This is the same situation as in Problem 1, except that the patient is the wife of a retired military man and has TRICARE Standard.

Outpatient Services: *TRICARE Standard*

	Bill/Allowable	**TRICARE payment**	**Patient Owes**
Consultation	$75	$_____	$_____

Inpatient services with separately billed professional charges

	Bill/Allowable	**TRICARE Payment**	**Patient Owes**
Salpingectomy	$600	$_____	$_____
Assistant surgeon	$120	$_____	$_____
Anesthesiologist	$400	$_____	$_____

Inpatient services billed by hospital

3-day stay (drugs, laboratory tests, operating room)	$2500	$_____	

| Total payment owed by patient to Dr. Caesar | | | $_____ |

Mathematical computations:

Problem 3. A TRICARE patient whose sponsor is a rank of E5 or above asks Dr. Caesar to accept assignment on her medical care, and Dr. Caesar agrees. She has not met her deductible. She is the wife of an active duty man. She has TRICARE Extra.

Dr. Caesar's bill:

Consultation	$50	Allowable:	$50
Complete blood cell count	20		20
Urinalysis	5		5
Blood serology and complement fixation	25		25
Posteroanterior and lateral chest radiograph	40		40
Electrocardiogram	35		30
Spirometry	40		40
Total	$215		$210

How much is Dr. Caesar's check from TRICARE Extra? $_____. The

patient owes the doctor $ _____. Dr. Caesar's

courtesy adjustment is $ _____.

  Mathematical computations:

ASSIGNMENT **14–4** ▸ **COMPLETE A CLAIM FORM FOR A TRICARE STANDARD CASE**

Performance Objective

Task: Complete a CMS-1500 (08-05) claim form for a TRICARE Standard case, post transactions to the financial accounting record, and define patient record abbreviations.

Conditions: Use the patient's record (Figure 14–1) and financial statement (Figure 14–2), one health insurance claim form (print from CD or Evolve website), a typewriter or computer, procedural and diagnostic code books, and appendices A and B in this *Workbook*.

Standards: Claim Productivity Measurement

         Time: _____ minutes

         Accuracy: _____

         (Note: The time element and accuracy criteria may be given by your instructor.)

Directions

1. Using optical character reader (OCR) guidelines, complete the CMS-1500 (08-05) claim form. If your instructor wants you to direct it to your local TRICARE fiscal intermediary, go to website http://www.tricare.osd.mil. Click on the area of the map you are residing in and then choose a state to access claims information for that state. Refer to Miss Rosa M. Sandoval's patient record for information and Appendix A to locate the fees to record on the claim and post to the financial statement. Date the claim May 31. Dr. Atrics is not accepting assignment on this TRICARE Standard case but is completing the claim for the patient's convenience. The family of this patient has not previously met its deductible.

2. Refer to Chapter 7 (Figure 7–12) of the *Handbook* for instructions on how to complete this claim form and to view a TRICARE template.

3. Use your *Current Procedural Terminology* (CPT) code book or Appendix A in this *Workbook* to determine the correct five-digit code number and modifiers for each professional service rendered. Use your Healthcare Common Procedure Coding System (HCPCS) Level II code book or refer to Appendix B in this *Workbook* for HCPCS procedure codes and modifiers.

4. On May 8, Miss Sandoval makes a partial payment of $20 by check (No. 4013). Record the proper information on the financial record but not on the claim form, and note the date you have billed TRICARE (May 31).

5. A Performance Evaluation Checklist may be reproduced from the "Instruction Guide to the *Workbook*" chapter if your instructor wishes you to submit it to assist with scoring and comments.

     After the instructor has returned your work to you, either make the necessary corrections and place your work in a three-ring notebook for future reference or, if you received a high score, place it in your portfolio for reference when applying for a job.

Abbreviations pertinent to this record:

pt	_____	ofc	_____
rt	_____	FU	_____
EPF	_____	retn	_____
yr(s)	_____	PO	_____
temp	_____	PF	_____
adv	_____	HX	_____
SF	_____	PX	_____
MDM	_____	wk	_____
c̄	_____	T	_____

1. Locate a financial accounting record (ledger).

   Note: Refer to the step-by-step procedures at the end of Chapter 3 in the *Handbook* and graphic examples Figures 3–16 and 10–3.

2. Insert the patient's name and address, including ZIP code in the box.

3. Enter the patient's personal data.

4. Ledger lines: Insert date of service (DOS), reference (CPT code number, check number, or dates of service for posting adjustments or when insurance was billed), description of the transaction, charge amounts, payments, adjustments, and running current balance. The posting date is the actual date the transaction is recorded. If the DOS differs from the posting date, list the DOS in the reference or description column.

   Note: A good bookkeeping practice is to take a red pen and draw a line across the financial accounting record (ledger) from left to right to indicate the last entry billed to the insurance company.

PATIENT RECORD NO. 14-4

Sandoval	Rosa	M	11-01-91	F	555-456-3322
LAST NAME	FIRST NAME	MIDDLE NAME	BIRTH DATE	SEX	HOME PHONE

209 West Maple Street	Woodland Hills	XY	12345	
ADDRESS	CITY	STATE	ZIP CODE	

CELL PHONE	PAGER NO.	FAX NO.	E-MAIL ADDRESS

994-XX-1164
PATIENT'S SOC. SEC. NO.   DRIVER'S LICENSE

Child—full time student (lives with mother)
PATIENT'S OCCUPATION   NAME OF COMPANY

ADDRESS OF EMPLOYER   PHONE

Hernan J. Sandoval (father)   Staff Sargeant – Grade 9 (active duty)
SPOUSE OR PARENT   OCCUPATION

United States Army   HHC 3rd Batt, 25th Infantry, APO New York, New York, 10030
EMPLOYER   ADDRESS   PHONE

TRICARE Standard   father (DOB 2/10/70)
NAME OF INSURANCE   INSURED OR SUBSCRIBER

886-XX-0999
POLICY/CERTIFICATE NO.   GROUP NO.

REFERRED BY: Maria Sandoval (mother)

DATE	PROGRESS NOTES
5-1-xx	New pt comes in complaining of pain in rt ear for 3 days. An EPF history was taken which
	revealed several ear infections (suppurative) over the past 3 yrs. An EPF exam revealed
	fluid and pus in rt ear. Temp 101°. Adv mother a myringotomy was necessary. Scheduled
	outpatient surg at College Hospital this afternoon. Imp: Acute rt suppurative otitis media
	(SF MDM).
	PA/llf *Pedro Atrics, MD*
5-1-xx	Pt admitted to outpatient surgery (College Hospital). Rt myringotomy c̄ aspiration
	performed. Pt did well. To be seen in ofc for FU in 2 days.
	PA/llf *Pedro Atrics, MD*
5-3-xx	Pt retns PO (PF HX/PX SF MDM). No pain rt ear. Pt progressing well. Retn in 1 wk.
	PA/llf *Pedro Atrics, MD*
5-8-xx	Pt retns PO (PF HX/PX SF MDM). T 98°, no fluid or pus in rt ear. No pain. Pt discharged,
	retn prn.
	PA/llf *Pedro Atrics, MD*

Figure 14–1

Acct No. 14-4

STATEMENT
Financial Account
COLLEGE CLINIC
4567 Broad Avenue
Woodland Hills, XY 12345-0001
Tel. 555-486-9002
Fax No. 555-487-8976

Rosa M. Sandoval
c/o Maria Sandoval
209 West Maple Street
Woodland Hills, XY 12345-0001

Phone No. (H) ___(555) 456-3322___ (W) _____ Birthdate ___11-9-91___

Primary Insurance Co. ___TRICARE Standard___ Policy/Group No. _886-XX-0999_

Secondary Insurance Co. _____ Policy/Group No. _____

DATE	REFERENCE	DESCRIPTION	CHARGES	CREDITS		BALANCE
				PYMNTS.	ADJ.	
20xx			BALANCE FORWARD ➔			
5-1-xx		NP OV				
5-1-xx		Myringotomy				
5-3-xx		PO OV				
5-8-xx		PO OV				

PLEASE PAY LAST AMOUNT IN BALANCE COLUMN ⬆

THIS IS A COPY OF YOUR FINANCIAL ACCOUNT AS IT APPEARS ON OUR RECORDS

Figure 14–2

ASSIGNMENT 14-5 ▸ COMPLETE A CLAIM FORM FOR A TRICARE
                               EXTRA CASE

Performance Objective

Task: Complete a CMS-1500 (08-05) claim form for a TRICARE Extra case, post transactions to the financial accounting record, and define patient record abbreviations.

Conditions: Use the patient's record (Figure 14–3) and financial statement (Figure 14–4), one health insurance claim form (print from CD or Evolve website), a typewriter or computer, procedural and diagnostic code books, and appendices A and B in this *Workbook*.

Standards: Claim Productivity Measurement

                   Time: _____ minutes

                   Accuracy: _____

                   (Note: The time element and accuracy criteria may be given by your instructor.)

Directions

1. Using OCR guidelines, complete the CMS-1500 (08-05) claim form. If your instructor wants you to direct it to your local TRICARE fiscal intermediary go to website http://www.tricare.osd.mil. Click on the area of the map you are residing in and then choose a state to access claims information for that state. Refer to Mrs. Darlene B. Drew's patient record for information and Appendix A to locate the fees to record on the claim and post to the financial statement. Date the claim February 3. Assume that the Nonavailability Statement (NAS) has been transmitted electronically so that the physician can treat the patient at College Hospital. Dr. Ulibarri is accepting assignment on this TRICARE Extra case. This patient met her deductible last November when seen by a previous physician.

2. Refer to Chapter 7 (Figure 7–12) of the *Handbook* for instructions on how to complete this claim form and to view a TRICARE template.

3. Use your CPT code book or Appendix A in this *Workbook* to determine the correct five-digit code number and modifiers for each professional service rendered. Use your HCPCS Level II code book or refer to Appendix B in this *Workbook* for HCPCS procedure codes and modifiers.

4. Record the proper information on the financial record and claim form and note the date when you have billed TRICARE Extra.

5. A Performance Evaluation Checklist may be reproduced from the "Instruction Guide to the *Workbook*" chapter if your instructor wishes you to submit it to assist with scoring and comments.

    After the instructor has returned your work to you, either make the necessary corrections and place your work in a three-ring notebook for future reference or, if you received a high score, place it in your portfolio for reference when applying for a job.

Abbreviations pertinent to this record:

Pt	_____	LC	_____
D	_____	MDM	_____
HX	_____	PF	_____
PX	_____	rec	_____
UA	_____	SF	_____
WBC	_____	C	_____
RBC	_____	M	_____
cc	_____	surg	_____
lab	_____	ofc	_____
Rx	_____	PO	_____
caps	_____	OV	_____
t.i.d.	_____	rtn	_____
Retn	_____	PRN	_____
Dx	_____		

1. Locate a financial accounting record (ledger).

   Note: Refer to the step-by-step procedures at the end of Chapter 3 in the *Handbook* and graphic examples Figures 3–16 and 10–3.

2. Insert the patient's name and address, including ZIP code in the box.

3. Enter the patient's personal data.

4. Ledger lines: Insert date of service (DOS), reference (CPT code number, check number, or dates of service for posting adjustments or when insurance was billed), description of the transaction, charge amounts, payments, adjustments, and running current balance. The posting date is the actual date the transaction is recorded. If the DOS differs from the posting date, list the DOS in the reference or description column.

   Note: A good bookkeeping practice is to take a red pen and draw a line across the financial accounting record (ledger) from left to right to indicate the last entry billed to the insurance company.

PATIENT RECORD NO. 14-5

Drew	Darlene	B	12-22-41	F	555-466-1002
LAST NAME	FIRST NAME	MIDDLE NAME	BIRTH DATE	SEX	HOME PHONE

720 Ganley Street,	Woodland Hills,	XY	12345
ADDRESS	CITY	STATE	ZIP CODE

555-320-9988	555-210-9400	555-466-1002	drew@wb.net
CELL PHONE	PAGER NO.	FAX NO.	E-MAIL ADDRESS

450-XX-3762	H0492188
PATIENT'S SOC. SEC. NO.	DRIVER'S LICENSE

Seamstress	J. B. Talon Company
PATIENT'S OCCUPATION	NAME OF COMPANY

2111 Ventura Road, Merck, XY 12346	555-733-0156
ADDRESS OF EMPLOYER	PHONE

Harry M. Drew	U.S. Navy Lieutenant Commander (L/C), Active Status
SPOUSE OR PARENT	OCCUPATION

Service #221-XX-0711 Social Security No. 221-XX-0711 Grade12	4-15-37
	BIRTH DATE

P.O. Box 2927, A.P.O., New York, New York 09194
ADDRESS

TRICARE Extra	67531	01-01-80
NAME OF INSURANCE	TRICARE EXTRA I.D. CARD NO.	EFFECTIVE DATE

REFERRED BY: James B. Jeffers, MD, 100 S. Broadway, Woodland Hills, XY 12345   Tax ID#77621074X

DATE	PROGRESS NOTES
1-13-xx	New pt comes in complaining of large sore in vagina causing extreme pain. Performed a
	D HX/PX. UA (non-automated with microscopy) loaded with WBCs and RBCs. Upon pelvic
	examination, a very tender mass is located in the paraurethral area (Skene's gland).
	I incised and drained the abscess and obtained 10 cc greenish pus; took culture and sent
	to lab. Pt feels much better. Rx Terramycin 30 caps 1 t.i.d. Retn in 5 days. Dx: Paraurethral
	abscess (LC/MDM).
	GU/llf *Gene Ulibarri, MD*
1-18-xx	Pt returns and a PF HX/PX performed. Abscess is filled with fluid again, opened, and a
	wick of Iodoform gauze placed to help with drainage. Rec daily sitz baths and outpatient
	hospitalization to remove gland. Culture results show pseudomonas organism.
	Arrangements made for surgery on the 24th, admit at 5:30 a.m., surgery at 7:30 a.m.
	(SF MDM).
	GU/llf *Gene Ulibarri, MD*
1-24-xx	Admit to College Hospital outpatient facility (C HX/PX M MDM). Surg: Excision of Skene's
	gland. To be seen in ofc next week for PO exam. Renewed Rx Terramycin.
	GU/llf *Gene Ulibarri, MD*
1-27-xx	PO OV (PF HX/PX SF/MDM). Pt doing well. No pain, urethral tissue and perineum looks
	healthy, healing well. Rtn PRN.
	GU/llf *Gene Ulibarri, MD*

Figure 14–3

Acct No.   14-5

STATEMENT
Financial Account
COLLEGE CLINIC
4567 Broad Avenue
Woodland Hills, XY 12345-0001
Tel. 555-486-9002
Fax No. 555-487-8976

Darlene B. Drew
720 Ganley Street
Woodland Hills, XY 12345

Phone No. (H)   555-466-1002   (W)   555-733-0156   Birthdate   12-22-41

Primary Insurance Co.   TRICARE Extra   Policy/Group No.   221-XX-0711

Secondary Insurance Co.   Policy/Group No.

DATE	REFERENCE	DESCRIPTION	CHARGES	CREDITS PYMNTS.	ADJ.	BALANCE
20xx		BALANCE FORWARD ➡				
1-13-xx		NP OV				
1-13-xx		UA				
1-13-xx		Drainage of Skene's gland abscess				
1-13-xx		Handling/Transport culture specimen				
1-18-xx		OV				
1-24-xx		Excision Skene's gland				
1-27-xx		PO OV				

PLEASE PAY LAST AMOUNT IN BALANCE COLUMN

THIS IS A COPY OF YOUR FINANCIAL ACCOUNT AS IT APPEARS ON OUR RECORDS

Figure 14–4

ASSIGNMENT 14–6 ▸ COMPLETE THREE CLAIM FORMS FOR A TRICARE STANDARD CASE

Performance Objective

Task: Complete three CMS-1500 (08-05) claim forms for a TRICARE Standard case, post transactions to the financial accounting record, and define patient record abbreviations.

Conditions: Use the patient's record (Figure 14–5) and financial statement (Figure 14–6), health insurance claim forms (print from CD or Evolve website), a typewriter or computer, procedural and diagnostic code books, and appendices A and B in this *Workbook*.

Standards: Claim Productivity Measurement

Time: _____ minutes

Accuracy: _____

(Note: The time element and accuracy criteria may be given by your instructor.)

Directions

1. This case requires three claim forms. Make photocopies of a CMS-1500 (08-05) claim form or print from CD or Evolve website. Using OCR guidelines, complete the CMS-1500 (08-05) claim forms. If your instructor wants you to direct them to your local TRICARE fiscal intermediary, go to website http://www.tricare.osd.mil. Click on the area of the map you are residing in and then choose a state to access claims information for that state. Refer to Mrs. Mae I. Abbreviate's patient record for information and Appendix A in this *Workbook* to locate the fees to record on the claim, and post them to the financial statement. Date the claims January 31. Dr. Coccidioides is not accepting assignment on this TRICARE Standard case but is completing the claim for the patient's convenience.

2. Refer to Chapter 7 (Figure 7–12) of the *Handbook* for instructions on how to complete these claim forms and to view a TRICARE template.

3. Use your CPT code book or Appendix A in this *Workbook* to determine the correct five-digit code number and modifiers for each professional service rendered. Use your HCPCS Level II code book or refer to Appendix B in this *Workbook* for HCPCS procedure codes and modifiers.

4. Record the proper information on the financial record and note the date when you have billed TRICARE.

5. A Performance Evaluation Checklist may be reproduced from the "Instruction Guide to the *Workbook*" chapter if your instructor wishes you to submit it to assist with scoring and comments.

After the instructor has returned your work to you, either make the necessary corrections and place your work in a three-ring notebook for future reference or, if you received a high score, place it in your portfolio for reference when applying for a job.

Abbreviations pertinent to this record:

NP	_____	F	_____
W	_____	P	_____
F	_____	R	_____
PE	_____	EENT	_____
CC	_____	GGE	_____
wk	_____	HC	_____
X	_____	MDM	_____
pt	_____	STAT	_____
PH	_____	CBC	_____
UCHD	_____	diff	_____
T & A	_____	WBC	_____
aet	_____	RTO	_____
Grav	_____	RTW	_____
Para1	_____	CT	_____
D & C	_____	dx	_____
DUB	_____	a.m.	_____
LMP	_____	D	_____
surg	_____	HX	_____
OS	_____	MC	_____
yr	_____	cm	_____
FH	_____	lt	_____
CA	_____	C & S	_____
L & W	_____	gm	_____
GB	_____	mg	_____
SH	_____	IM	_____
PX	_____	retn	_____
ht	_____	ofc	_____
wt	_____	OV	_____
lbs	_____	PF	_____
BP	_____	SF	_____
T	_____	HC	_____

Additional Coding

1. Refer to Mrs. Abbreviate's medical record, abstract information, and code procedures that would be billed by outside providers.

Site	*Description of Service*	*Code*
a. College Hospital Radiology	_____	_____
b. College Hospital Laboratory	_____	_____
c. College Hospital Laboratory	_____	_____
d. College Hospital Radiology	_____	_____
e. College Hospital Microbiology	_____	_____
f. College Hospital Radiology	_____	_____

2. Use your diagnostic code book and code the symptoms that the patient complained of on January 14, 20xx.

Symptom	*Code*
a. _____	_____
b. _____	_____
c. _____	_____
d. _____	_____

3. Locate a financial accounting record (ledger).

   Note: Refer to the step-by-step procedures at the end of Chapter 3 in the *Handbook* and graphic examples Figures 3–16 and 10–3.

4. Insert the patient's name and address, including ZIP code in the box.

5. Enter the patient's personal data.

6. Ledger lines: Insert date of service (DOS), reference (CPT code number, check number, or dates of service for posting adjustments or when insurance was billed), description of the transaction, charge amounts, payments, adjustments, and running current balance. The posting date is the actual date the transaction is recorded. If the DOS differs from the posting date, list the DOS in the reference or description column.

   Note: A good bookkeeping practice is to take a red pen and draw a line across the financial accounting record (ledger) from left to right to indicate the last entry billed to the insurance company.

PATIENT RECORD NO. 14-6

Abbreviate	Mae	I		01-02-42	F	555-986-7667
LAST NAME	FIRST NAME	MIDDLE NAME		BIRTH DATE	SEX	HOME PHONE

4667 Symbol Road	Woodland Hills	XY	12345
ADDRESS	CITY	STATE	ZIP CODE

555-740-3300		555-986-7667	abbreviate@wb.net
CELL PHONE	PAGER NO.	FAX NO.	E-MAIL ADDRESS

865-XX-2311	E0598247
PATIENT'S SOC. SEC. NO.	DRIVER'S LICENSE

administrative assistant	U. R. Wright Company
PATIENT'S OCCUPATION	NAME OF COMPANY

6789 Abridge Road, Woodland Hills, XY 12346	555-988-7540
ADDRESS OF EMPLOYER	PHONE

Shorty S. Abbreviate	Staff Sargeant, Grade 12 (Active Duty)
SPOUSE OR PARENT	OCCUPATION

United States Army	HHC, 2nd Batt., 27th Infantry, APO New York, New York, 10030	PHONE
EMPLOYER	ADDRESS	

TRICARE Standard	husband (DOB 3/25/40)
NAME OF INSURANCE	INSURED OR SUBSCRIBER

023-XX-7866	
POLICY/CERTIFICATE NO.	GROUP NO.

REFERRED BY: Jane B. Accurate (friend)

Figure 14–5a

DATE	PROGRESS NOTES No. 14-6
1-14-xx	NP, 45-year-old W F in for complete PE. CC: Recent onset of flu-like symptoms of
	approximate 2 wk duration, including cough; chest pain X 2 days. Pt states beginning to
	cough up moderate amounts of greenish sputum with blood streaks, fatigue, fever, and chills.
	Comprehensive history includes PH: UCHD, T & A aet 6, Grav 1 Para 1, D & C aet 41 for
	DUB, LMP 12-18-XX, surg on OS after accident last yr. FH: Father expired of kidney CA aet
	63; mother L & W after GB surg in 1999; no siblings. SH: Pt admits to past alcohol abuse,
	denies alcohol use in last 6 months. No smoking, denies drug abuse. Comprehensive PX:
	Ht 5' 7", wt 150 lbs, BP 150/80, T 100.5 F, P 88, R 18; EENT ō except OS opaque;
	chest, rales scattered bilaterally, pt is dyspneic. Abdomen soft, nontender.
	GGE (HC MDM). Pt would like to avoid hospitalization if at all possible. Sent to College
	Hospital for STAT chest x-ray (2 views) and laboratory tests (electrolyte panel and complete
	CBC, automated with diff WBC. RTO tomorrow morning for test results. Disability from work began Jan. 13
	Completed disability form for work; estimated RTW, 2 weeks.
	BC/llf *Brady Coccicioides, MD*
1-14-xx	Call received from hospital radiology department: Chest x-rays revealed probable lung
	abscess in left lower lobe; inconclusive. Ordered STAT CT of thorax without contrast for
	more definitive dx. Contacted pt and recommended she have CT done this evening.
	RTO tomorrow a.m.
	BC/llf *Brady Coccicioides, MD*
1-15-xx	Pt returns to office for test results (D HX/PX MC/MDM). CT reveals lung abscess of
	3.0 cm in lt lower lobe. Pt able to produce sputum for C & S (Gram stain smear), sent to
	College Hospital laboratory, microbiology department. Rocephin (Ceftriaxone sodium)
	1 gm ($5 per 250 mg and 1000 mg = 1 gm) given IM in office, instructed pt to retn to ofc daily
	for Rocephin injections; reevaluate on Friday.
	BC/llf *Brady Coccicioides, MD*
1-16-xx	Rocephin 1 gm IM ordered by Dr. Coccicioides; administered by medical assistant in left
	gluteus maximus.
	BC/llf *Ali Marie Hobkins, CMA*
1-17-xx	Rocephin 1 gm IM ordered by Dr. Coccicioides; administered by medical assistant in right
	gluteus maximus.
	BC/llf *Ali Marie Hobkins, CMA*
1-18-xx	Pt returns for reevaluation (OV PF HX/PX SF MDM). Culture revealed streptococcal
	pneumoniae. Administered Rocephin 1 gm IM. Will continue daily injections.
	Arrangements made for house call over weekend.
	BC/llf *Brady Coccicioides, MD*
1-19-xx	HC Saturday (PF HX/PX SF MDM). Rocephin 1 gm IM. Pt states she is feeling much
	better, fatigue gone, cough decreased, afebrile. Ordered repeat chest x-ray (2 views) at
	College Hospital Monday. RTO Monday afternoon.
	BC/llf *Brady Coccicioides, MD*
1-21-xx	OV (PF HX/PX SF MDM). Repeat chest x-ray negative except few residual shadows.
	No injection today, start oral antibiotics. Pt to return in 1 wk for f/u or call sooner if
	symptoms reappear. Estimated RTW, 1/28/XX.
	BC/llf *Brady Coccicioides, MD*

Figure 14–5b

STATEMENT
Financial Account
COLLEGE CLINIC
4567 Broad Avenue
Woodland Hills, XY 12345-0001
Tel. 555-486-9002
Fax No. 555-487-8976

Mae I. Abbreviate
4667 Symbol Road
Woodland Hills, XY 12345

Phone No. (H) ___555-986-7667___ (W) ___555-988-7540___ Birthdate __01/02/42__

Primary Insurance Co. ___TRICARE Standard___ Policy/Group No. 023-XX-7866

Secondary Insurance Co._____ Policy/Group No._____

DATE	REFERENCE	DESCRIPTION	CHARGES	CREDITS		BALANCE
				PYMNTS.	ADJ.	
20xx			BALANCE FORWARD ➔			
1-14-xx		NP OV				
1-15-xx		OV				
1-15-xx		Injection AB				
1-15-xx		Rocefin 1 gm				
1-16-xx		Injection AB				
1-16-xx		Rocefin 1 gm				
1-17-xx		Injection AB				
1-17-xx		Rocefin 1 gm				
1-18-xx		OV				
1-18-xx		Injection AB				
1-18-xx		Rocefin 1 gm				
1-19-xx		HC				
1-19-xx		Injection AB				
1-19-xx		Rocefin 1 gm				
1-21-xx		OV				

PLEASE PAY LAST AMOUNT IN BALANCE COLUMN

THIS IS A COPY OF YOUR FINANCIAL ACCOUNT AS IT APPEARS ON OUR RECORDS

Figure 14–6

ASSIGNMENT FOR TRICARE CASE 7 ONSCREEN COMPLETION OF CMS-1500 (08-05) INSURANCE CLAIM FORM

Performance Objective

Task: Enter transactions from patient's onscreen encounter form (superbill) and complete block-by-block onscreen health insurance claim form

Conditions: Onscreen encounter form (superbill) and computer

Standards: Time: _____ minutes

                  Accuracy: _____

                  (Note: The time element and accuracy criteria may be given by your instructor.)

Directions. Before attempting the assignment, refer to *Workbook* Appendix C and follow the instructions provided to familiarize yourself with the Student Software Challenges section of the software. Then insert the CD that accompanies the *Workbook* into the computer disk drive.

1. For this assignment, follow the instructions for entering data into the onscreen CMS-1500 (08-05) health insurance claim form, completing blocks 1 through 33 for Case 7.

2. Use your CPT code book or Appendix A in this *Workbook* to determine the correct five-digit code number and modifiers for each professional service rendered.

3. A Performance Evaluation Checklist may be reproduced from the "Instruction Guide to the *Workbook*" chapter if your instructor wishes you to submit it to assist with scoring and comments.

4. Print a hard copy of the completed health insurance claim form.

5. After the instructor has returned your work to you, either make the necessary corrections and place your work in a three-ring notebook for future reference, or, if you received a high score, place it in your portfolio for reference when applying for a job.

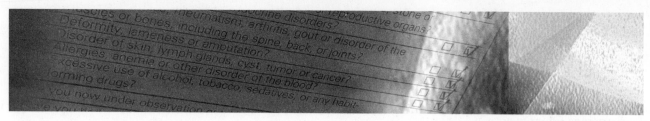

Workers'
Compensation

KEY TERMS

Your instructor may wish to select some words pertinent to this chapter for a test. For definitions of the terms, further study, and/or reference, the words, phrases, and abbreviations may be found in the glossary at the end of the Handbook. *Key terms for this chapter follow.*

accident

adjudication

by report (BR)

claims examiner

compromise and release (C and R)

deposition

ergonomic

extraterritorial

Federal Employees' Compensation Act (FECA)

fee schedule

injury

insurance adjuster

lien

medical service order

nondisability (ND) claim

occupational illness (or disease)

Occupational Safety and Health Administration (OSHA)

permanent and stationary (P and S)

permanent disability (PD)

petition

second-injury fund

sequelae

sub rosa films

subsequent-injury fund (SIF)

temporary disability (TD)

third-party liability

third-party subrogation

waiting period (WP)

work hardening

Workers' Compensation Appeals Board (WCAB)

workers' compensation (WC) insurance

KEY ABBREVIATIONS

See how many abbreviations and acronyms you can translate and then use this as a handy reference list. Definitions for the key abbreviations are located near the back of the Handbook *in the glossary.*

AME _____

BR _____

C and R _____

ERISA _____

FECA _____

HMO _____

IAIABC _____

IME _____

LHWCA _____

MSDS _____

ND _____

OSHA _____

P and S _____

PD _____

PPO _____

QME _____

ROM _____

SIF _____

TD _____

WC _____

WCAB _____

WP _____

PERFORMANCE OBJECTIVES

The student will be able to:

- Define and spell the key terms and key abbreviations for this chapter, given the information from the *Handbook* glossary, within a reasonable time period and with enough accuracy to obtain a satisfactory evaluation.
- After reading the chapter, answer the fill-in-the-blanks, multiple choice, and true/false review questions with enough accuracy to obtain a satisfactory evaluation.
- Given a list of common medical abbreviations and symbols that appear in chart notes, fill in the correct meaning of each abbreviation within a reasonable time period and with enough accuracy to obtain a satisfactory evaluation.

- Given the patients' medical chart notes, ledger cards, and blank insurance forms, complete each workers' compensation form for billing, within a reasonable time period and with enough accuracy to obtain a satisfactory evaluation.
- Given the patients' medical chart notes, ledger cards, and blank insurance claim forms, complete each CMS-1500 (08-05) Health Insurance Claim Form for submission to a workers' compensation insurance company within a reasonable time period and with enough accuracy to obtain a satisfactory evaluation.
- Using the Mock Fee Schedule in Appendix A in this *Workbook*, correctly post payments, adjustments, and balances on the patients' ledger cards within a reasonable time period and with enough accuracy to obtain a satisfactory evaluation.

STUDY OUTLINE

History
   Workers' Compensation Statutes
   Workers' Compensation Reform
Workers' Compensation Laws and Insurance
   Purposes of Workers' Compensation Laws
   Self-Insurance
   Managed Care
Eligibility
   Industrial Accident
   Occupational Illness
Coverage
   Federal Laws

State Laws
State Disability and Workers' Compensation
Benefits
Types of State Claims
   Nondisability Claim
   Temporary Disability Claim
   Permanent Disability Claim
Fraud and Abuse
Occupational Safety and Health Administration Act of 1970
   Background
   Coverage

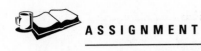

ASSIGNMENT 15-1 ► REVIEW QUESTIONS

Part I Fill in the Blank

Review the objectives, key terms, glossary definitions of key terms, chapter information, and figures before completing the following review questions.

1. Name two kinds of statutes under workers' compensation.

P18

a. _federal comp laws_

b. _State comp laws_

2. An unexpected, unintended event that occurs at a particular time and place, causing injury to an individual not of his or her own making, is called a/an

P20

accident

3. Maria Cardoza works in a plastics manufacturing company and inhales some fumes that cause bronchitis. Because this condition is associated with her employment, it is called a/an

P20

occupational illness or disease

4. Name the federal workers' compensation acts that cover workers.

a. _Workmens comp law of the District of Columbia_

b. _Federal coal mine Health & Safety act_

c. _Federal Comp Employees Comp Act_

d. _Longshoremens & Harbor Workers Comp act_

5. State compensation laws that require each employer to accept its provisions and provide for specialized benefits for employees who are injured at work are called

State workers Comp insurance

6. State compensation laws that may be accepted or rejected by the employer are known as

P21

compulsory

7. State five methods used for funding workers' compensation.

a. _monopolistic state_

b. _provincial fund_

c. _territorial fund_

P21

d. _competitive state fund_

e. _private insurance company_

8. Who pays the workers' compensation insurance premiums? *Company*

9. What is the time limit in your state for submitting the employers' and/or physicians' report on an industrial accident?

   w/in 7 days

10. When an employee with a preexisting condition is injured at work and the injury produces a disability greater than what would have been caused by the second injury alone, the benefits are derived from a/an

    2nd injury fund.

11. Name jobs that may not be covered by workers' compensation insurance.

    a. *Army*

    b. *Navy*

    c. *Marines*

    d. *Coast Guard*

    e. *Air line pilot*

    f. *Singer*

12. What is the minimum number of employees per business needed in your state for workers' compensation statutes to become effective? *1*

13. What waiting period must elapse in your state before workers' compensation payments begin? *7 days*

14. List five types of workers' compensation benefits.

    a. *Medical treatment*

    b. *Temporary disability indemnity*

    c. *Permanent disability indemnity*

    d. *Death benefits for Survivors*

    e. *rehab benefits*

15. Who can treat an industrial injury?

    Dr approved by workmans Comp Dr

16. What are three types of workers' compensation claims and the differences among them?

    a. *Nondisability claim - involves minor injury, the patient has been seen by a Dr & is allowed to continue to work*

[handwritten margin note: P525-526]

b. temporary disability - a worker has been injured on the job ~~is unallowed &~~ is unable ~~to~~ work for a set period of time

c. permanent disability - a worker has been injured on the job & is unable & not allowed medically to ever return to work

17. Weekly temporary disability payments are based on

[handwritten margin note: P527] ~~the job they were~~ the rating of the case ~~doing when they became disabled~~

18. After suffering an industrial injury, Mr. Fields is in a treatment program in which he is given real work tasks for building strength and endurance. This form of therapy is

[handwritten margin note: P526] called _work hardening_ .

19. When an industrial case reaches the time for rating the disability, this is accomplished

by _the workers comp board_ .

20. May an injured person appeal his or her case if he or she is not satisfied with the

rating? _yes_   If so, to whom does he or she appeal? _WCAB_

[handwritten margin note: P527] or _Industrial Accident Commission_

21. When fraud or abuse is suspected in a workers' compensation case, the physician

should report the situation to ~~Department~~ _workmans comp insurance carrier_

22. Explain third-party subrogation

to substitute 1 person for another

23. When an individual suffers a work-related injury or illness, the employer must

complete and send a form called a/an _Employers Report of Occupational Injury or illness form_ ~~employees claim for workers comp benefits~~
to the insurance company and workers' compensation state offices, and if the employee
is sent to a physician's office for medical care, the employer must complete a form called

a/an _medical service order_, which authorizes the physician to treat the employee.

Part II Multiple Choice

Choose the best answer.

24. Employers are required to meet health and safety standards for their employees under federal and state statutes known as

    a. Occupational Safety and Health Administration (OSHA) Act of 1970

    b. Health Insurance Portability and Accountability Act (HIPAA)

    c. Clinical Laboratory Improvement Amendment (CLIA)

    d. Employee Retirement Income Security Act (ERISA)

25. The process of carrying on a lawsuit is called

    a. lien

    b. litigation

    c. deposition

    d. adjudication

26. A proceeding during which an attorney questions a witness who answers under oath but not in open court is called a/an

    a. subpoena

    b. subrogation

    c. petition

    d. deposition

27. The legal promise of a patient to satisfy a debt to the physician from proceeds received from a litigated case is termed a/an

    a. medical service order

    b. subpoena

    c. lien

    d. promissory note

28. When a physician treats an industrial injury, he or she must complete a First Treatment Medical Report or Doctor's First Report of Occupational Injury or Illness and send it to the following:

    a. insurance carrier

    b. employer

    c. state workers' compensation office

    d. all of the above

Part III True/False

Write "T" or "F" in the blank to indicate whether you think the statement is true or false.

___T___ 29. The first thing an employee should do after he or she is injured on the job is to notify his or her employer or immediate supervisor.

___F___ 30. A roofer takes his girlfriend to a roofing job and she is injured. She is covered under workers' compensation insurance.

___T___ 31. A stamped physician's signature is acceptable on the Doctor's First Report of Occupational Injury or Illness form.

___F___ 32. In a workers' compensation case, bills should be submitted monthly or at the time of termination of treatment, and a claim becomes delinquent after a time frame of 45 days.

___T___ 33. If an individual seeks medical care for a workers' compensation injury from another state, the state's regulations are followed in which the injured person's claim was originally filed.

ASSIGNMENT **15–2** ▸ **COMPLETE A DOCTOR'S FIRST REPORT OF OCCUPATIONAL INJURY OR ILLNESS FORM FOR A WORKERS' COMPENSATION CASE**

Performance Objective

Task:	Complete a Doctor's First Report of Occupational Injury or Illness form and define patient record abbreviations.
Conditions:	Use the patient's record (Figure 15–1), a Doctor's First Report of Occupational Injury or Illness form (Figure 15–2), and a typewriter or computer.
Standards:	Claim Productivity Measurement

Time: _____ minutes

Accuracy: _____

(Note: The time element and accuracy criteria may be given by your instructor.)

Directions

1. Complete the Doctor's First Report of Occupational Injury or Illness form (Figure 15–2) for this nondisability type of claim.

2. Define abbreviations found in the patient's medical record.

After the instructor has returned your work to you, either make the necessary corrections and place your work in a three-ring notebook for future reference or, if you received a high score, place it in your portfolio for reference when applying for a job.

Abbreviations pertinent to this record:

Apt	_____	CT	_____
Lt	_____	Neg	_____
pt	_____	MC	_____
ED	_____	MDM	_____
Hosp	_____	DC	_____
ER	_____	PD	_____
C	_____	FU	_____
HX	_____	Wks	_____
PX	_____	Approx	_____
c/o	_____	RTW	_____
L	_____	WC	_____

PATIENT RECORD NO. 15-2-3

Hiranuma	Glen	M	12-24-45	M	555-467-3383
LAST NAME	FIRST NAME	MIDDLE NAME	BIRTH DATE	SEX	HOME PHONE

4372 Hanley Avenue	Woodland Hills	XY	12345
ADDRESS	CITY	STATE	ZIP CODE

555-908-3433		555-467-3383		hiranuma@wb.net
CELL PHONE	PAGER NO.	FAX NO.		E-MAIL ADDRESS

558-XX-9960	U3402189
PATIENT'S SOC. SEC. NO.	DRIVER'S LICENSE

house painter	Pittsburgh Paint Company (commercial painting company)
PATIENT'S OCCUPATION	NAME OF COMPANY

3725 Bonfeld Avenue, Woodland Hills, XY 12345	555-486-9070
ADDRESS OF EMPLOYER	PHONE

Esme M. Hiranuma	homemaker
SPOUSE OR PARENT	OCCUPATION

EMPLOYER	ADDRESS	PHONE

State Compensation Insurance Fund, 14156 Magnolia Boulevard, Torres, XY 12349
NAME OF INSURANCE

016-2432-211
POLICY/CERTIFICATE NO.   GROUP NO.

REFERRED BY: Pittsburgh Paint Company

DATE	PROGRESS NOTES
5-22-xx	At 9:30 a.m. this ♂ house painter was painting an apt ceiling (apt located at 3540 W. 87th Street, Woodland Hills, XY 12345, County of Woodland Hills) when he slipped and fell from a tall ladder landing on his head and lt side of body; brief unconsciousness for approximately 15 minutes. Employer was notified by coworker and pt was sent to College Hosp ED. I was called to the hosp at request of employer and saw pt in ER at 5 p.m. (performed a C HX/PX). Pt c/o L shoulder pain and swelling; L leg and hip pain; neck and head pain. X-rays were taken of lt hip (complete), lt femur (2 views), and cervical spine (3 views) as well as CT of brain (without contrast)—all neg. I admitted pt for overnight stay in hosp for concussion. Applied sling for L shoulder sprain. Cleaned and dressed L hip and leg abrasions (MC/MDM). Plan to DC 5/23/xx. No PD expected. Pt to FU in 2 wks. Approx. RTW 6/6 xx. Prepared WC report.
	GP/llf *Gerald Practon, MD*
5-23-xx	Pt's HA gone. Vital signs normal. Discharged home. RTO 1 wk.
	GP/llf *Gerald Practon, MD*

Figure 15–1

DOCTOR'S FIRST REPORT OF OCCUPATIONAL INJURY OR ILLNESS

Within 5 days of initial examination, for every occupational injury or illness, send 2 copies of this report to the employers' workers' compensation insurance carrier or the self-insured employer. Failure to file a timely doctor's report may result in assessment of a civil penalty. In the case of diagnosed or suspected pesticide poisoning, send a copy of this report to Division of Labor Statistics and Research.

1. **INSURER NAME AND ADDRESS**

2. **EMPLOYER NAME**
    Policy No.

3. Address   No. and Street   City   Zip

4. Nature of business(e.g., food manufacturing, building construction, retailer of women's clothes)

5. **PATIENT NAME** (first, middle initial, last name)   6. Sex ☐Male ☐Female   7. Date of Birth   Mo.   Day   Yr.

8. Address   No. and Street   City   Zip   9. Telephone Number

10. Occupation (Specific job title)   11. Social Security Number

12. Injured at: No. and Street   City   County

13. Date and hour of injury or onset or illness   Mo.   Day   Yr.   Hour ____a.m____p.m

14. Date last worked   Mo.   Day   Yr.

15. Date and hour of first examination or treatment   Mo.   Day   Yr.   Hour ____a.m____p.m

16. Have you (or your office) previously treated patient?   ☐Yes   ☐No

Patient please complete this portion, if able to do so. Otherwise, doctor please complete immediately. Inability or failure of a patient to complete this portion shall not affect his/her rights to workers' compensation under the Labor Code. **17. DESCRIBE HOW THE ACCIDENT OR EXPOSURE HAPPENED** (Give specific object, machinery or chemical.)

18. **SUBJECTIVE COMPLAINTS** (Describe fully.)

19. **OBJECTIVE FINDINGS**
    A. Physical examination
    B. X-ray and laboratory results (State if none or pending.)

20. **DIAGNOSIS** (If occupational illness specify etiologic agent and duration of exposure.) Chemical or toxic compound involved?   ICD - 9 Code   ☐Yes ☐No

21. Are your findings and diagnosis consistent with patient's account of injury or onset of illness?   ☐Yes ☐No If "no" please explain

22. Is there any other current condition that will impede or delay patient's recovery?   ☐ Yes   ☐ No   If "yes" please explain

23. **TREATMENT REQUIRED**

24. If further treatment required, specify treatment plan/estimated duration.

25. If hospitalized as inpatient, give hospital name and location   Date admitted   Mo.   Day   Yr.   Estimated stay

26. **WORK STATUS** –Is patient able to perfom usual work?   ☐ Yes   ☐ No
    If "no," date when patient can return to: Regular work___/___/
    Modified work___/___/   Specify restrictions

Doctor's Signature _____   License Number _____
Doctor's Name and Degree_____   IRS Number_____
Address_____   Telephone Number_____

Figure 15–2

ASSIGNMENT 15–3 ▸ COMPLETE A CLAIM FORM FOR A WORKERS' COMPENSATION CASE

Performance Objectives

Task: Complete a CMS-1500 (08-05) claim form for a workers' compensation case and post transactions to the financial accounting record.

Conditions: Use the patient's record (Figure 15–1) and financial statement (Figure 15–3), a CMS-1500 claim form (print from CD or Evolve website), a typewriter or computer, procedural and diagnostic code books, and Appendix A in this *Workbook*.

Standards: Claim Productivity Measurement

Time: _____ minutes

Accuracy: _____

(Note: The time element and accuracy criteria may be given by your instructor.)

Directions

1. Using optical character reader (OCR) guidelines, complete a CMS-1500 (08-05) claim form and direct it to the proper workers' compensation carrier. Refer to Mr. Glen M. Hiranuma's patient record for information and Appendix A in this *Workbook* to locate the fees to record on the claim, and post them to the financial statement. Date the claim May 24 of the current year.

2. Refer to Chapter 7 (Figure 7–14) of the *Handbook* for instructions on how to complete this claim form and a workers' compensation template.

3. Use your CPT code book or Appendix A in this *Workbook* to determine the correct five-digit code number and modifiers for each professional service rendered. Use your HCPCS Level II code book or refer to Appendix B in this *Workbook* for HCPCS procedure codes and modifiers. Note: In your state, a workers' compensation fee schedule may be available with this information.

4. Record the proper information on the financial record and claim form, and note the date you have billed the workers' compensation.

5. A Performance Evaluation Checklist may be reproduced from the "Instruction Guide to the *Workbook*" chapter if your instructor wishes you to submit it to assist with scoring and comments.

After the instructor has returned your work to you, either make the necessary corrections and place your work in a three-ring notebook for future reference or, if you received a high score, place it in your portfolio for reference when applying for a job.

Additional Coding

1. Refer to Mr. Glen M. Hiranuma's medical record, abstract information, and code procedures that would be billed by outside providers.

Site	Description of Service	Code
a. College Hospital Radiology	_____	_____
b. College Hospital Radiology	_____	_____
c. College Hospital Radiology	_____	_____
d. College Hospital Radiology	_____	_____

2. Locate a financial accounting record (ledger).

   Note: Refer to the step-by-step procedures at the end of Chapter 3 in the *Handbook* and graphic examples Figures 3–16 and 10–3.

3. Insert the patient's name and address, including ZIP code in the box.

4. Enter the patient's personal data.

5. Ledger lines: Insert date of service (DOS), reference (CPT code number, check number, or dates of service for posting adjustments or when insurance was billed), description of the transaction, charge amounts, payments, adjustments, and running current balance. The posting date is the actual date the transaction is recorded. If the DOS differs from the posting date, list the DOS in the reference or description column.

   Note: A good bookkeeping practice is to take a red pen and draw a line across the financial accounting record (ledger) from left to right to indicate the last entry billed to the insurance company.

Acct No. 15-2-3

STATEMENT
Financial Account
COLLEGE CLINIC
4567 Broad Avenue
Woodland Hills, XY 12345-0001
Tel. 555-486-9002
Fax No. 555-487-8976

Workers' Compensation

State Compensation Insurance Fund
14156 Magnolia Boulevard
Torres, CY 12349-0218

Patient's Name___Glen M. Hiranuma___

Social Security No. 558-XX-9960

Date of Injury ___5-22-xx___ Employer___Pittsburgh Paint Company___

Policy No. _016-2432-211_

Phone No. (H)_555-467-3383_ Phone No. (W)____555-486-9070___

Claim No._____unassigned_____

DATE	REFERENCE	DESCRIPTION	CHARGES	CREDITS PYMNTS.	ADJ.	BALANCE
20xx			BALANCE FORWARD →			
5-22-xx		Hospital Admit				
5-22-xx		WC Report				
5-23-xx		Discharge				

PLEASE PAY LAST AMOUNT IN BALANCE COLUMN

THIS IS A COPY OF YOUR FINANCIAL ACCOUNT AS IT APPEARS ON OUR RECORDS

Figure 15–3

ASSIGNMENT **15–4** ► **COMPLETE A DOCTOR'S FIRST REPORT OF OCCUPATIONAL INJURY OR ILLNESS FORM FOR A WORKERS' COMPENSATION CASE**

Performance Objective

Task: Complete a Doctor's First Report of Occupational Injury or Illness form and define patient record abbreviations.

Conditions: Use the patient's record (Figure 15–4), a Doctor's First Report of Occupational Injury or Illness form (Figure 15–5), and a typewriter or computer.

Standards: Claim Productivity Measurement

Time: _____ minutes

Accuracy: _____

(Note: The time element and accuracy criteria may be given by your instructor.)

Directions

1. Complete the Doctor's First Report of Occupational Injury or Illness form for this temporary disability type of claim. Refer to Carlos A. Giovanni's patient record for November 11 through November 15.

2. Define abbreviations found in the patient's medical record.

After the instructor has returned your work to you, either make the necessary corrections and place your work in a three-ring notebook for future reference or, if you received a high score, place it in your portfolio for reference when applying for a job.

Abbreviations pertinent to this record:

pt	Patient	H	
ER		MDM	
C		TD	
HX		RTW	
PX		approx	
CT		HV	
R		EPF	
tr		M	
adm		PO	

DC	_____	PF	_____
Hosp	_____	SF	_____
OV	_____	X	_____
LC	_____	adv	_____
HA	_____	trt	_____
BP	_____	reg	_____
RTO	_____	W	_____
Wks	_____	Cons	_____

PATIENT RECORD NO. 15-4-5

Giovanni	Carlos	A	10-24-45	M	555-677-3485
LAST NAME	FIRST NAME	MIDDLE NAME	BIRTH DATE	SEX	HOME PHONE

89 Beaumont Court	Woodland Hills	XY	12345
ADDRESS	CITY	STATE	ZIP CODE

	555-230-7788	555-677-3485	giovannic@wb.net
CELL PHONE	PAGER NO.	FAX NO.	E-MAIL ADDRESS

556-XX-9699	Y0394876
PATIENT'S SOC. SEC. NO.	DRIVER'S LICENSE

TV repairman	Giant Television Co. (TV repair company)
PATIENT'S OCCUPATION	NAME OF COMPANY

8764 Ocean Avenue, Woodland Hills, XY 12345	555-647-8851
ADDRESS OF EMPLOYER	PHONE

Maria B. Giovanni	homemaker
SPOUSE OR PARENT	OCCUPATION

EMPLOYER	ADDRESS	PHONE

State Compensation Insurance Fund, 600 S. Lafayette Park Place, Ehrlich, XY 12350
NAME OF INSURANCE

57780	
POLICY/CERTIFICATE NO.	GROUP NO.

REFERRED BY: Giant Television Company

Figure 15–4

DATE	PROGRESS NOTES

Patient: Giovanni, Carlos A.   Patient Record No. 15-04-05

11-11-xx — Pt referred to College Hospital ER by employer for workers' compensation injury. I was called in as on-call neurosurgeon to evaluate the pt. Pt states that today at 2 p.m. he fell from the roof of a private home while installing an antenna at 2231 Duarte St., Woodland Hills, XY 12345 in Woodland Hills County. He describes the incident as follows: "When I was attaching the base of an antenna, the weight of the antenna shifted and knocked me off the roof." Pt complains of head pain and indicates brief loss of consciousness. I performed a C HX/PX. Complete skull x-rays showed fractured skull. CT of head/brain (without contrast) indicates well-defined R. subdural hematoma. Pt suffering from cerebral concussion; no open wound. Tr plan: Adm pt to College Hospital (5 p.m.) and schedule R infratentorial craniotomy to evacuate hematoma. (H/MDM). Obtained authorization and prepared Dr.'s First Report.
AP/llf   *Astro Parkinson, MD*

11-12-xx — Performed R infratentorial craniotomy and evacuated subdural hematoma. Pt stable and returned to room; will be seen daily. TD: Estimated RTW 1-15-xx. Possible cranial defect & head disfigurement resulting. Pt to be hospitalized for approx 2 weeks.
AP/llf   *Astro Parkinson, MD*

11-13-xx — HV (EPF HX/PX M/MDM). Pt improving; recommend consult with Dr. Graff for cranial defect. Authorization obtained from adjuster (Steve Burroughs) at State Comp.
AP/llf   *Astro Parkinson, MD*

11-14-xx — Pt seen in cons by Dr. Cosmo Graff who stated he does not recommend correcting PO cranial defect. Both Dr. Graff and I explained how the defect resulted from the injury; there may be some improvement over time. Pt states he is grateful to be alive (EPF HX/PX M/MDM).
AP/llf   *Astro Parkinson, MD*

11-15-xx thru 11-29-xx — Daily HV (EPF HX/PX M/MDM). Pt progressing appropriately; no complications have occurred.
AP/llf   *Astro Parkinson, MD*

11-30-xx — DC from hosp. Permanent cranial defect resulting from fracture and surgery. RTO 1 wk.
AP/llf   *Astro Parkinson, MD*

12-7-xx — OV (EPF HX/PX LC/MDM) Pt doing very well. No HA or visual disturbances, BP 120/80, alert and oriented. He is anxious to return to work. Pt cautioned about maintaining low activity level until released. RTO 2 wks.
AP/llf   *Astro Parkinson, MD*

12-21-xx — OV (PF HX/PX SF/MDM). Pt continues to improve. Suggested he start a walking program 3 x wk and monitor symptoms. May do light activity and lifting (10 lbs). Adv to call if any symptoms return. RTO 10 days.
AP/llf   *Astro Parkinson, MD*

12-29-xx — OV (PF HX/PX SF/MDM). Pt did not experience any symptoms with increased activity. No further trt necessary. Pt will increase activity and call if any problems occur. Pt scheduled to resume reg W on 1-15-xx. Final report submitted to workers' compensation carrier.
AP/llf   *Astro Parkinson, MD*

Figure 15–4, cont'd

DOCTOR'S FIRST REPORT OF OCCUPATIONAL INJURY OR ILLNESS

Within 5 days of initial examination, for every occupational injury or illness, send 2 copies of this report to the employers' workers' compensation insurance carrier or the self-insured employer. Failure to file a timely doctor's report may result in assessment of a civil penalty. In the case of diagnosed or suspected pesticide poisoning, send a copy of this report to Division of Labor Statistics and Research.

1. INSURER NAME AND ADDRESS

2. EMPLOYER NAME

Policy No.

3. Address   No. and Street   City   Zip

4. Nature of business(e.g., food manufacturing, building construction, retailer of woman's clothes)

5. PATIENT NAME (first, middle initial, last name)	6. Sex ☐Male ☐Female	7. Date of mo. Day Yr. Birth
8. Address No. and Street City Zip		9. Telephone Number
10. Occupation (Specific job title)		11. Social Security Number
12. Injured at: No. and Street City		County
13. Date and hour of injury or onset or illness Mo. Day Yr. Hour ____a.m____p.m		14. Date last worked Mo. Day Yr.
15. Date and hour of first examination or treatment Mo. Day Yr. Hour ____a.m____p.m		16. Have you (or your office) previously treated patient? ☐ Yes ☐ No

Patient please complete this portion, if able to do so. Otherwise, doctor please complete immediately. Inability or failure of a patient to complete this portion shall not affect his/her rights to workers' compensation under the Labor Code.
17. DESCRIBE HOW THE ACCIDENT OR EXPOSURE HAPPENED (Give specific object, machinery or chemical.)

18. SUBJECTIVE COMPLAINTS (Describe fully.)

19. OBJECTIVE FINDINGS

A. Physical examination

B. X-ray and laboratory results (State if none or pending.)

20. DIAGNOSIS (if occupational illness specify etiologic agent and duration of exposure.) Chemical or toxic compound involved?   ICD - 9 Code   ☐ Yes ☐No

21. Are your findings and diagnosis consistent with patient's account of injury or onset of illness?   ☐ Yes ☐ No If "no" please explain

22. Is there any other current condition that will impede or delay patient's recovery?   ☐ Yes   ☐ No   If "yes" please explain

23. TREATMENT REQUIRED

24. If further treatment required, specify treatment plan/estimated duration.

25. If hospitalized as inpatient, give hospital name and location   Date admitted   Mo.   Day   Yr.   Estimated stay

26. WORK STATUS –is patient able to perfom usual work?   ☐ Yes   ☐ No
If "no," date when patient can return to: Regular work___/___/
Modified work___/___/   Specify restrictions

Doctor's Signature _____   License Number _____
Doctor's Name and Degree_____   IRS Number_____
Address _____   Telephone Number _____

Figure 15–5

ASSIGNMENT 15-5 ▸ COMPLETE A CLAIM FORM FOR A WORKERS' COMPENSATION CASE

Performance Objective

Task: Complete a CMS-1500 (08-05) claim form for a workers' compensation case and post transactions to the financial accounting record.

Conditions: Use the patient's record (Figure 15–4) and financial statement (Figure 15–6), a CMS-1500 (08-05) claim form (print from CD or Evolve website), a typewriter or computer, procedural and diagnostic code books, and Appendix A in this *Workbook*.

Standards: Claim Productivity Measurement

                Time: _____ minutes

                Accuracy: _____

                (Note: The time element and accuracy criteria may be given by your instructor.)

Directions

1. Using OCR guidelines, complete a CMS-1500 (08-05) claim form for November dates of service and direct it to the correct workers' compensation carrier for this temporary disability workers' compensation claim. Refer to Mr. Carlos A. Giovanni's patient record for information and Appendix A in this *Workbook* to locate the fees to record on the claim and post to the financial statement. Date the claim November 30 of the current year.

   Note: A progress report is being submitted with this claim; services for December will be billed on a separate claim (see Assignment 15–6).

2. Refer to Chapter 7 (Figure 7–14) of the *Handbook* for instructions on how to complete this claim form and a workers' compensation template.

3. Use your CPT code book or Appendix A in this *Workbook* to determine the correct five-digit code number and modifiers for each professional service rendered. Use your HCPCS Level II code book or refer to Appendix B in this *Workbook* for HCPCS procedure codes and modifiers.

4. Record the proper information on the financial record and claim form, and note the date you have billed the workers' compensation insurance carrier.

5. A Performance Evaluation Checklist may be reproduced from the "Instruction Guide to the *Workbook*" chapter if your instructor wishes you to submit it to assist with scoring and comments.

   After the instructor has returned your work to you, either make the necessary corrections and place your work in a three-ring notebook for future reference or, if you received a high score, place it in your portfolio for reference when applying for a job.

Additional Coding

1. Refer to Mr. Giovanni's medical record, abstract information, and code procedures that would be billed by outside providers.

Site	Description of Service	Code
a. College Hospital Radiology	_____	_____
b. College Hospital Radiology	_____	_____

2. Locate a financial accounting record (ledger).

   Note: Refer to the step-by-step procedures at the end of Chapter 3 in the *Handbook* and graphic examples Figures 3–16 and 10–3.

3. Insert the patient's name and address, including ZIP code in the box.

4. Enter the patient's personal data.

5. Ledger lines: Insert date of service (DOS), reference (CPT code number, check number, or dates of service for posting adjustments or when insurance was billed), description of the transaction, charge amounts, payments, adjustments, and running current balance. The posting date is the actual date the transaction is recorded. If the DOS differs from the posting date, list the DOS in the reference or description column.

   Note: A good bookkeeping practice is to take a red pen and draw a line across the financial accounting record (ledger) from left to right to indicate the last entry billed to the insurance company.

Acct No. ___15-5___

STATEMENT
Financial Account
COLLEGE CLINIC
4567 Broad Avenue
Woodland Hills, XY 12345-0001
Tel. 555-486-9002
Fax No. 555-487-8976

Workers' Compensation

State Compensation Insurance Fund
14156 Magnolia Boulevard
Torres, CY 12349-0218

Patient's Name___Carlos A. Giovanni_____   Social Security No. ___556-XX9699___

Date of Injury___11-11-20xx___ Employer ___Giant Television Company_____   Policy No. ___57780_____

Phone No. (H)_555-677-3485____ Phone No. (W) _____555-647-8851_____   Claim No. ___unassigned_____

DATE	REFERENCE	DESCRIPTION	CHARGES	CREDITS		BALANCE
				PYMNTS.	ADJ.	
20xx		BALANCE FORWARD ➡				
11-11-xx		Hospital admit				
11-11-xx		WC Report				
11-12-xx		Craniotomy				
11-13 to 11-29-xx		HV				
11-30-xx		Discharge				
12-7-xx		OV				
12-21-xx		OV				
12-29-xx		OV				
12-29-xx		Medical Report				

PLEASE PAY LAST AMOUNT IN BALANCE COLUMN

THIS IS A COPY OF YOUR FINANCIAL ACCOUNT AS IT APPEARS ON OUR RECORDS

Figure 15–6

ASSIGNMENT 15–6 ▸ COMPLETE A CLAIM FORM FOR A WORKERS' COMPENSATION CASE

Performance Objective

Task: Complete a CMS-1500 (08-05) claim form for a workers' compensation case and post transactions to the financial accounting record.

Conditions: Use the patient's record (Figure 15–4) and financial statement (Figure 15–6), a CMS-1500 (08-05) claim form (print from CD or Evolve website), a typewriter or computer, procedural and diagnostic code books, and Appendix A in this *Workbook*.

Standards: Claim Productivity Measurement

Time: _____ minutes

Accuracy:_____

(Note: The time element and accuracy criteria may be given by your instructor.)

Directions

1. Using OCR guidelines, complete a CMS-1500 (08-05) claim form for December services and direct it to the correct workers' compensation carrier for this temporary disability workers' compensation claim. Refer to Mr. Carlos A. Giovanni's patient record for information and Appendix A in this *Workbook* to locate the fees to record on the claim, and post them to the financial statement. Date the claim December 29 of the current year.

2. Refer to Chapter 7 (Figure 7–14) of the *Handbook* for instructions on how to complete this claim form and a workers' compensation template.

3. Use your CPT code book or Appendix A in this *Workbook* to determine the correct five-digit code number and modifiers for each professional service rendered. Use your HCPCS Level II code book or refer to Appendix B in this *Workbook* for HCPCS procedure codes and modifiers.

4. Record the proper information on the financial record and claim form, and note the date you have billed the workers' compensation insurance carrier.

5. A Performance Evaluation Checklist may be reproduced from the "Instruction Guide to the *Workbook*" chapter if your instructor wishes you to submit it to assist with scoring and comments.

After the instructor has returned your work to you, either make the necessary corrections and place your work in a three-ring notebook for future reference or, if you received a high score, place it in your portfolio for reference when applying for a job.

6. Ledger lines: Insert date of service (DOS), reference (CPT code number, check number, or dates of service for posting adjustments or when insurance was billed), description of the transaction, charge amounts, payments, adjustments, and running current balance. The posting date is the actual date the transaction is recorded. If the DOS differs from the posting date, list the DOS in the reference or description column.

Note: A good bookkeeping practice is to take a red pen and draw a line across the financial accounting record (ledger) from left to right to indicate the last entry billed to the insurance company.

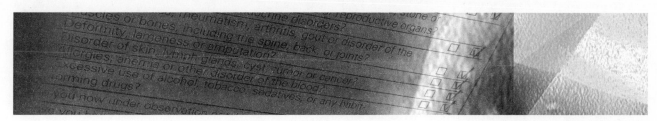

Disability Income Insurance and Disability Benefits Programs

KEY TERMS

Your instructor may wish to select some words pertinent to this chapter for a test. For definitions of the terms, further study, and/or reference, the words, phrases, and abbreviations may be found in the glossary at the end of the Handbook. *Key terms for this chapter follow.*

Some of the insurance terms presented in this chapter are shown marked with an asterisk (*) and may seem familiar from previous chapters. However, their meanings may or may not have a slightly different connotation when referring to disability income insurance. Key terms for this chapter follow.

accidental death and dismemberment

Armed Services Disability

benefit period*

Civil Service Retirement System (CSRS)

consultative examiner (CE)

cost-of-living adjustment

Disability Determination Services (DDS)

disability income insurance

double indemnity

exclusions*

Federal Employees Retirement System (FERS)

future purchase option

guaranteed renewable*

hearing

long-term disability insurance

noncancelable clause*

partial disability*

reconsideration

regional office (RO)

residual benefits*

residual disability

short-term disability insurance

Social Security Administration (SSA)

Social Security Disability Insurance (SSDI) program

State Disability Insurance (SDI)

supplemental benefits

Supplemental Security Income (SSI)

temporary disability*

temporary disability insurance (TDI)

total disability*

unemployment compensation disability (UCD)

Veterans Affairs (VA) disability program

Veterans Affairs (VA) outpatient clinic card

voluntary disability insurance

waiting period*

waiver of premium*

KEY ABBREVIATIONS

See how many abbreviations and acronyms you can translate and then use this as a handy reference list. Definitions for the key abbreviations are located near the back of the Handbook *in the glossary.*

AIDS _____

CSRS _____

CE _____

DDS _____

FERS _____

HIV _____

OASDHI _____

RO _____

SDI _____

SSA _____

SSDI _____

SSI _____

TDI _____

UCD _____

VA _____

PERFORMANCE OBJECTIVES

The student will be able to:

■ Define and spell the key terms and key abbreviations for this chapter, given the information from the *Handbook* glossary, within a reasonable time period, and with enough accuracy to obtain a satisfactory evaluation.

■ After reading the chapter, answer the fill-in-the-blank, multiple choice, and true/false review questions with enough accuracy to obtain a satisfactory evaluation.

■ Fill in the correct meaning of each abbreviation, given a list of common medical abbreviations and symbols that appear in chart notes, within a reasonable time period and with enough accuracy to obtain a satisfactory evaluation.

■ Complete each state disability form, given the patients' medical chart notes and blank state disability forms, within a reasonable time period and with enough accuracy to obtain a satisfactory evaluation.

STUDY OUTLINE

Disability Claims
History
Disability Income Insurance
   Individual
   Group
Federal Disability Programs
   Workers' Compensation
   Disability Benefit Programs
State Disability Insurance
   Background
   State Programs

Funding
Eligibility
Benefits
Time Limits
Medical Examinations
Restrictions
Voluntary Disability Insurance
Claims Submission Guidelines
   Disability Income Claims
Conclusion

ASSIGNMENT 16–3 ▶ COMPLETE TWO STATE DISABILITY INSURANCE FORMS

Performance Objective

Task: Complete two state disability insurance forms and define patient record abbreviations.

Conditions: Use the patient's record (Figure 16–4), a Doctor's Certificate form (Figure 16–5), a Physician's Supplementary Certificate form (Figure 16–6), and a typewriter or computer.

Standards: Time: _____ minutes

                 Accuracy: _____

                 (Note: The time element and accuracy criteria may be given by your instructor.)

Directions

1. Assume that the Claim Statement of Employee has been completed satisfactorily by Mr. Fred E. Thorndike (Figure 16–4). Complete the Doctor's Certificate form (Figure 16–5) and date it December 2. In completing this portion of the assignment, look at the first entry made by Dr. Practon on November 25 only.

2. Mr. Thorndike returns to see Dr. Practon on December 7, at which time his disability leave needs to be extended. Complete the Physician's Supplementary Certificate form (Figure 16–6) by referring to the entry made during the second visit, and date the certificate December 7. Remember that this is not a claim for payment to the physician, and so no ledger card has been furnished for this patient.

3. Refer to Chapter 16 and Figures 16–4 and 16–5 of the *Handbook* to assist you in completing these forms.

   After the instructor has returned your work to you, either make the necessary corrections and place your work in a three-ring notebook for future reference or, if you received a high score, place it in your portfolio for reference when applying for a job.

Abbreviations pertinent to this record:

pt	_____	wk	_____
SDI	_____	est	_____
PE	_____	FU	_____
wks	_____	c̄	_____
dx	_____	CXR	_____
Cont	_____	reg	_____
RTO	_____		

PATIENT RECORD NO. 16-3

Thorndike	Fred	E	02-17-44	M	555-465-7820
LAST NAME	FIRST NAME	MIDDLE NAME	BIRTH DATE	SEX	HOME PHONE

5784 Helen Street	Woodland Hills	XY	12345
ADDRESS	CITY	STATE	ZIP CODE

555-432-7744	555-320-5500	555-466-7820	thorndike@wb.net
CELL PHONE	PAGER NO.	FAX NO.	E-MAIL ADDRESS

549-XX-8721	M00430548
PATIENT'S SOC. SEC. NO.	DRIVER'S LICENSE

salesman Payoll No. 6852	Easy on Paint Company
PATIENT'S OCCUPATION	NAME OF COMPANY

4586 West 20th Street, Woodland Hills, XY 12345	555-467-8898
ADDRESS OF EMPLOYER	PHONE

Jennifer B. Thorndike	homemaker
SPOUSE OR PARENT	OCCUPATION

EMPLOYER	ADDRESS	PHONE

Pacific Mutual Insurance Company,120 South Main Street, Merck, XY 12346
NAME OF INSURANCE

6709	Fred E. Thorndike
POLICY/CERTIFICATE NO.	GROUP NO.	INSURED OR SUBSCRIBER

REFERRED BY: John Diehl (Friend)

DATE	PROGRESS NOTES
11-25-xx	On or about 11-3-xx, pt began to have chest pain and much coughing. On 11-24-xx, pt too ill to work and
	decided to file for SDI benefits. Pt states illness is not work connected and he does not receive sick pay.
	PE: Pt examined and complained of productive cough of 3 wks duration and chest pain. Chest x-rays
	confirmed dx-mucopurulent chronic bronchitis. Cont home rest and prescribed antibiotic medication. RTO
	12-7-xx. Pt will be capable of returning to wk 12-8-xx.
	GP/mtf Gerald Practon, MD
12-07-xx	Est pt returns for F/U c bronchitis. Chest pain improved. Still running low grade temp c̄ productive cough.
	F/U CXR shows clearing. Recommended bed rest x 7d. Will extend disability to 12-15-xx at which time pt
	can resume reg work. No complications anticipated.
	GP/mtf Gerald Practon, MD

Figure 16–4

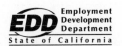

Employment Development Department
State of California

Claim for Disability Insurance Benefits – Doctor's Certificate

TYPE or PRINT with BLACK INK.

34. PATIENT'S FILE NUMBER	35. PATIENT'S SOCIAL SECURITY NO.	36. PATIENT'S LAST NAME	

37. DOCTOR'S NAME AS SHOWN ON LICENSE	38. DOCTOR'S TELEPHONE NUMBER ( )	39. DOCTOR'S STATE LICENSE NO.

40. DOCTOR'S ADDRESS – NUMBER AND STREET, CITY, STATE, COUNTRY (IF NOT USA), ZIP CODE. POST OFFICE BOX NUMBER IS NOT ACCEPTED AS THE SOLE ADDRESS

41. THIS PATIENT HAS BEEN UNDER MY CARE AND TREATMENT FOR THIS MEDICAL PROBLEM

FROM _____ / _____ / _____ TO _____ / _____ / _____ AT INTERVALS OF ☐ DAILY ☐ WEEKLY ☐ MONTHLY ☐ AS NEEDED

42. AT ANY TIME DURING YOUR ATTENDANCE FOR THIS MEDICAL PROBLEM, HAS THE PATIENT BEEN INCAPABLE OF PERFORMING HIS/HER REGULAR OR CUSTOMARY WORK? ☐ NO – SKIP TO THE DOCTOR'S CERTIFICATION SECTION ☐ YES – ENTER DATE DISABILITY BEGAN: _____ / _____ / _____	43. DATE YOU RELEASED OR ANTICIPATE RELEASING PATIENT TO RETURN TO HIS/HER REGULAR / CUSTOMARY WORK ("UNKNOWN," "INDEFINITE," ETC., NOT ACCEPTED.) _____ / _____ / _____

44. ICD9 DISEASE CODE, PRIMARY (REQUIRED UNLESS DIAGNOSIS NOT YET OBTAINED) _____ . _____	45. ICD9 DISEASE CODE(S), SECONDARY _____ . ____, _____ . ____, _____ . ____

46. DIAGNOSIS (REQUIRED) – IF NO DIAGNOSIS HAS BEEN DETERMINED, ENTER OBJECTIVE FINDINGS OR A DETAILED STATEMENT OF SYMPTOMS

47. FINDINGS – STATE NATURE, SEVERITY, AND EXTENT OF THE INCAPACITATING DISEASE OR INJURY. INCLUDE ANY OTHER DISABLING CONDITIONS

48. TYPE OF TREATMENT / MEDICATION RENDERED TO PATIENT	49. IF PATIENT WAS HOSPITALIZED, PROVIDE DATES OF ENTRY AND DISCHARGE _____ / _____ / _____ TO _____ / _____ / _____

50. DATE AND TYPE OF SURGERY / PROCEDURE PERFORMED OR TO BE PERFORMED _____ / _____ / _____	ICD9 PROCEDURE CODE(S)

51. IF PATIENT IS NOW PREGNANT OR HAS BEEN PREGNANT, WHAT DATE DID PREGNANCY TERMINATE OR WHAT DATE DO YOU EXPECT DELIVERY? _____ / _____ / _____	52. IF PREGNANCY IS / WAS ABNORMAL, STATE THE ABNORMAL AND INVOLUNTARY COMPLICATION CAUSING MATERNAL DISABILITY

53. BASED ON YOUR EXAMINATION OF PATIENT, IS THIS DISABILITY THE RESULT OF "OCCUPATION," EITHER AS AN "INDUSTRIAL ACCIDENT" OR AS AN "OCCUPATIONAL DISEASE"? (INCLUDE SITUATIONS WHERE PATIENT'S OCCUPATION HAS AGGRAVATED PRE-EXISTING CONDITIONS.) ☐ YES ☐ NO	54. ARE YOU COMPLETING THIS FORM FOR THE SOLE PURPOSE OF REFERRAL / RECOMMENDATION TO AN ALCOHOLIC RECOVERY HOME OR DRUG-FREE RESIDENTIAL FACILITY AS INDICATED BY THE PATIENT IN QUESTION 23? ☐ YES ☐ NO	55. WOULD DISCLOSURE OF THIS INFORMATION TO YOUR PATIENT BE MEDICALLY OR PSYCHOLOGICALLY DETRIMENTAL? ☐ YES ☐ NO

Doctor's Certification and Signature (REQUIRED): Having considered the patient's regular or customary work, I certify under penalty of perjury that, based on my examination, this Doctor's Certificate truly describes the patient's disability (if any) and the estimated duration thereof.

I further certify that I am a _____ | _____ licensed to practice in the State of _____ .
(TYPE OF DOCTOR)   (SPECIALTY, IF ANY)

► _____   ► _____
ORIGINAL SIGNATURE OF ATTENDING DOCTOR – RUBBER STAMP IS NOT ACCEPTABLE   DATE SIGNED

Under sections 2116 and 2122 of the California Unemployment Insurance Code, it is a violation for any individual who, with intent to defraud, falsely certifies the medical condition of any person in order to obtain disability insurance benefits, whether for the maker or for any other person, and is punishable by imprisonment and/or a fine not exceeding $20,000. Section 1143 requires additional administrative penalties.

DE 2501 Rev. 77 (3-06) **(INTERNET)**

Figure 16–5

NOTICE OF FINAL PAYMENT

The information contained in your claim for Disability Insurance indicates that you are now able to work, therefore, this is the final check that you will receive on this claim.

IF YOU ARE **STILL** DISABLED: You should complete the Claimant's Certification portion of this form and contact your doctor immediately to have him/her complete the Physician's Supplementary Certificate below.

IF YOU BECOME DISABLED **AGAIN:** File a new Disability Insurance claim form.

IF YOU ARE UNEMPLOYED AND AVAILABLE FOR WORK: Report to the nearest Unemployment Insurance office of the Department for assistance in finding work and to determine your entitlement to Unemployment Insurance Benefits.

This determination is final unless you file an appeal within twenty (20) days from the date of the mailing of this notification. You may appeal by giving a detailed statement as to why you believe the determination is in error. All communications regarding this Disability Insurance claim should include your Social Security Account Number and be addressed to the office shown.

- -

CLAIMANT'S CERTIFICATION

I certify that I continue to be disabled and incapable of doing my regular work, and that I have reported all wages, Worker's Compensation benefits and other monies received during the claim period to the Employment Development Department.

ENTER YOUR SOCIAL SECURITY NUMBER ___549___ ___XX___ ___8721___

Sign Your Name_____   **Date Signed**_____
            Fred E. Thorndike   December 6, 20XX

PHYSICIAN'S SUPPLEMENTARY CERTIFICATE

	Department Use Only	

1. Are you still treating patient?_____ Date of last treatment_____ , 20___ .
2. What present condition continues to make the patient disabled?
_____
_____
_____

3. Date patient recovered, or will recover sufficiently (even if under treatment) to be able to perform his/her regular and customary work_____ , 20_____. Please enter a specific or estimated recovery date.
4. Would the disclosure of this information to your patient be medically or psychologically detrimental to the patient?
Yes ☐   No ☐

I hereby certify that the above statements in my opinion truly describe the claimant's condition and the estimated duration thereof.

Doctor's Signature_____

_____ , 20 ____
            Date   Phone Number_____

DE 2525XX Rev. 13 (3-86)   – Versión en español en el dorso –

Figure 16–6

ASSIGNMENT 16–4 ▸ COMPLETE A STATE DISABILITY INSURANCE FORM

Performance Objective

Task: Complete a state disability insurance form and define patient record abbreviations.

Conditions: Use the patient's record (Figure 16–7), a Doctor's Certificate form (Figure 16–8), and a typewriter or computer.

Standards: Time: _____ minutes

Accuracy: _____

(Note: The time element and accuracy criteria may be given by your instructor.)

Directions

1. Assume that the Claim Statement of Employee has been completed satisfactorily by Mr. James T. Fujita (Figure 16–7). Complete the Doctor's Certificate form
(Figure 16–8) and date it December 15. Remember that this is not a claim for payment to the physician, and so no ledger card has been furnished for this patient.

2. Refer to Chapter 16 and Figure 16–4 of the *Handbook* to assist you in completing this form.

After the instructor has returned your work to you, either make the necessary corrections and place your work in a three-ring notebook for future reference or, if you received a high score, place it in your portfolio for reference when applying for a job.

Abbreviations pertinent to this record:

pt _____   imp _____

exam _____   wk _____

hx _____   SDI _____

neg _____   wk _____

WBC _____

PATIENT RECORD NO. 16-4

Fujita	James	T	03-27-34	M	555-677-2881
LAST NAME	FIRST NAME	MIDDLE NAME	BIRTH DATE	SEX	HOME PHONE

3538 South A Street	Woodland Hills	XY		12345
ADDRESS	CITY	STATE		ZIP CODE

555-499-6556	555-988-4100	555-677-2881	fujita@wb.net
CELL PHONE	PAGER NO.	FAX NO.	E-MAIL ADDRESS

567-XX-8898	M4387931
PATIENT'S SOC. SEC. NO.	DRIVER'S LICENSE

electrician Payoll No. 8834	Macy Electric Company
PATIENT'S OCCUPATION	NAME OF COMPANY

2671 North C Street, Woodland Hills, XY 12345	555-677-2346
ADDRESS OF EMPLOYER	PHONE

Mary J. Fujita	homemaker
SPOUSE OR PARENT	OCCUPATION

EMPLOYER	ADDRESS	PHONE

Atlantic Mutual Insurance Company, 111 South Main Street, Woodland Hills, XY 12345
NAME OF INSURANCE

F20015		James T. Fujita
POLICY/CERTIFICATE NO.	GROUP NO.	INSURED OR SUBSCRIBER

REFERRED BY: Cherry Hotta (aunt)

DATE	PROGRESS NOTES
12-07-XX	Today pt could not go to work and came for exam complaining of pain in abdomen, nausea, and no vomiting. Pt
	has hx of mesentery adenopathy. Exam neg except abdomen showed tenderness all over with voluntary guarding.
	WBC 10,000. Imp: Mesenteric adenitis. Advised strict bed rest at home and bland diet. To return in 1 wk. Will file
	for SDI benefits. Pt states illness is not work connected and he receives sick leave pay of $150/wk.
	GI/mtf *Gaston Input, MD*
12-15-xx	Exam showed normal nontender abdomen. No nausea. Pt tolerating food well. WBC 7,500. Pt will be capable of
	returning to work 12-22-xx.
	GI/mtf *Gaston Input, MD*

Figure 16–7

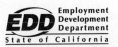

EDD
Employment
Development
Department
State of California

Claim for Disability Insurance Benefits – Doctor's Certificate

TYPE or PRINT with BLACK INK.

34. PATIENT'S FILE NUMBER	35. PATIENT'S SOCIAL SECURITY NO.	36. PATIENT'S LAST NAME

37. DOCTOR'S NAME AS SHOWN ON LICENSE	38. DOCTOR'S TELEPHONE NUMBER ( )	39. DOCTOR'S STATE LICENSE NO.

40. DOCTOR'S ADDRESS – NUMBER AND STREET, CITY, STATE, COUNTRY (IF NOT USA), ZIP CODE. POST OFFICE BOX NUMBER IS NOT ACCEPTED AS THE SOLE ADDRESS

41. THIS PATIENT HAS BEEN UNDER MY CARE AND TREATMENT FOR THIS MEDICAL PROBLEM

FROM ___/___/___ TO ___/___/___ AT INTERVALS OF ☐ DAILY ☐ WEEKLY ☐ MONTHLY ☐ AS NEEDED

42. AT ANY TIME DURING YOUR ATTENDANCE FOR THIS MEDICAL PROBLEM, HAS THE PATIENT BEEN INCAPABLE OF PERFORMING HIS/HER REGULAR OR CUSTOMARY WORK? ☐ NO – SKIP TO THE DOCTOR'S CERTIFICATION SECTION ☐ YES – ENTER DATE DISABILITY BEGAN: ___/___/___	43. DATE YOU RELEASED OR ANTICIPATE RELEASING PATIENT TO RETURN TO HIS/HER REGULAR / CUSTOMARY WORK ("UNKNOWN," "INDEFINITE," ETC., NOT ACCEPTED.) ___/___/___

44. ICD9 DISEASE CODE, PRIMARY (REQUIRED UNLESS DIAGNOSIS NOT YET OBTAINED) ___.___	45. ICD9 DISEASE CODE(S), SECONDARY ___.___, ___.___, ___.___

46. DIAGNOSIS (REQUIRED) – IF NO DIAGNOSIS HAS BEEN DETERMINED, ENTER OBJECTIVE FINDINGS OR A DETAILED STATEMENT OF SYMPTOMS

47. FINDINGS – STATE NATURE, SEVERITY, AND EXTENT OF THE INCAPACITATING DISEASE OR INJURY. INCLUDE ANY OTHER DISABLING CONDITIONS

48. TYPE OF TREATMENT / MEDICATION RENDERED TO PATIENT	49. IF PATIENT WAS HOSPITALIZED, PROVIDE DATES OF ENTRY AND DISCHARGE ___/___/___ TO ___/___/___

50. DATE AND TYPE OF SURGERY / PROCEDURE PERFORMED OR TO BE PERFORMED ___/___/___	ICD9 PROCEDURE CODE(S)

51. IF PATIENT IS NOW PREGNANT OR HAS BEEN PREGNANT, WHAT DATE DID PREGNANCY TERMINATE OR WHAT DATE DO YOU EXPECT DELIVERY? ___/___/___	52. IF PREGNANCY IS / WAS ABNORMAL, STATE THE ABNORMAL AND INVOLUNTARY COMPLICATION CAUSING MATERNAL DISABILITY

53. BASED ON YOUR EXAMINATION OF PATIENT, IS THIS DISABILITY THE RESULT OF "OCCUPATION," EITHER AS AN "INDUSTRIAL ACCIDENT" OR AS AN "OCCUPATIONAL DISEASE"? (INCLUDE SITUATIONS WHERE PATIENT'S OCCUPATION HAS AGGRAVATED PRE-EXISTING CONDITIONS.) ☐ YES ☐ NO	54. ARE YOU COMPLETING THIS FORM FOR THE SOLE PURPOSE OF REFERRAL / RECOMMENDATION TO AN ALCOHOLIC RECOVERY HOME OR DRUG-FREE RESIDENTIAL FACILITY AS INDICATED BY THE PATIENT IN QUESTION 23? ☐ YES ☐ NO	55. WOULD DISCLOSURE OF THIS INFORMATION TO YOUR PATIENT BE MEDICALLY OR PSYCHOLOGICALLY DETRIMENTAL? ☐ YES ☐ NO

Doctor's Certification and Signature (REQUIRED): Having considered the patient's regular or customary work, I certify under penalty of perjury that, based on my examination, this Doctor's Certificate truly describes the patient's disability (if any) and the estimated duration thereof.

I further certify that I am a _____ _____ licensed to practice in the State of _____ .
(TYPE OF DOCTOR)   (SPECIALTY, IF ANY)

► _____   ► _____
ORIGINAL SIGNATURE OF ATTENDING DOCTOR – RUBBER STAMP IS NOT ACCEPTABLE   DATE SIGNED

Under sections 2116 and 2122 of the California Unemployment Insurance Code, it is a violation for any individual who, with intent to defraud, falsely certifies the medical condition of any person in order to obtain disability insurance benefits, whether for the maker or for any other person, and is punishable by imprisonment and/or a fine not exceeding $20,000. Section 1143 requires additional administrative penalties.

DE 2501 Rev. 77 (3-06) **(INTERNET)**

Figure 16–8

ASSIGNMENT 16–5 ▸ COMPLETE TWO STATE DISABILITY INSURANCE FORMS

Performance Objective

Task: Complete two state disability insurance forms and define patient record abbreviations.

Conditions: Use the patient's record (Figure 16–9), a Doctor's Certificate form (Figure 16–10), a Request for Additional Medical Information form (Figure 16–11), and a typewriter or computer.

Standards: Time: _____ minutes

Accuracy: _____

(Note: The time element and accuracy criteria may be given by your instructor.)

Directions

1. Mr. Jake J. Burrows (Figure 16–9) has previously applied for state disability benefits. After 2 months, he is referred to another doctor for further care. Complete the form (Figure 16–10) and date it June 25. You will notice that this form is almost identical to the Doctor's Certificate and is mailed to the claimant to secure the certification of a new physician or to clarify a specific claimed period of disability. In completing this part of the assignment, look at the first three entries on the patient record only.

2. Complete the Request for Additional Medical Information form (Figure 16–11) by looking at the last entry on Mr. Burrows' record, and date the report July 15. Remember that this is not a claim for payment to the physician, and so no ledger card has been furnished for this patient.

3. Refer to Chapter 16 and Figures 16–4 and 16–6 of the *Handbook* to assist you in completing these forms.

After the instructor has returned your work to you, either make the necessary corrections and place your work in a three-ring notebook for future reference or, if you received a high score, place it in your portfolio for reference when applying for a job.

Abbreviations pertinent to this record:

pt _____   hosp _____

c̄ _____   approx _____

C5/6 _____   retn _____

imp _____   RTO _____

adm _____   wks _____

PATIENT RECORD NO. 16-5

Burrows	Jake	J	04-26-50	M	555-478-9009
LAST NAME	FIRST NAME	MIDDLE NAME	BIRTH DATE	SEX	HOME PHONE

319 Barry Street	Woodland Hills	XY	12345	
ADDRESS	CITY	STATE	ZIP CODE	

555-765-9080	555-542-0979	555-478-9009		burrows@wb.net
CELL PHONE	PAGER NO.	FAX NO.		E-MAIL ADDRESS

457-XX-0801	D0453298
PATIENT'S SOC. SEC. NO.	DRIVER'S LICENSE

assembler	Convac Electronics Company
PATIENT'S OCCUPATION	NAME OF COMPANY

3440 West 7th Street, Woodland Hills, XY 12345	555-467-9008
ADDRESS OF EMPLOYER	PHONE

3440 West 7th Street, Woodland Hills, XY 12345   555-467-9008
ADDRESS OF EMPLOYER   PHONE

Jane B. Burrows	homemaker
SPOUSE OR PARENT	OCCUPATION

EMPLOYER	ADDRESS	PHONE

Blue Shield	Jake J. Burrows
NAME OF INSURANCE	INSURED OR SUBSCRIBER

T8471811A	53553AT
POLICY/CERTIFICATE NO.	GROUP NO.

REFERRED BY: Clarence Butler, MD, 300 Sixth Street, Woodland Hills, XY 12345   NPI# 620114352X

DATE	PROGRESS NOTES
6-02-xx	Pt. Referred by Dr. Butler. Pt states on 4-19-xx was wrestling c̄ son and jerked his neck the wrong way.
	2 days later had much pain and muscle spasm in the cervical region. X-rays show degenerated disk C5/6.
	Exam: limited range of neck motion and limited abduction both arms. Imp: Degenerated cervical disk C5/6.
	Pt unable to work as of this date. Myelogram ordered. Return for test results.
	RS/mtf *Raymond Skeleton, MD*
6-24-xx	Myelogram positive at C5/6. Scheduled for surgery the following day.
	RS/mtf *Raymond Skeleton, MD*
6-25-xx	Pt adm to College Hospital for disk excision and anterior cervical fusion at C5/6. Pt will be discharged from
	hosp on 6-29-xx. Approx date of retn to work 8-15-xx.
	RS/mtf *Raymond Skeleton, MD*
6-26 to	Pt seen daily in hospital. Discharged 6-29. RTO 2 weeks.
6-29-xx	RS/mtf *Raymond Skeleton, MD*
7-15-xx	Pt has some restriction of cervical motion. No muscle spasm. Very little cervical pain. Pt to be seen in
	2 wks. To retn to work 8-15-xx.
	RS/mtf *Raymond Skeleton, MD*

Figure 16–9

In order that any disability insurance to which you may be entitled may be paid without undue delay, please have the physician who treats or treated you during the period indicated below complete this form and return it to us at his earliest convenience.

Para que cualquier beneficio del Segurdo de Incapacidad a que Ud. pueda tener derecho a recibir sea pagado sin demoras excesivas, haga el favor de hacer que el médico que le atiende o atiendó, durante el período indicado abajo, complete este formulario y que lo regrese a nuestra oficina cuanto antes.

Henry B. Garcia
_____
Disability Insurance Program Representative

6-2 thru 7-25-XX
_____
Period Dates - Feches del Periodo

457-XX-0801
_____
S.S.A. – No. Des S.S.

	Month	Day	Year		Month	Day	Year		

1. I attended the patient for the present medical problem from: To: At intervals of:

2. History:
   State the nature, severity and the bodily extent of the incapacitating disease or injury.
   Findings:
   Dianosis:
   Type of treatment and/or medication rendered to patient:

3. Diagnosis confirmed by: (*Specify type of test or X-ray*)

4. Is this patient now pregnant or has she been pregnant since the date of treatment as reported above?   Yes ☐ No ☐   If "Yes", date pregnancy terminated or future EDC:

   Is the pregnancy normal?   Yes ☐ No ☐   If "No", state the abnormal and involuntary complication causing maternal disability:

5. Operation: Date performed: ☐   Type of

   Date to be performed: ☐   Operation:

6. Has the patient at any time during your attendance for this medical problem, been incapable of performing his/her regular work?   Yes ☐ No ☐   If "Yes", the disability commenced on:

7. APPROXIMATE date, based on your examination of patient, disability (if any) should end or has ended sufficiently to permit the patient to resume regular or customary work. Even if considerable question exists, make *SOME* "estimate." This is a requirement of the Code, and the claim will be delayed if such date is not entered. Such answers as "Indefinite" or "don't know" will not suffice.   (ENTER DATE)

8. Based on your examination of patient, is this disability the result of "occupation" either as an "industrial accident" or as an "occupational disease?" (This should include aggravation of pre-existing conditions by occupation.)   Yes ☐ No ☐

9. Have you reported this *OR A CONCURRENT DISABILITY* to any insurance carrier as a Workers' Compensation Claim?   Yes ☐ No ☐   If "Yes," to whom?

10. Was or is patient confined as a registered bed patient in a hospital?   Yes ☐ No ☐
    Was patient treated in the surgical unit of a hospital or surgical unit?   Yes ☐ No ☐
    If "Yes," please provide name and address:

11. Date and hour entered as a registered bed patient and discharged pursuant to your orders:

ENTERED		STILL CONFINED	DISCHARGED	
on , 20 , at	A.M. P.M.	on , 20	on , 20 , at	A.M. P.M.

12. Would the disclosure of this information to your patient be medically or psychologically detrimental to the patient?   Yes ☐ No ☐

I hereby certify that, based on my examination, the above statements truly descibe the patient's disability (if any) and the estimated duration thereof, and that I am a _____ licensed to practice by the State of _____
(TYPE OF DOCTOR)

_____   _____
PRINT OR TYPE DOCTOR'S NAME AS SHOWN ON LICENSE   SIGNATURE OF ATTENDING DOCTOR

( )

NO. AND STREET   CITY   ZIP CODE   STATE LICENSE NUMBER   TELEPHONE NUMBER   DATE OF SIGNING THIS FORM

Certification may be made by a licensed physician and surgeon, osteopath, chiropractor, dentist, podiatrist, optometrist, designated psychologist, or an authorized medical officer of a United States Government facility. All items on this sheet must be completed.

Figure 16–10

STATE OF CALIFORNIA
EMPLOYMENT DEVELOPMENT DEPARTMENT

**REQUEST FOR ADDITIONAL
MEDICAL INFORMATION**

457-XX-0801   – Our file No,
Jake J. Burrows   – Your patient
                          – Regular or Customary Work

Raymond Skeleton, M.D.
4567 Broad Avenue
Woodland Hills, XY 12345

The original basic information and estimate of duration of your patient's disability have been carefully evaluated. At the present time, the following additional information based upon the progress and present condition of this patient is requested. This will assist the Department in determining eligibilty for further disability insurance benefits. Return of the completed form as soon as possible will be appreciated.

WM. C. SCHMIDT, M.D., MEDICAL DIRECTOR

CLAIMS EXAMINER   *DOCTOR: Please complete either part A or B, date and sign.*

PART A   IF YOUR PATIENT HAS RECOVERED SUFFICIENTLY TO BE ABLE TO RETURN TO HIS/HER REGULAR OR CUSTOMARY WORK LISTED ABOVE, PLEASE GIVE THE DATE, _____ 20 _____

PART B   THIS PART REFERS TO PATIENT WHO IS STILL DISABLED.

Are you still treating the patient? Yes ☐ No ☐   _____ 20 _____ .
                                                          DATE OF LAST TREATMENT

What are the medical circumstances which continue to make your patient disabled?
_____
_____
_____

What is your present estimate of the date your patient will be able to perform his/her regular or customary work listed above?   Date _____ 20 _____ .

Further comments: _____
_____
_____

Would the disclosure of this information to your patient be medically or physically detrimental to the patient? Yes ☐ No ☐

Date _____ 20 _____   _____
                                                DOCTOR'S SIGNATURE

ENCLOSED IS A STAMPED PREADDRESSED ENVELOPE FOR YOUR CONVENIENCE.

DE 2547 Rev. 17 (4-84)

Figure 16–11

ASSIGNMENT 16–6 ▸ COMPLETE A STATE DISABILITY INSURANCE FORM

Performance Objective

Task: Complete a state disability insurance form and define patient record abbreviations.

Conditions: Use the patient's record (Figure 16–12), a Doctor's Certificate form (Figure 16–13), and a
                   typewriter or computer.

Standards: Time: _____ minutes

                   Accuracy: _____

                   (Note: The time element and accuracy criteria may be given by your instructor.)

Directions

1. Mr. Vincent P. Michael (Figure 16–12) is applying for state disability benefits. Complete the Doctor's Certificate
   form (Figure 16–13) and date it September 21. Assume that the Claim Statement of Employee has been
   completed satisfactorily by Mr. Michael. Remember that this is not a claim for payment to the physician, and so
   no ledger card has been furnished for this patient.

2. Refer to Chapter 16 and Figure 16–4 of the *Handbook* to assist you in completing this form.

   After the instructor has returned your work to you, either make the necessary corrections and place your work in
a three-ring notebook for future reference or, if you received a high score, place it in your portfolio for reference
when applying for a job.

Abbreviations pertinent to this record:

pt _____   imp _____

exam _____   CVA _____

L _____   adv _____

ESR _____   retn _____

mm _____   wk _____

hr _____   approx _____

PATIENT RECORD NO. 16-6

Michael	Vincent	P	05-17-45	M	555-567-9001
LAST NAME	FIRST NAME	MIDDLE NAME	BIRTH DATE	SEX	HOME PHONE

1529 1/2 Thompson Boulevard	Woodland Hills	XY	12345	
ADDRESS	CITY	STATE	ZIP CODE	

555-398-5677	555-311-0098	555-567-9001	michael@wb.net
CELL PHONE	PAGER NO.	FAX NO.	E-MAIL ADDRESS

562-XX-8888	E0034578
PATIENT'S SOC. SEC. NO.	DRIVER'S LICENSE

assembler "A"	Burroughs Corporation
PATIENT'S OCCUPATION	NAME OF COMPANY

5411 North Lindero Canyon Road, Woodland Hills, XY 12345	555-560-9008
ADDRESS OF EMPLOYER	PHONE

Helen J. Michael	homemaker
SPOUSE OR PARENT	OCCUPATION

EMPLOYER	ADDRESS	PHONE

Blue Shield	Vincent P. Michael
NAME OF INSURANCE	INSURED OR SUBSCRIBER

T8411981A	677899AT
POLICY/CERTIFICATE NO.	GROUP NO.

REFERRED BY: Robert T. Smith (friend)

DATE	PROGRESS NOTES
9-20-xx	Pt complains of having had the flu, headache, dizziness, and of being tired. Pt unable to go to work today. Exam
	shows weakness of L hand. Pt exhibits light dysphasia and confusion. Chest x-ray shows cardiomegaly and slight
	pulmonary congestion. ESR 46 mm/hr. Imp: Post flu syndrome, transient ischemic attack, possible CVA.
	Prescribed medication for congestion and adv pt to take aspirin 1/day. Pt to stay off work and retn in 1 wk. Approx
	date of retn to work 10-16-xx.
	BC/mtf *Brady Coccidioides, MD*

Figure 16–12

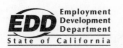
Employment
Development
Department
State of California

Claim for Disability Insurance Benefits – Doctor's Certificate

TYPE or PRINT with BLACK INK.

34. PATIENT'S FILE NUMBER	35. PATIENT'S SOCIAL SECURITY NO.	36. PATIENT'S LAST NAME

37. DOCTOR'S NAME AS SHOWN ON LICENSE	38. DOCTOR'S TELEPHONE NUMBER ( )	39. DOCTOR'S STATE LICENSE NO.

40. DOCTOR'S ADDRESS – NUMBER AND STREET, CITY, STATE, COUNTRY (IF NOT USA), ZIP CODE. POST OFFICE BOX NUMBER IS NOT ACCEPTED AS THE SOLE ADDRESS

41. THIS PATIENT HAS BEEN UNDER MY CARE AND TREATMENT FOR THIS MEDICAL PROBLEM

FROM ____/____/____ TO ____/____/____ AT INTERVALS OF ☐ DAILY ☐ WEEKLY ☐ MONTHLY ☐ AS NEEDED

42. AT ANY TIME DURING YOUR ATTENDANCE FOR THIS MEDICAL PROBLEM, HAS THE PATIENT BEEN INCAPABLE OF PERFORMING HIS/HER REGULAR OR CUSTOMARY WORK?

☐ NO – SKIP TO THE DOCTOR'S CERTIFICATION SECTION   ☐ YES – ENTER DATE DISABILITY BEGAN: ____/____/____

43. DATE YOU RELEASED OR ANTICIPATE RELEASING PATIENT TO RETURN TO HIS/HER REGULAR / CUSTOMARY WORK ("UNKNOWN," "INDEFINITE," ETC., NOT ACCEPTED.) ____/____/____

44. ICD9 DISEASE CODE, PRIMARY (REQUIRED UNLESS DIAGNOSIS NOT YET OBTAINED) ____.____

45. ICD9 DISEASE CODE(S), SECONDARY ____.____, ____.____, ____.____

46. DIAGNOSIS (REQUIRED) – IF NO DIAGNOSIS HAS BEEN DETERMINED, ENTER OBJECTIVE FINDINGS OR A DETAILED STATEMENT OF SYMPTOMS

47. FINDINGS – STATE NATURE, SEVERITY, AND EXTENT OF THE INCAPACITATING DISEASE OR INJURY. INCLUDE ANY OTHER DISABLING CONDITIONS

48. TYPE OF TREATMENT / MEDICATION RENDERED TO PATIENT

49. IF PATIENT WAS HOSPITALIZED, PROVIDE DATES OF ENTRY AND DISCHARGE ____/____/____ TO ____/____/____

50. DATE AND TYPE OF SURGERY / PROCEDURE PERFORMED OR TO BE PERFORMED ____/____/____

ICD9 PROCEDURE CODE(S)

51. IF PATIENT IS NOW PREGNANT OR HAS BEEN PREGNANT, WHAT DATE DID PREGNANCY TERMINATE OR WHAT DATE DO YOU EXPECT DELIVERY? ____/____/____

52. IF PREGNANCY IS / WAS ABNORMAL, STATE THE ABNORMAL AND INVOLUNTARY COMPLICATION CAUSING MATERNAL DISABILITY

53. BASED ON YOUR EXAMINATION OF PATIENT, IS THIS DISABILITY THE RESULT OF "OCCUPATION," EITHER AS AN "INDUSTRIAL ACCIDENT" OR AS AN "OCCUPATIONAL DISEASE"? (INCLUDE SITUATIONS WHERE PATIENT'S OCCUPATION HAS AGGRAVATED PRE-EXISTING CONDITIONS.)
☐ YES ☐ NO

54. ARE YOU COMPLETING THIS FORM FOR THE SOLE PURPOSE OF REFERRAL / RECOMMENDATION TO AN ALCOHOLIC RECOVERY HOME OR DRUG-FREE RESIDENTIAL FACILITY AS INDICATED BY THE PATIENT IN QUESTION 23?
☐ YES ☐ NO

55. WOULD DISCLOSURE OF THIS INFORMATION TO YOUR PATIENT BE MEDICALLY OR PSYCHOLOGICALLY DETRIMENTAL?
☐ YES ☐ NO

Doctor's Certification and Signature (REQUIRED): Having considered the patient's regular or customary work, I certify under penalty of perjury that, based on my examination, this Doctor's Certificate truly describes the patient's disability (if any) and the estimated duration thereof.

I further certify that I am a _____ _____ licensed to practice in the State of _____ .
(TYPE OF DOCTOR)   (SPECIALTY, IF ANY)

► _____
ORIGINAL SIGNATURE OF ATTENDING DOCTOR – RUBBER STAMP IS NOT ACCEPTABLE

► _____
DATE SIGNED

Under sections 2116 and 2122 of the California Unemployment Insurance Code, it is a violation for any individual who, with intent to defraud, falsely certifies the medical condition of any person in order to obtain disability insurance benefits, whether for the maker or for any other person, and is punishable by imprisonment and/or a fine not exceeding $20,000. Section 1143 requires additional administrative penalties.

DE 2501 Rev. 77 (3-06) **(INTERNET)**

Figure 16–13

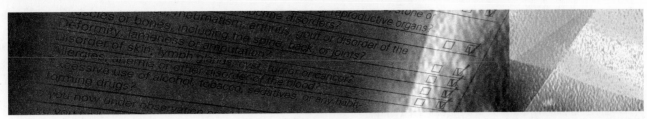

Hospital Billing

KEY TERMS

Your instructor may wish to select some words pertinent to this chapter for a test. For definitions of the terms, further study, and/or reference, the words, phrases, and abbreviations may be found in the glossary at the end of the Handbook. *Key terms for this chapter follow.*

admission review

ambulatory payment classifications (APCs)

appropriateness evaluation protocols (AEPs)

capitation

case rate

charge description master (CDM)

charges

clinical outliers

code sequence

comorbidity

cost outlier

cost outlier review

day outlier review

diagnosis-related groups (DRGs)

DRG creep

DRG validation

elective surgery

grouper

inpatient

International Classification of Diseases, Ninth Revision, Clinical Modification (ICD-9-CM)

looping

major diagnostic categories (MDCs)

outpatient

percentage of revenue

per diem

preadmission testing (PAT)

principal diagnosis

procedure review

Quality Improvement Organization (QIO) program

readmission review

scrubbing

stop loss

transfer review

Uniform Bill (UB-04) CMS-1450 paper or electronic claim form

utilization review (UR)

KEY ABBREVIATIONS

See how many abbreviations and acronyms you can translate and then use this as a handy reference list. Definitions for the key abbreviations are located near the back of the Handbook *in the glossary.*

AEPs _____

AHA _____

AHIMA _____

APCs _____

APGs _____

ASCs _____

ASHD _____

AVGs _____

CDM _____

CMHCs _____

CMS _____

CMS-1450 _____

CPT _____

DDE _____

DRGs _____

ED _____

EDI

FL _____

GAO _____

HIM _____

HSI _____

ICD-9-CM _____

ICD-10-CM _____

JCAHO _____

LOS _____

MCDs _____

NF _____

OPPS _____

PAT _____

PPS _____

QIO _____

RHIA _____

RHIT _____

RN _____

TEFRA _____

UB-04 _____

UR _____

PERFORMANCE OBJECTIVES

The student will be able to:

- Define and spell the key terms and key abbreviations for this chapter, given the information from the *Handbook* glossary, within a reasonable time period and with enough accuracy to obtain a satisfactory evaluation.
- Answer the fill-in-the-blank, mix and match, multiple choice, and true/false review questions after reading the chapter, with enough accuracy to obtain a satisfactory evaluation.
- Given computer-generated UB-04 claim forms, state the reasons why claims may be either rejected or delayed or why incorrect payment is received; state these reasons within a reasonable time period and with enough accuracy to obtain a satisfactory evaluation.

- Analyze, edit, and insert entries on computer-generated UB-04 claim forms so that payment will be accurate, within a reasonable time period and with enough accuracy to obtain a satisfactory evaluation.
- Answer questions about the UB-04 claim form to become familiar with the data it contains, within a reasonable time period and with enough accuracy to obtain a satisfactory evaluation.
- Answer questions about the UB-04 claim form to learn which hospital departments input data for different blocks on this form, within a reasonable time period and with enough accuracy to obtain a satisfactory evaluation.

ASSIGNMENT 17-2 ▸ LOCATE AND SEQUENCE DIAGNOSTIC CODES FOR CONDITIONS

Performance Objective

Task: Locate the correct diagnostic code for each diagnosis listed for five cases.

Conditions: Use a pen or pencil and the ICD-9-CM diagnostic code book.

Standards: Time: _____ minutes

                  Accuracy: _____

                  (Note: The time element and accuracy criteria may be given by your instructor.)

Directions. These cases point out the value of proper versus improper coding with regard to correct sequence and inclusion of specific codes that indicate the variance of payment. Assign the correct ICD-9-CM code numbers. Note that the same case was assigned different DRG codes, thereby listing different principal and secondary hospital diagnoses, and that the DRG payment for each is substantially different. Also note the difference in the major diagnostic category (MDC).

CASE 1

Age: 12   Sex: Male

MDC: Four diseases and disorders of the respiratory system

DRG: Code 98: Bronchitis and asthma, age 0 to 17

Principal Diagnosis

Asthma w/o status asthmaticus_____

Secondary Diagnoses

Pneumonia, organism NOS _____

Otitis media NOS _____

DRG Payment: $2705

MDC: Four diseases and disorders of the respiratory system

DRG: Code 91: Simple pneumonia and pleurisy, age 0 to17

Principal Diagnosis

Pneumonia, organism not otherwise

   specified (NOS) _____

Secondary Diagnoses

Asthma w/o status asthmaticus _____

Otitis media NOS _____

DRG Payment: $3246

CASE 2

Age: 77   Sex: Male

MDC: Five diseases and disorders of the circulatory system

DRG: Code 138: Cardiac arrhythmia and conduction disorders, age >69 and/or chief complaint (CC)

MDC: Four diseases and disorders of the circulatory respiratory system

DRG: Code 83: Major chest trauma, age >69 and/or CC

Principal Diagnosis

Atrial fibrillation _____

Secondary Diagnoses

Fracture (Fx) six ribs—closed _____

Transcerebral ischemia NOS _____

Syncope and collapse _____

Fx scapula NOS—closed _____

Fall not elsewhere classifiable

     (NEC) and NOS _____

         Procedures

         Contrast cerebral arteriogram _____

         Computed axial tomographic (CAT) scan of head _____

         Diagnostic (Dx) ultrasonography—heart _____

         Physical therapy NEC _____

DRG Payment: $5882

Principal Diagnosis

Fx six ribs—closed _____

Secondary Diagnoses

Atrial fibrillation _____

Transcerebral ischemia NOS _____

Syncope and collapse _____

Fx scapula NOS—closed _____

Fall NEC and NOS _____

DRG Payment: $6206

Note: Because this is a hospital case, ICD-9-CM Volume 3 should be used to code the procedures. However, Volume 3 is not used in the medical office.

CASE 3

Age: 42   Sex: Male
MDC: Nineteen mental diseases and disorders

DRG: Code 426: Depressive neuroses

Principal Diagnosis

Neurotic depression _____

Secondary Diagnoses

Acute myocardial infarction anterior wall

     NEC _____

Chest pain NOS _____

Heart disease NOS _____

Paranoid personality _____

MDC: Five diseases and disorders of the circulatory
     system
DRG: Code 122: Circulatory disorders with
     ami w/o cv comp disch alive

Principal Diagnosis

Acute myocardial infarction anterior wall

     NEC _____

Secondary Diagnoses

Neurotic depression _____

Chest pain NOS _____

Heart disease NOS _____

Paranoid personality _____

Procedures

Dx ultrasound—heart _____

Other resp procedures _____

DRG Payment: $6007   *DRG Payment:* $8637

Note: Because this is a hospital case, ICD-9-CM Volume 3 should be used to code the procedures. However, as mentioned, Volume 3 is not used in the medical office.

CASE 4

Age: 65   Sex: Male
MDC: Five diseases and disorders of the circulatory
    system
DRG: Code 468: Unrelated OR proc

MDC: Twelve diseases and disorders of the male
    reproductive system
DRG: Code 336: Transurethral prostatectomy,
    age >69 and/or CC

Principal Diagnosis

Hypertensive heart disease NOS_____

Principal Diagnosis

Malig neopl prostate _____

Secondary Diagnoses

Hematuria _____

Hyperplasia of prostate _____

Hemiplegia NOS _____

Late eff cerebrovasc dis _____

Malig neopl prostate _____

Secondary Diagnoses

Hematuria _____

Hypertensive heart disease NOS_____

Hemiplegia NOS _____

Late eff cerebrovasc dis _____

Hyperplasia of prostate _____

Procedures

Transurethral prostatect _____

Urethral dilation _____

Cystoscopy NEC _____

Intravenous pyelogram _____

Nephrotomogram NEC _____

DRG Payment: $13,311   *DRG Payment:* $6377

Note: Because this is a hospital case, ICD-9-CM Volume 3 should be used to code the procedures. However, as mentioned, Volume 3 is not used in the medical office.

CASE 5

Age: 62   Sex: Female
MDC: Six diseases and disorders of the digestive system
DRG: Code 188: Other digestive system diagnoses, age >69 and/or CC

Principal Diagnosis

Descending colon inj—closed _____

Secondary Diagnoses

Liver injury NOS—closed _____

Open wnd knee/leg—compl _____

Firearm accident NOS _____

No procedures performed

DRG Payment: $4710

MDC: Seven diseases and disorders of the hepatobiliary system and pancreas
DRG: Code 205: Disorders of the liver exc malig, cirr, alc hepa, age >69 and/or CC

Principal Diagnosis

Liver injury NOS—closed _____

Secondary Diagnoses

Atrial fibrillation _____

Urin tract infection NOS _____

Descending colon inj—closed _____

Open wnd knee/leg—compl _____

Firearm accident NOS _____

E. coli infect NOS _____

DRG Payment: $6847

ASSIGNMENT 17–3 ▸ IDENTIFY HOSPITAL DEPARTMENTS THAT INPUT DATA FOR THE UB-04 CLAIM FORM

Performance Objective

Task: Answer questions about the hospital departments that supply data for the UB-04 claim form.

Conditions: Use an ink pen.

Standards: Time: _____ minutes

                Accuracy: _____

                (Note: The time element and accuracy criteria may be given by your instructor.)

Directions. Depending on your instructor's preference, you may complete this exercise with or without notes or other material.

You have become familiar with the information in all 86 blocks of the UB-04 claim form. This assignment will help you learn which of six hospital departments input information into the computer system to be printed out in the various blocks.

This assignment will enhance your understanding of how multiple employees in a large facility take part in helping produce a completed UB-04 claim form. It will also increase your understanding of where errors and omissions originate so that you may amend them when you start the editing and correction process. Answer the following questions.

1. Which department is responsible for inputting the charges for a blood test?

_____

2. Which department is responsible for inputting an insurance certificate or subscriber number?

_____

3. Which department is responsible for inputting the procedure codes?

_____

4. Which department is responsible for inputting the patient's name and address?

_____

5. Which department is responsible for inputting the diagnostic codes?

_____

ASSIGNMENT 17–4 ▸ STUDY UB-04 CLAIM FORM BLOCK OR FIELD FORM LOCATOR (FL) DATA

Performance Objective

Task: Answer questions about the UB-04 claim form blocks.

Conditions: Use an ink pen.

Standards: Time: _____ minutes

                   Accuracy: _____

                   (Note: The time element and accuracy criteria may be given by your instructor.)

Directions. Depending on your instructor's preference, you may complete this exercise with or without notes or other material.

You have learned about a number of reimbursement methods, confidentiality issues, evaluation protocols, and the utilization review process. This information is necessary for processing an insurance claim to obtain maximum reimbursement. To the UB-04 claim form, you must become familiar with the data it contains, including codes and the location of various types of information. Answer the following questions.

1. In FL 4, state the correct billing codes for

   a. Inpatient services _____

   b. Outpatient services _____

2. What is listed in FL 7? _____

   _____

3. What insurance carriers or programs require FL 9 to be completed? _____

   _____

4. What format is required in FL 10 for the patient's date of birth? _____

5. If a patient was in the hospital for the delivery of a premature infant, what code would be used in FL 15?

   _____

6. If a patient was discharged from inpatient care at 2:15 PM, how would this be noted in FL 16?

   _____

7. What is the correct code to use in FL 17 if a patient was discharged to a home hospice situation?

   _____

8. If neither the patient nor spouse was employed, what code would be used to indicate this in FL 18 through 28?

   _____

9. State the reason for the codes used in FL 31 through 34.

_____

_____

10. What revenue code must be shown on all bills as a final entry and in what block or field form locator (FL) does it occur?

_____

ASSIGNMENT 17-5 ▸ UB-04 CLAIM FORM QUESTIONS ABOUT EDITING

Performance Objective

Task: Answer questions about editing the blocks on the UB-04 claim form.

Conditions: Use an ink pen.

Standards: Time: _____ minutes

                Accuracy: _____

                (Note: The time element and accuracy criteria may be given by your instructor.)

Directions. You are now ready to learn more about the critical editing process for determining errors and omissions on the UB-04 claim form. This important skill may help you secure a job in the claims processing department. Refer to Figure 17–4 in the *Handbook* and, at the end of the chapter, the procedure for editing a UB-04 paper or electronic claim form, and answer the questions.

1. Where does the editing process begin on the UB-04 claim form? _____

_____

2. What block/field(s) form locator (FL) must be filled in when insurance information on the UB-04 claim form is verified?

_____

3. What block/field form locator (FL) should the principal diagnostic code appear in?

_____

4. For an inpatient claim, if FL 43 lists the hospital room, FL 44 lists the per-day rate, and FL 46 lists the number of hospital days, what other block/field form locator (FL) is used to verify this claim for accuracy?

_____

5. Besides room rate and number of inpatient days, what is another important factor in reviewing the services shown in FL 42 through 46?

_____

_____

6. For outpatient claims, what other item/items is/are shown besides the date, description of the service rendered, and fee?

_____

7. Where can an insurance editor check when there is doubt about a service shown on a UB-04 claim form?

_____

8. Which block/field form locator (FL) should show the estimated amount due from the insurance company?

_____

ASSIGNMENT 17–6 ▸ LOCATE ERRORS ON A COMPUTER-GENERATED
UB-04 CLAIM FORM

Performance Objective

Task: Locate the blocks on the computer-generated insurance claim form that need completion of missing information or have data that need to be corrected before submission to the insurance company.

Conditions: Use Mary J. Torre's completed insurance claim (Figure 16–1), the checklist for editing a UB-04 claim form, and a red ink pen.

Standards: Time: _____ minutes

Accuracy: _____

(Note: The time element and accuracy criteria may be given by your instructor.)

Directions. Refer to Figure 17–5 in the *Handbook* to employ the step-by-step approach while editing the computer-generated UB-04 claim form (Figure 17–1). Use the checklist to help you when reviewing the claim form. Locate the blocks on the claim form that need completion of missing information or that have data to be corrected before submission to the insurance company. Highlight all errors you discover. Insert all corrections and missing information in red. If you cannot locate the necessary information but know it is mandatory, write "NEED" in the corresponding form locator block/field.

In addition, you notice that the second line entry for pharmacy shows a total of $6806. However, you know from reviewing the case that one injection of a drug known as TPA (revenue code 259 and fee $5775), which dissolves clots and opens vessels when a patient has a myocardial infarction, was not broken out of the fee. Hand write this final entry. On line 2, cross out the total charge $6806 and insert the correct pharmacy-reduced amount.

Checklist for Editing a Uniform Bill (UB-04) Claim Form: Mary J. Torre

Steps	Form Locator Blocks/Fields
1	FL 1 _____ and 5 _____
2	FL 4: Inpatient _____ Outpatient _____
3	FL 8b_____, 38 _____, 58 _____
	and 59 _____
4	FL 10 _____
5	FL 8b _____ and 11 _____
6	FL 50 _____, 60 _____, 61 _____
	62 _____, and 65 _____
7	FL 67 _____ and 69 _____
8	FL 74 _____ _____ and 74 a-e _____
9	FL 76 _____
10	FL 6 _____, 12 _____, and 32 _____

11   **Inpatient:** FL 42–47: 13 _____

16 _____, and 46 _____

12   FL 47 _____

13   FL 42 _____ and 46 _____

14   **Outpatient:** FL 43 _____, 44 _____

and 45 _____

15   Detailed record to be checked

16   FL 42 _____, 43 _____, and 47 _____

17   FL 55 _____

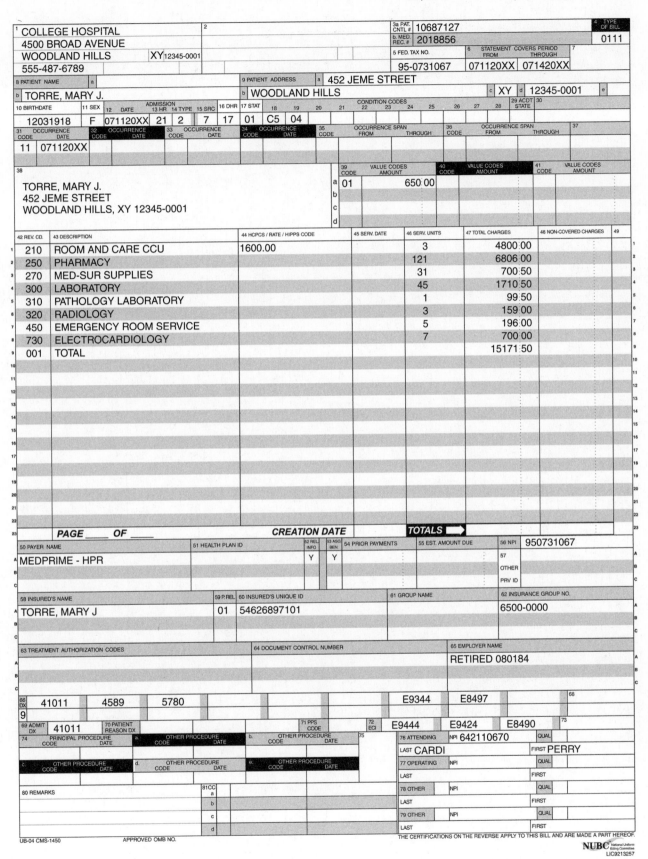

¹ COLLEGE HOSPITAL 4500 BROAD AVENUE WOODLAND HILLS XY 12345-0001 555-487-6789	²		3a PAT. CNTL # 10687127			4 TYPE OF BILL
			b. MED. REC. # 2018856			0111
			5 FED. TAX NO.	6 STATEMENT COVERS PERIOD FROM THROUGH		7
			95-0731067	071120XX 071420XX		

8 PATIENT NAME	a	9 PATIENT ADDRESS	a 452 JEME STREET				
b TORRE, MARY J.		b WOODLAND HILLS			c XY	d 12345-0001	e

10 BIRTHDATE	11 SEX	12 DATE ADMISSION 13 HR 14 TYPE 15 SRC	16 DHR	17 STAT	18 19 20 21 CONDITION CODES 22 23 24 25 26 27 28	29 ACDT STATE	30
12031918	F	071120XX 21 2 7	17	01	C5 04		

31 OCCURRENCE CODE DATE	32 OCCURRENCE CODE DATE	33 OCCURRENCE CODE DATE	34 OCCURRENCE CODE DATE	35 OCCURRENCE SPAN CODE FROM THROUGH	36 OCCURRENCE SPAN CODE FROM THROUGH	37
11 071120XX						

38		39 CODE VALUE CODES AMOUNT	40 CODE VALUE CODES AMOUNT	41 CODE VALUE CODES AMOUNT
TORRE, MARY J. 452 JEME STREET WOODLAND HILLS, XY 12345-0001	a	01 650 00		
	b			
	c			
	d			

42 REV. CD.	43 DESCRIPTION	44 HCPCS / RATE / HIPPS CODE	45 SERV. DATE	46 SERV. UNITS	47 TOTAL CHARGES	48 NON-COVERED CHARGES	49
1 210	ROOM AND CARE CCU	1600.00		3	4800 00		1
2 250	PHARMACY			121	6806 00		2
3 270	MED-SUR SUPPLIES			31	700 50		3
4 300	LABORATORY			45	1710 50		4
5 310	PATHOLOGY LABORATORY			1	99 50		5
6 320	RADIOLOGY			3	159 00		6
7 450	EMERGENCY ROOM SERVICE			5	196 00		7
8 730	ELECTROCARDIOLOGY			7	700 00		8
9 001	TOTAL				15171 50		9
10							10
11							11
12							12
13							13
14							14
15							15
16							16
17							17
18							18
19							19
20							20
21							21
22							22
23	PAGE ___ OF ___	CREATION DATE		TOTALS ➡			23

50 PAYER NAME	51 HEALTH PLAN ID	52 REL INFO	53 ASG BEN	54 PRIOR PAYMENTS	55 EST. AMOUNT DUE	56 NPI 950731067	
A MEDPRIME - HPR		Y	Y			57	A
B						OTHER	B
C						PRV ID	C

58 INSURED'S NAME	59 P.REL	60 INSURED'S UNIQUE ID	61 GROUP NAME	62 INSURANCE GROUP NO.	
A TORRE, MARY J	01	54626897101		6500-0000	A
B					B
C					C

63 TREATMENT AUTHORIZATION CODES	64 DOCUMENT CONTROL NUMBER	65 EMPLOYER NAME	
A			A
B		RETIRED 080184	B
C			C

66 DX	41011	4589	5780				E9344	E8497		68	
9											
69 ADMIT DX	41011	70 PATIENT REASON DX			71 PPS CODE	72 ECI	E9444	E9424	E8490	73	

74 PRINCIPAL PROCEDURE CODE DATE	a. OTHER PROCEDURE CODE DATE	b. OTHER PROCEDURE CODE DATE	75	76 ATTENDING NPI 642110670	QUAL
c. OTHER PROCEDURE CODE DATE	d. OTHER PROCEDURE CODE DATE	e. OTHER PROCEDURE CODE DATE		LAST CARDI FIRST PERRY	
				77 OPERATING NPI	QUAL
				LAST FIRST	

80 REMARKS	81CC a	78 OTHER NPI	QUAL
	b	LAST FIRST	
	c	79 OTHER NPI	QUAL
	d	LAST FIRST	

UB-04 CMS-1450   APPROVED OMB NO.   THE CERTIFICATIONS ON THE REVERSE APPLY TO THIS BILL AND ARE MADE A PART HEREOF.

NUBC National Uniform Billing Committee LIC9213257

Figure 17–1

ASSIGNMENT 17-7 ▸ LOCATE ERRORS ON A COMPUTER-GENERATED UB-04 CLAIM FORM

Performance Objective

Task: Locate the Form Locator blocks/fields on the computer-generated insurance claim form that need completion of missing information or have data that need to be corrected before submission to the insurance company.

Conditions: Use Henry M. Cosby's completed insurance claim (Figure 17–2), the checklist for editing a UB-04 claim form, and a red ink pen.

Standards: Time: _____ minutes

Accuracy: _____

(Note: The time element and accuracy criteria may be given by your instructor.)

Directions. Refer to Figure 17–5 in the *Handbook* to employ the step-by-step approach while editing the computer-generated UB-04 claim form (Figure 17–2). Use the checklist to help you when reviewing the claim form. Locate the Form Locator blocks/fields on the claim form that need completion of missing information or that have data to be corrected before submission to the insurance company. Highlight all errors you discover. Insert all corrections and missing information in red. If you cannot locate the necessary information but know it is mandatory, write "NEED" in the corresponding Form Locator block/field. State the reason or reasons why the claim may be rejected or delayed or why incorrect payment may be generated because of one or more errors discovered.

Checklist for Editing a Uniform Bill (UB-04) Claim Form: Henry M. Cosby
Steps   *Form Locator Blocks/Fields*

1   FL 1 _____ and 5 _____

2   FL 4: Inpatient _____ Outpatient _____

3   FL 8b _____, 38 _____, 58 _____

 and 59 _____

4   FL 10 _____

5   FL 8b _____ and 11 _____

6   FL 50 _____, 60 _____, 61 _____

 62 _____ and 65 _____

7   FL 67 _____ and 69 _____

8   FL 74 _____ _____ and 74 a-e _____

9   FL 76 _____

10   FL 6 _____, 12 _____, and 32 _____

11   **Inpatient:** FL 42–47: 13 _____,

       16 _____, and 46 _____

12   FL 47 _____

13   FL 42 _____ and 46 _____

14   **Outpatient:** FL 43 _____, 44 _____,

      and 45 _____

15   Detailed record to be checked

16   FL 42 _____, 43 _____, and 47 _____

17   FL 55 _____

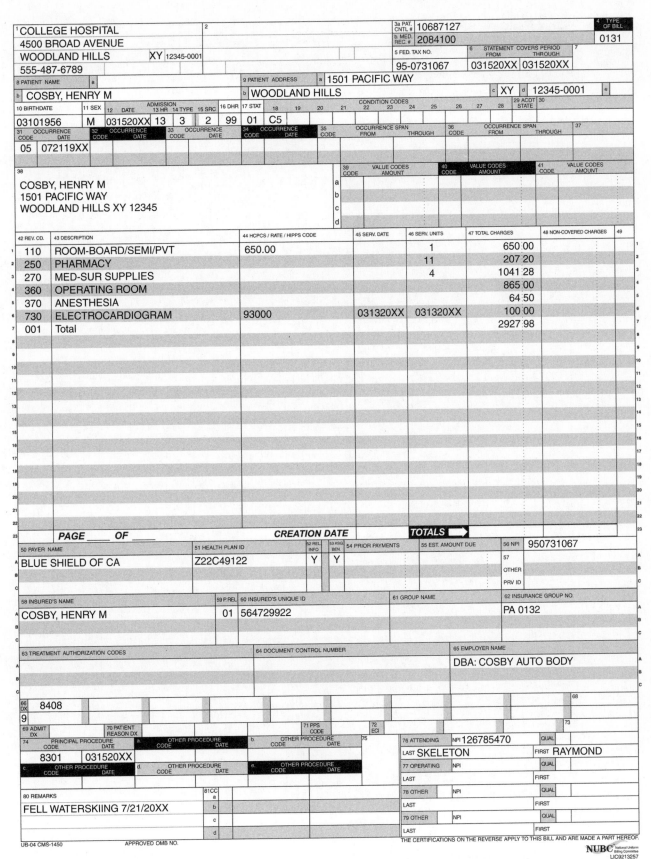

Figure 17–2

ASSIGNMENT 17–8 ▸ LOCATE ERRORS ON A COMPUTER-GENERATED UB-04 CLAIM FORM

Performance Objective

Task: Locate the blocks on the computer-generated insurance claim form that need completion of missing information or have data that need to be corrected before submission to the insurance company.

Conditions: Use Harold M. McDonald's completed insurance claim (Figure 17–3), the checklist for editing a UB-04 claim form, and a red ink pen.

Standards: Time: _____ minutes

Accuracy: _____

(Note: The time element and accuracy criteria may be given by your instructor.)

Directions. Refer to Figure 17–5 in the *Handbook* to employ the step-by-step approach while editing the computer-generated UB-04 claim form (Figure 17–3). Use the checklist to help you when reviewing the claim form. Locate the blocks on the claim form that need completion of missing information or that have data to be corrected before submission to the insurance company. Highlight all errors you discover. Insert all corrections and missing information in red. If you cannot locate the necessary information but know it is mandatory, write "NEED" in the corresponding block.

You notice that the seventh CPT/Healthcare Common Procedure Coding System (HCPCS) code 43450 for operating room is missing. On hospital claims, the entry for operating room is usually blank and must be handwritten in, because this is the code for the surgical procedure.

Checklist for Editing a Uniform Bill (UB-04) Claim Form: Harold M. McDonald

Steps   *Form Locator Block/Fields*

1   FL 1 _____ and 5 _____

2   FL 4: Inpatient _____ Outpatient _____

3   FL 8b _____, 38 _____, 58 _____,

     and 59 _____

4   FL 10 _____

5   FL 8b _____ and 11 _____

6   FL 50 _____, 60 _____, 61 _____,

     62 _____, and 65 _____

7   FL 67 _____ and 69 _____

8   FL 74 _____ _____ and 74 a-e _____

9   FL 76 _____

10   FL 6 _____, 12 _____, and 32 _____

11   **Inpatient:** FL 42–47: 13 _____,

       16 _____, and 46 _____

12   FL 47 _____

13   FL 42 _____ and 46 _____

14   **Outpatient:** FL 43 _____, 44 _____,

       and 45 _____

15   Detailed record to be checked

16   FL 42 _____, 43 _____, and 47 _____

17   FL 55 _____

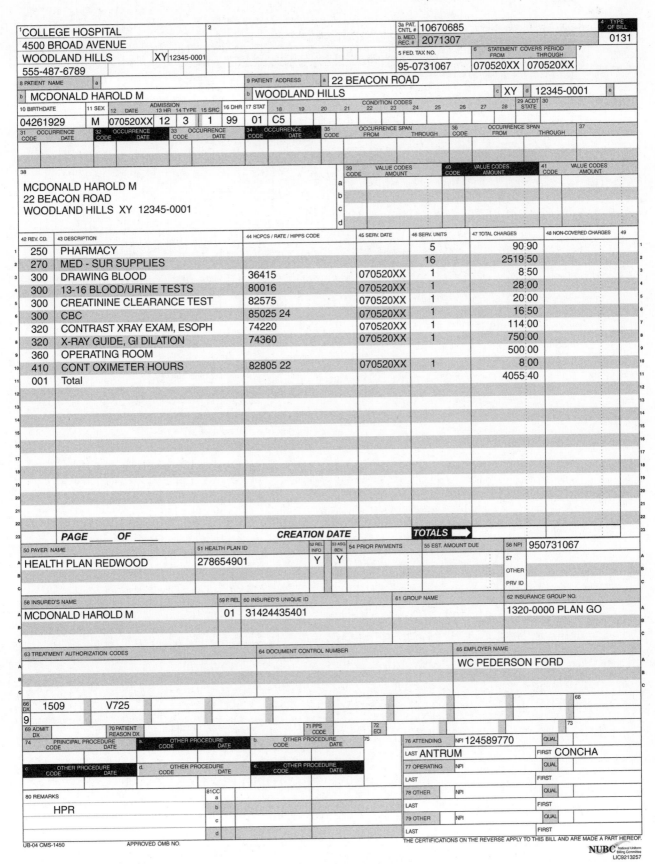

Figure 17–3

ASSIGNMENT **17–9** ▸ **LOCATE ERRORS ON A COMPUTER-GENERATED UB-04 CLAIM FORM**

Performance Objective

Task: Locate the blocks on the computer-generated insurance claim form that need completion of missing information or have data that need to be corrected before submission to the insurance company.

Conditions: Use Pedro Martinez's completed insurance claim (Figure 17–4), the checklist for editing a UB-04 claim form, and a red ink pen.

Standards: Time: _____ minutes

               Accuracy: _____

               (Note: The time element and accuracy criteria may be given by your instructor.)

Directions. Refer to Figure 17–5 in the *Handbook* to employ the step-by-step approach while editing the computer-generated UB-04 claim form (Figure 17–4). Use the checklist to help you when reviewing the claim form. Locate the blocks on the claim form that need completion of missing information or that have data to be corrected before submission to the insurance company. Highlight all errors you discover. Insert all corrections and missing information in red. If you cannot locate the necessary information but know it is mandatory, write "NEED" in the corresponding block. Then write a list of reasons why the claim may be rejected or delayed or why incorrect payment may be generated because of errors discovered.

Checklist for Editing a Uniform Bill (UB-04) Claim Form: Pedro Martinez

Steps	*Form Locator Block/Fields*
1	FL 1 _____ and 5 _____
2	FL 4: Inpatient _____ Outpatient _____
3	FL 8b _____, 38 _____, 58 _____, and 59 _____
4	FL 10 _____
5	FL 8b _____ and 11 _____
6	FL 50 _____, 60 _____, 61 _____, 62 _____ and 65 _____
7	FL 67 _____ and 69 _____
8	FL 74 _____ _____ and 74 a-e _____
9	FL 76 _____
10	FL 6 _____, 12 _____, and 32 _____

11   **Inpatient:** FL 42–47: 13 _____,

          16 _____, and 46 _____

12   FL 47 _____

13   FL 42 _____ and 46 _____

14   **Outpatient:** FL 43 _____, 44 _____,

          and 45 _____

15   Detailed record to be checked

16   FL 42 _____, 43 _____, and 47 _____

17   FL 55 _____

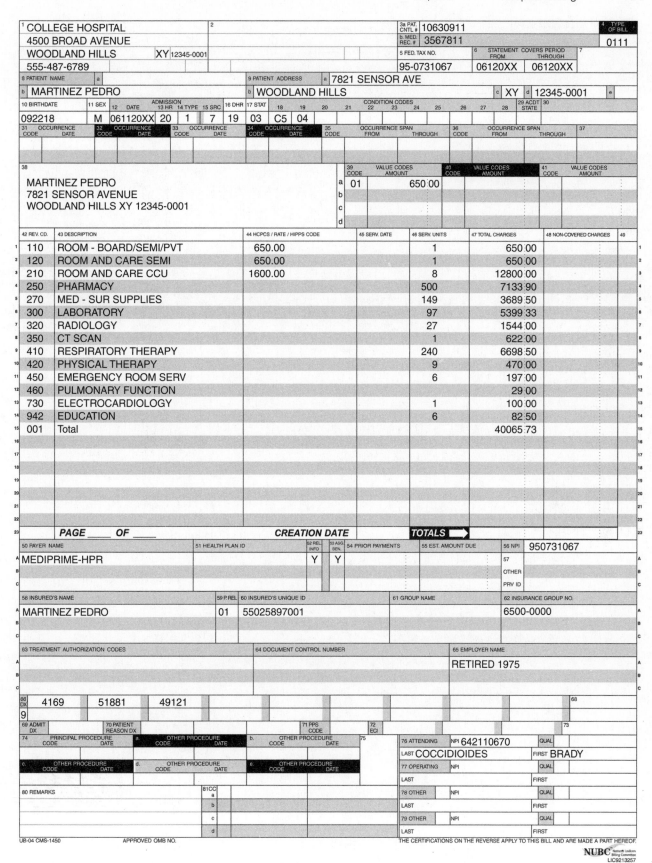

Figure 17–4

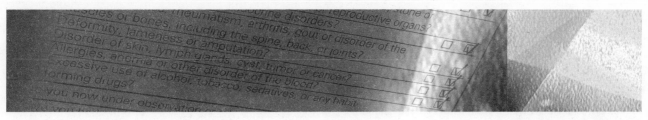

Seeking a Job and Attaining Professional Advancement

KEY TERMS

Your instructor may wish to select some words pertinent to this chapter for a test. For definitions of the terms, further study, and/or reference, the words, phrases, and abbreviations may be found in the glossary at the end of the Handbook. Key terms for this chapter follow.

alien

application form

blind mailing

business associate agreement

certification

Certified Coding Specialist (CCS)

Certified Coding Specialist-Physician (CCS-P)

Certified Medical Assistant (CMA)

Certified Medical Billing Specialist (CMBS)

Certified Professional Coder (CPC, CPC-A, CPC-H)

chronologic resume

claims assistance professional (CAP)

combination resume

continuing education

cover letter

electronic claims processor (ECP)

employment agency

functional resume

interview

mentor

National Certified Insurance and Coding Specialist (NCICS)

networking

portfolio

Professional Association of Health Care Office Managers (PAHCOM)

Registered Medical Assistant (RMA)

Registered Medical Coder (RMC)

registration

resume

self-employment

service contract

KEY ABBREVIATIONS

See how many abbreviations and acronyms you can translate and then use this as a handy reference list. Definitions for the key abbreviations are located near the back of the Handbook *in the glossary.*

AAPC _____

AHIMA _____

CAP _____

CCAP _____

CCS _____

CCS-P _____

CECP _____

CMA _____

CMBS _____

CMRS _____

CPC, CPC-A, CPC-H _____

ECP _____

EEOC _____

HRS _____

INS _____

NCICS _____

PAHCOM _____

RMA _____

RMC _____

PERFORMANCE OBJECTIVES

The student will be able to:

- Define and spell the key terms and key abbreviations for this chapter, given the information from the *Handbook* glossary, within a reasonable time period and with enough accuracy to obtain a satisfactory evaluation.
- After reading the chapter, answer the fill-in-the-blanks, multiple choice, and true/false review questions with enough accuracy to obtain a satisfactory evaluation.
- Research information in preparation for typing a resume, given a worksheet to complete, within a reasonable time period and with enough accuracy to obtain a satisfactory evaluation.
- Type an accurate resume in attractive format, using plain typing paper, within a reasonable time period, to obtain a satisfactory evaluation.

- Compose and type a letter of introduction to go with the resume and place it in a typed envelope, using one sheet of plain typing paper and a number 10 envelope, within a reasonable time period, to obtain a satisfactory evaluation.
- Complete an application form for a job, given an application for position form, within a reasonable time period and with enough accuracy to obtain a satisfactory evaluation.
- Compose and type a follow-up thank-you letter and place it in a typed envelope, using one sheet of plain typing paper and a number 10 envelope, within a reasonable time period, to obtain a satisfactory evaluation.
- Access the Internet and visit websites to research and/or obtain data, within a reasonable time period and with enough accuracy to obtain a satisfactory evaluation.

STUDY OUTLINE

Employment Opportunities
　Insurance Billing Specialist
　Claims Assistance Professional
Job Search
　Online Job Search
　Job Fairs
　Application
　Letter of Introduction
　Resume
　Interview
　Follow-up Letter

Self-Employment
　Setting Up an Office
　Finances to Consider
　Marketing, Advertising, Promotion, and Public
　　Relations
　Documentation
　Mentor and Business Incubator Services
　Networking
Procedure: Creating an Electronic Resume

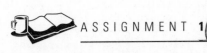 ASSIGNMENT 18-1 ▸ REVIEW QUESTIONS

Part I Fill in the Blank

Review the objectives, key terms, glossary definitions of key terms, chapter information, and figures before completing the following review questions.

1. You have just completed a 1-year medical insurance billing course at a college. Name some preliminary job search contacts to make on campus.

   a. job placement personnel
   b. classmates
   c. instructors
   d. school counselors

2. Name skills that may be listed on an application form or in a resume when a person is seeking a position as an insurance billing specialist.

   a. list typing w.p.m.
   b. computer equipment operated
   c. experience in medical software programs
   d. accurate procedure & diagnostic coding
   e. experience expertise in insurance claims completion + submission
   f. knowledge of medical terminology + insurance terminology

3. A question appears on a job application form about salary. Two ways in which to handle this question are

   a. negotiable   y write
   b. a flexible

4. State the chief purpose of a cover letter when a resume is sent to a prospective employer.

   introduction of the person sending the resume

5. List the items to be compiled in a portfolio.

   a. letters of recommendation
   b. school diplomas
   c. name & addresses of references
   d. social security card
   e. neatly typed insurance claim forms w/evidence of coding experience

f. degrees

g. transcripts

h. Certificates

i extra copies of the resume

j. other related items related to prior education & work experience

6. You are being interviewed for a job and the interviewer asks this question: "What is your religious preference?" How would you respond?

Forgive me for being rude, but I ~~dont think~~ that's not pertanent to my job qualifications ~~or a job interview~~

7. If a short period of time elapses after an interview and the applicant has received no word from the prospective employer, what follow-up steps may be taken?

P.641   a. write a follow up letter, thanks for the interview + restate your interest in the job

b. send email

8. If an individual creates a billing company and coding services are to be part of the offerings, the coding professional should have what type of professional status?

Certified Professional coder

9. Hugh Beason was the owner of XYZ Medical Reimbursement Service. A fire occurred, damaging some of the equipment and part of the office premises and requiring him to stop his work for a month so that repairs could be made. What type/types of insurance would be helpful for this kind of problem?

Property insurance

10. Gwendolyn Stevens has an insurance billing company and is attending a professional meeting where she has given business cards to a few attendees. Give two reasons for using this business marketing strategy.

a. Potential for new clients

b. spread the word about her business

11. State the difference between *certification* and *registration*.

a. Certification: a statement issued by a board or association verifying that a person meets professional standards

b. Registration: entry into an official registry or record that lists names of persons in an occupation who've satisfied specific requirements or gotten a certain level of education + paying a fee

12. Name some ways an insurance billing specialist may seek to keep knowledge current.

    a. _net_

    b. _continuous education_

    c. _Coworkers_

    d. _read books_

13. Jerry Hahn is pursuing a career as a claims assistance professional. When he markets his business, the target

    P630 audience should be _those who need a professional claims assistant_
    hospital patients that need help w/insurance issues

14. Jennifer Inouye has been hired as a coding specialist by a hospital and needs to keep documentation when working. This may consist of

    a. _Name of patient_

    b. _whats wrong w/them_

    c. _Oro primary care physician_

15. Give the names of at least two national organizations that certify billers and coders.

    a. _American Association of Medical Billers in LA or V_

    b. _American Association of Professional coders_
    academy

Part II Multiple Choice

Choose the best answer.

16. A resume format that emphasizes work experience dates is known as

    a. functional

    b. combination

    c. business

    d. chronologic

17. When an individual plans to start an insurance billing company, he or she should have enough funds to operate the business for a period of

    a. 6 months or more

    P644

    b. 18 months or more

    c. 1 year or more

    d. 2 years

18. Under HIPAA regulations, if a physician has his insurance billing outsourced to a person, this individual is

known as a/an _____ because he or she uses and discloses individuals' identifiable health information.

   a. billing specialist

   (b) business associate

   c. outside contractor

   d. outside vendor

19. When insurance billing is outsourced to a company, a document should be created, signed, and notarized by both parties known as a

   a. contract agreement

   b. business agreement

   (c) service contract

   d. legal contract

20. A guide who offers advice, criticism, and guidance to an inexperienced person to help him or her reach a goal is known as a/an

   (a) mentor

   b. counselor

   c. associate

   d. instructor

Part III True/False

Write "T" or "F" in the blank to indicate whether you think the statement is true or false.

__T__ 21. A resume format that stresses job skills is known as functional.

__T__ 22. When job applicants have similar skills and education, surveys have shown that hiring by employers has been based on bilingual skills.

__T__ 23. Enhancing knowledge and keeping up to date are responsibilities of an insurance billing specialist.

__F__ 24. Professional status of an insurance billing specialist may be obtained by passing a national examination for an CMRS.

__F__ 25. Professional status of a claims assistance professional may be obtained by passing a national examination as a CCS.

ASSIGNMENT 18–2 ▸ CONSULT A RESUME WORKSHEET

Performance Objective

Task: Complete a worksheet in preparation for typing your resume.

Conditions: Use one sheet of plain typing paper and a computer or typewriter.

Standards: Time: _____ minutes

               Accuracy: _____

               (Note: The time element and accuracy criteria may be given by your instructor.)

Directions. Complete a worksheet in preparation for typing your resume. Some of the information requested on the worksheet should not appear on the resume but should be available if you are asked to provide it.

1. Insert title of personal data sheet.

2. Insert heading: name, address, telephone number, and so on.

3. Select one of three formats for data.

4. Insert heading and data for education information.

5. Insert heading and data for skill information.

6. Insert heading and data for employment information.

7. Insert reference information.

8. Print worksheet.

9. Ask a classmate to review and comment on worksheet.

ASSIGNMENT **18–3** ▶ **TYPE A RESUME**

Performance Objective

Task: Respond to a job advertisement and type a resume by abstracting data from your worksheet devel-
                       oped in Assignment 18–2.

Conditions: Use one sheet of plain typing paper, a newspaper advertisement (Figure 18–1), and a computer or
                       typewriter.

Standards: Time: _____ minutes

                       Accuracy: _____

                       (Note: The time element and accuracy criteria may be given by your instructor.)

Directions. An advertisement appeared in your local newspaper (Figure 18–1). You decide to apply for the position.
Abstract data that you think are relevant from your information worksheet, and type a resume in rough draft. Ask
the instructor for suggestions to improve the rough draft. Refer to Chapter 18 and Figure 18–6 in the *Handbook* to
help organize your resume into an attractive format before you type the final copy.

1. Insert title of personal data sheet from worksheet.

2. Insert heading: name, address, telephone number, and so on.

3. Select one of three formats for data.

4. Insert heading and data for education information.

5. Insert heading and data for skill information.

6. Insert heading and data for employment information.

7. Insert reference information.

8. Proofread resume.

9. Print resume.

MEDICAL INSURANCE CODING/REIMBURSEMENT SPECIALIST

Mid-Atlantic Clinic, a 20-physician, multi-specialty group practice in Chicago, Illinois, has a need for a coding and reimbursement specialist. Knowledge of medical terminology, CPT and ICD-9-CM coding systems, Medicare regulations, third-party insurance reimbursement and physician billing procedures required. Proficiency in the interpretation and coding of procedural and diagnostic codes is strongly preferred. Successful candidates must have excellent communication and problem-solving skills. This position offers a competitive salary and superior benefits. Please send resume to:

George B. Pason, Personnel Director
Mid-Atlantic Clinic
1230 South Main Street
Chicago, IL 60611

Figure 18–1

ASSIGNMENT **18-4** ▸ **COMPLETE A COVER LETTER**

Performance Objective

Task: Compose a cover letter to accompany your resume.

Conditions: Use one sheet of plain typing paper, a number 10 envelope, and a computer or typewriter.

Standards: Time: _____ minutes

                 Accuracy: _____

                 (Note: The time element and accuracy criteria may be given by your instructor.)

Directions. Compose a cover letter introducing yourself, and type a rough draft. Consult the instructor for suggestions. Type the cover letter on plain bond paper in a form that can be mailed. Refer to the sample letter in Chapter 18 and Figure 18–5 in the *Handbook* as a guide to help organize your thoughts. Type the name and address of the employer on a number 10 envelope, and insert the letter with the resume from Assignment 18–3.

ASSIGNMENT 18–5 ▸ COMPLETE A JOB APPLICATION FORM

Performance Objective

Task:　　　　Complete a job application form by using data from your resume.

Conditions:　Use application form (Figures 18–2, *A* and *B*), your resume, and computer or typewriter.

Standards:　Time: _____ minutes

　　　　　　Accuracy: _____

　　　　　　(Note: The time element and accuracy criteria may be given by your instructor.)

Directions. Assume that the employer asked you to come to his or her place of business to complete an application form and make an appointment for an interview. Using your data and resume, complete an application form (Figures 18–2, *A* and *B*).

APPLICATION FOR POSITION/ Medical or Dental Office
AN EQUAL OPPORTUNITY EMPLOYER

(In answering questions, use extra blank sheet if necessary)

No employee, applicant, or candidate for promotion training or other advantage shall be discriminated against (or given preference) because of race, color, religion, sex, age, physical handicap, veteran status, or national origin.
PLEASE READ CAREFULLY AND WRITE OR PRINT ANSWERS TO ALL QUESTIONS. DO NOT TYPE

Date of application

A. PERSONAL INFORMATION

Name- Last   First   Middle   Social Security No.   Area Code/Phone No. ( )

Present Address: -Street   (Apt. #)   City   State   Zip   How long at this address?

Previous Address: -Street   City   State   Zip   Person to notify in case of Emergency or Accident - Name:

From: To: Address: Telephone:

B. EMPLOYMENT INFORMATION

For what position are you applying?   ☐ Full-time ☐ Part-time ☐ Either   Date available for employment?:   Wage/Salary Expectations:

List hrs./days you prefer to work: List any hrs./days you are not available: (Except for times required for religious practices or observances)   Can you work overtime, if necessary? ☐ Yes ☐ No

Are you employed now? ☐ Yes ☐ No   If so, may we inquire of your present employer?: ☐ No ☐ Yes, If yes: Name of employer: Phone number: ( )

Have you ever been bonded?: ☐ Yes ☐ No   If required for position, are you bondable? ☐ Yes ☐ No ☐ Uncertain   Have you applied for a position with this office before? ☐ No ☐ Yes, If yes, when?:

Referred by/ or where did you hear of this job?:

Can you, upon employment, submit verification of your legal right to work in the United States? ☐ Yes ☐ No
Submit proof that you meet legal age requirement for employment? ☐ Yes ☐ No   Language(s) applicant speaks or writes (if use of a language other than English is relevant to the job for which applicant is applying):

C. EDUCATIONAL HISTORY

Name and address of schools attended (Include current)	Dates From	Dates Thru	Highest grade/level completed	Diploma/degree(s) obtained/areas of study:
High school				
College				Degree/Major
Post graduate				Degree/Major
Other				Course/Diploma/License Certificate

Specific training, education, or experiences which will assist you in the job for which you have applied:

Future educational plans:

D. SPECIAL SKILLS

CHECK BELOW THE KINDS OF WORK YOU HAVE DONE:

☐ BLOOD COUNTS	☐ DENTAL ASSISTANT	☐ MEDICAL INSURANCE FORMS	☐ RECEPTIONIST
☐ BOOKKEEPING	☐ DENTAL HYGIENIST	☐ MEDICAL TERMINOLOGY	☐ TELEPHONES
☐ COLLECTIONS	☐ FILING	☐ MEDICAL TRANSCRIPTION	☐ TYPING
☐ COMPOSING LETTERS	☐ INJECTIONS	☐ NURSING	☐ STENOGRAPHY
☐ COMPUTER INPUT	☐ INSTRUMENT STERILIZATION	☐ PHLEBOTOMY (Draw Blood)	☐ URINALYSIS
OFFICE EQUIPMENT USED: ☐ COMPUTER	☐ DICTATING EQUIPMENT	☐ POSTING	☐ X-RAY
		☐ WORD PROCESSOR	☐ OTHER:

Other kinds of tasks performed or skills that may be applicable to position: Typing speed: Shorthand speed:

RM NO. 72-110 ©1976 BIBBERO SYSTEMS INC. PETALUMA, CA (MB-CO) # 2-5 (REV. 10/92)
REORDER CALL 800-BIBBERO (800) 242-2376

(PLEASE COMPLETE OTHER SIDE)

Figure 18–2a

E. EMPLOYMENT RECORD

LIST MOST RECENT EMPLOYMENT FIRST

May we contact your previous Employer(s) for a reference? ☐ yes ☐ no

1) Employer

Work performed. Be specific.

Address   Street   City   State   Zip code

Phone number (   )

Type of business | Dates | Mo. | Yr. | Mo. | Yr.
From   To

Your position | Hourly rate/Salary
Starting   Final

Supervisor's name

Reason for leaving

2) Employer

Work performed. Be specific:

Address   Street   City   State   Zip code

Phone number (   )

Type of business | Dates | Mo. | Yr. | Mo. | Yr.
From   To

Your position | Hourly rate/Salary
Starting   Final

Supervisor's name

Reason for leaving

3) Employer

Work performed. Be specific:

Address   Street   City   State   Zip code

Phone number (   )

Type of business | Dates | Mo. | Yr. | Mo. | Yr.
From   To

Your position | Hourly rate/Salary
Starting   Final

Supervisor's name

Reason for leaving

F. REFERENCES: FRIENDS/ACQUAINTANCES NON-RELATED

1) Name   Address   Telephone Number (☐Work ☐Home)   Occupation   Years acquainted

2) Name   Address   Telephone Number (☐Work ☐Home)   Occupation   Years acquainted

Please feel free to add any information which you feel will help us consider you for employment.

READ THE FOLLOWING CAREFULLY, THEN SIGN AND DATE THE APPLICATION

I certify that all answers given by me on this application are true, correct and complete to the best of my knowledge. I acknowledge notice that the information contained in this application is subject to check. I agree that, if hired, my continued employment may be contingent upon the accuracy of that information. If employed, I further agree to comply with company/office rules and regulations.

Signature _____   Date: _____

RM NO. 72-110   ©1976 BIBBERO SYSTEMS INC.   PETALUMA, CA (MB-CO) # 6-7 (REV. 4/92)

TO REORDER CALL 800-BIBBERO (800) 242-2376

ASSIGNMENT 18–6 ▸ **PREPARE A FOLLOW-UP THANK-YOU LETTER**

Performance Objective

Task: Prepare a follow-up thank-you letter after the interview, sending it to the interviewer.

Conditions: Use one sheet of plain typing paper, a number 10 envelope, and a computer or typewriter.

Standards: Time: _____ minutes

                    Accuracy: _____

                    (Note: The time element and accuracy criteria may be given by your instructor.)

Directions. After the interview, you decide to send a follow-up thank-you letter to the person who interviewed you. Type a letter and address a number 10 envelope. Refer to Chapter 18 and Figure 18–12 in the *Handbook* to help organize your thoughts.

ASSIGNMENT 18–7 ▸ VISIT WEB SITES FOR JOB OPPORTUNITIES

Performance Objective

Task: Access the Internet and visit several websites of the World Wide Web.

Conditions: Use a computer with printer and/or a pen or pencil to make notes.

Standards: Time: _____ minutes

                Accuracy: _____

(Note: The time element and accuracy criteria may be given by your instructor.)

Directions. For active weblinks to the following resources, visit the Evolve website online at: http://evolve. elsevier.com/Fordney/handbook. If you have access to the Internet, visit the World Wide Web and do some job searching. After obtaining the website data, take them to share for class discussion. Note that some sites may not be accessible if you attempt to visit them during peak hours.

1. Visit the American Association of Medical Assistants' website, and click on "AAMA Job Source." See whether there are any new job opportunities in your state. Print a hard copy of the names, addresses, and telephone numbers of participating employers near your region while you remain online.
2. Connect to the Allied Health Opportunities for Healthcare Professionals' website. Click on "Employment Opportunities." After you get to that screen, click on "Allied Health Opportunities," and at the next screen, click on "Medical Assistants" or "Health Information Management Professionals." Then see whether you can locate any listings for billing or coding positions. Print out some of the listings that appeal to you, and take them to class for discussion.
3. Check out an online resource, hcPro's Health Information Management Supersite. This site has job postings for many medical job titles for people involved in health information management. Click on the Career Center under the Interactive site features to see job postings. Then click on "HIM Job Listings." Enter a job title, such as "coder" or "biller," to do a search, and see whether you can locate any job openings. Print some of these listings to share and discuss during class.
4. Visit the JustCoding website and click the link to the Coding Career Center. Then click on "Search for a Job" under the "For Employees" heading. Enter a key word, such as "coder," and see whether you can obtain any search results. Print some of these listings to share and discuss during class.
5. Access the Internet and use a search engine (Yahoo, Excite, AltaVista). Key in "Yahoo insurance billers" to search for job opportunities. See whether you can locate any jobs that are in your region or state. List three website addresses that you find and take them to share for class discussion.

ASSIGNMENT 18–8 ▸ CRITICAL THINKING

Performance Objective

Task: Write a paragraph describing the benefits of becoming certified in this field.

Conditions: Use a computer with printer and/or a pen or pencil.

Standards: Time: _____ minutes

               Accuracy: _____

               (Note: The time element and accuracy criteria may be given by your instructor.)

Directions. Write a paragraph or two describing why you would like to become certified in this field, and incorporate a numbered list of benefits. Make sure grammar, punctuation, and spelling are correct.

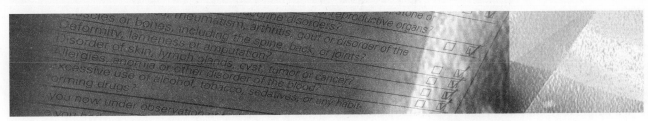

Tests

TEST 1: PROCEDURE (E/M AND MEDICINE SECTIONS) AND DIAGNOSTIC PROCEDURE CODE TEST

Directions. Using a *Current Procedural Terminology* (CPT) code book or Appendix A in this *Workbook*, insert the correct code numbers and modifiers for each service rendered. Give a brief description for each professional service rendered, although this is not needed for completing the CMS-1500 (08-05) claim form.

An optional exercise is to abstract the pertinent data from each case, then use the *International Classification of Diseases, Ninth Revision, Clinical Modification* (ICD-9-CM) code book to insert the diagnosis code.

Insert year of the CPT code book used

_____

Insert year of the ICD-9-CM code book used

_____

1. Dr. Input sees a new patient, Mrs. Post, in the office for acute abdominal distress. The physician spends approximately 1 hour obtaining a comprehensive history and physical examination with high-complexity decision making. Several diagnostic studies are ordered, and Mrs. Post is given an appointment to return in 1 week.

Description

_____ CPT # _____

_____ ICD # _____

2. Mr. Nakahara, an established patient, sees Dr. Practon in the office on January 11 for a reevaluation of his diabetic condition. Dr. Practon takes a detailed history and performs a detailed examination. Decision making is moderately complex.

Description

_____ CPT # _____

_____ ICD # _____

3. Dr. Cardi sees Mrs. Franklin for a follow-up office visit for her hypertension. A problem-focused history and examination of her cardiovascular system are obtained and reveal a blood pressure of 140/100. Decision making is straightforward, with medication being prescribed. The patient is advised to return in 2 weeks to have her blood pressure checked by the nurse. Mrs. Franklin returns 2 weeks later, and the nurse checks her blood pressure.

Description

_____ CPT # _____

_____ ICD # _____

_____ CPT # _____

_____ ICD # _____

4. Dr. Skeleton receives a call at 7 PM from Mrs. Snyder. Her husband, a patient of Dr. Skeleton's, has been very ill for 2 hours with profuse vomiting. Dr. Skeleton goes to their home to see Mr. Snyder and spends considerable time obtaining a detailed history and examination. The medical decision making is of a highly complex nature. The physician administers an injection of prochlorperazine (Compazine).

Description

_____ CPT # _____

_____ CPT # _____

_____ ICD # _____

5. Dr. Cutis sees an established patient, a registered nurse, for determination of pregnancy. A detailed history and examination are obtained, with moderate-complexity medical decision making. A Papanicolaou smear is taken, a blood sample is drawn, and the specimens are sent to an independent laboratory for a qualitative human chorionic gonadotropin (hCG) test. The patient also complains of something she has discovered under her armpit. On examination, there is a furuncle of the left axilla, which is incised and drained during this visit. The laboratory requires CPT coding on the laboratory requisition. List how these laboratory procedures would appear on the requisition sheet. The Papanicolaou smear is processed according to the Bethesda System and under physician supervision.

Professional Service Rendered by Dr. Cutis

_____ CPT # _____

_____ CPT # _____

_____ CPT # _____

_____ CPT # _____

_____ ICD # _____

_____ ICD # _____

Laboratory Service on Requisition Sheet

_____ CPT # _____

_____ CPT # _____

6. Dr. Antrum makes a house call on Betty Mason, an established patient, for a problem-focused history of acute otitis media. A problem-focused examination is performed, with straightforward medical decision making. While there, Dr. Antrum also sees Betty's younger sister, Sandra, whom she has seen previously in the office, for acute tonsillitis. A problem-focused history and examination are performed with low-complexity decision making. In addition to the examinations, Dr. Antrum gives both children injections of penicillin.

Professional Service Rendered to Betty

_____ CPT # _____

_____ CPT # _____

_____ ICD # _____

Professional Service Rendered to Sandra

_____ CPT # _____

_____ CPT # _____

_____ ICD # _____

7. Two weeks later, Dr. Antrum is called to the emergency department at College Hospital at 2 AM on Sunday to see Betty Mason for recurrent chronic otitis media with suppuration. A problem-focused history and examination are performed with straightforward decision making. Dr. Antrum administers a second injection of penicillin.

Description

_____ CPT # _____

_____ CPT # _____

_____ ICD # _____

8. While at the hospital, Dr. Antrum is asked to see another patient in the emergency department, who is new to her. A problem-focused history is taken. She performs a problem-focused examination and straightforward decision making for an intermediate 3.5-cm laceration of the scalp. The laceration is sutured, and the patient is advised to come to the office in 4 days for a dressing change. Four days later, the patient comes into the office for a dressing change by the nurse.

Description

_____   CPT # _____

_____   CPT # _____

_____   CPT # _____

_____   ICD # _____

9. Dr. Menter, a psychiatrist, sees the following patients in the hospital. Code each procedure.
   Ms. Blake: Consultation, expanded problem-focused history and examination and straightforward decision making; referred by Dr. Practon   CPT # _____

   Mrs. Clark: Group psychotherapy (50 min)   CPT # _____

   Mrs. Samson: Group psychotherapy (50 min)   CPT # _____

   Mr. Shoemaker: Group psychotherapy (50 min)   CPT # _____

   Miss James: Individual psychotherapy (25 min)   CPT # _____

10. Dr. Input, a gastroenterologist, sees Mrs. Chan in the hospital at the request of Dr. Practon for an esophageal ulcer. In addition to the detailed history and examination and the low-complexity decision making, Dr. Input performs an esophageal intubation and washings, and prepares slides for cytology. Two days later, he sees Mrs. Chan in follow-up inpatient consultation and obtains a problem-focused interval history and examination with low-complexity decision making. He performs a gastric intubation and collects washings for cytologic evaluation for a gastric ulcer.

Description

_____   CPT # _____

_____   CPT # _____

_____   ICD # _____

_____   CPT # _____

_____   CPT # _____

_____   ICD # _____

11. Mrs. Galati, a new patient, goes to Dr. Cardi because of chest pain (moderate to severe), weakness, fatigue, and dizziness. Dr. Cardi takes a comprehensive history and performs a comprehensive examination, including electrocardiography (ECG) with interpretation and report, followed by treadmill ECG. He also performs a vital capacity test and dipstick urinalysis, and draws blood for triiodothyronine (T_3) testing and for analysis by sequential multiple analyzer computer (SMAC) (16 panel tests, including complete blood cell count [CBC]), which are sent to and billed by a laboratory. Medical decision making is of high complexity.

Description

_____	CPT # _____
_____	CPT # _____
_____	CPT # _____
_____	CPT # _____
_____	CPT # _____
_____	CPT # _____
_____	ICD # _____
_____	ICD # _____
_____	ICD # _____

12. Jake Wonderhill has not had his eyes examined by Dr. Lenser for about 5 years. He is seen by Dr. Lenser, who performs the following ophthalmologic procedures in addition to a comprehensive eye examination: fluorescein angioscopy and electroretinography. Mr. Wonderhill receives a diagnosis of retinitis pigmentosa.

Description

_____	CPT # _____
_____	CPT # _____
_____	CPT # _____
_____	ICD # _____

13. Dr. Practon is making rounds at the College Hospital and answers an urgent call on 3rd Floor East. He performs resuscitation on Mr. Sanchez for cardiac arrest and orders the patient taken to the critical care unit. Chest radiographs, laboratory work, blood gas measurements, and ECG are performed. The physician is detained 2 hours in constant attendance on the patient.

Description

_____	CPT # _____
_____	CPT # _____
_____	ICD # _____

14. Mrs. Powers, a new patient, sees Dr. Skeleton for low sciatica. Dr. Skeleton takes a detailed history and performs a detailed examination of the patient's lower back and extremities. Medical decision making is of low complexity. Diathermy (30 minutes) is given. The next day the patient comes in for therapeutic exercises in the Hubbard tank (30 minutes).

Description

_____ CPT # _____

_____ CPT # _____

_____ ICD # _____

_____ CPT # _____

_____ ICD # _____

15. a. Mrs. Garcia, a new patient, is seen by Dr. Caesar for occasional vaginal spotting (detailed history/examination and low-complexity decision making). The doctor determines that the bleeding is coming from the cervix and asks her to return in 3 days for cryocauterization of the cervix. During the initial examination, Mrs. Garcia asks for an evaluation for possible infertility. Dr. Caesar advises her to wait 2 to 3 weeks and make an appointment for two infertility tests.
    b. When the patient returns in 3 days for cryocauterization, the doctor also takes a wet mount for bacteria/fungi, which is sent to and billed by a laboratory.
    c. Three weeks later, an injection procedure for hysterosalpingography and endometrial biopsy are performed.

Description

a. _____ CPT # _____

   _____ ICD # _____

b. _____ CPT # _____

   _____ CPT # _____

   _____ ICD # _____

c. _____ CPT # _____

   _____ CPT # _____

   _____ ICD # _____

Multiple Choice. After reading the boxed codes with descriptions, select the answer/answers that is/are best in each case.

59120	surgical treatment of ectopic pregnancy; tubal or ovarian, requiring salpingectomy and/or oophorectomy, abdominal or vaginal approach.
59121	tubal or ovarian, without salpingectomy and/or oophorectomy
59130	abdominal pregnancy
59135	interstitial, uterine pregnancy requiring total hysterectomy
59136	interstitial, uterine pregnancy with partial resection of uterus
59140	cervical, with evacuation

16. In regard to this section of CPT codes, which of the following statements is true about codes 59120 through 59140? Mark all that apply.

    a. They refer to abdominal hysterotomy.

    b. They involve laparoscopic treatment of ectopic pregnancy.

    c. They refer to treatment of ectopic pregnancy by surgery.

    d. They involve tubal ligation.

17. In regard to this section of CPT codes, for treatment of a tubal ectopic pregnancy, necessitating oophorectomy, the code to select is

    a. 59121

    b. 59120

    c. 59135

    d. 59136

    e. 59130

18. In regard to this section of CPT codes, for treatment of an ectopic pregnancy (interstitial, uterine) requiring a total hysterectomy, the code/codes to select is/are

    a. 59135

    b. 59135 and 59120

    c. 59120

    d. 59130 and 59120

    e. 59121

TEST 2: PROCEDURE CODE WITH MODIFIERS AND DIAGNOSTIC CODE TEST

Match the description given in the right column with the procedure code/modifier combination in the left column. Write the letter in the blank.

Procedure with Modifier   *Description*

1. 99245–21 _____   a. Dr. Practon assisted Dr. Caesar with a total abdominal hysterectomy and bilateral salpingo-oophorectomy.

2. 99204–57 _____   b. Dr. Skeleton interprets a thoracolumbar x-ray film that was taken at College Hospital.

3. 58150–80 _____   c. Mrs. Ulwelling saw Dr. Antrum for an office visit as a new patient, and she recommended that the patient undergo a laryngoscopy, with stripping of vocal cords to be done the following day.

4. 32440–55 _____   d. Mrs. Gillenbach walked through a plate glass window and underwent a rhinoplasty, performed by Dr. Graff on February 16, 20xx. On February 26, 20xx, she came to see Dr. Graff for a consultation regarding reconstructive surgery on her right leg.

5. 72080–26 _____   e. Mr. Mercado was seen by Dr. Langerhans in the office for a complicated diabetic consultation. A comprehensive history and examination were obtained, with high-complexity medical decision making; however, the physician spent a total of 2 hours with the patient.

6. 29425–58 _____   f. Dr. Cutler performed a bilateral orchiopexy (inguinal approach) on baby Kozak.

7. 54640–50 _____   g. Dr. Skeleton applied a short leg walking cast to Mrs. Belchere's right leg 4 weeks after his initial treatment of her fractured tibia.

8. 99253–24 _____   h. Dr. Cutler went on vacation, and Dr. Coccidioides took care of Mrs. Ash during the postoperative period after her total pneumonectomy.

Directions. Using a *Current Procedural Terminology* (CPT) code book or Appendix A in this *Workbook*, insert the correct code numbers and modifiers for each service rendered. Give a brief description for each professional service rendered, although this is not needed for completing the CMS-1500 (08-05) claim form.

9. Dr. Input performs a gastrojejunostomy for carcinoma in situ of the duodenum and calls in Dr. Scott to administer the anesthesia and Dr. Cutler to assist. This intraperitoneal surgery takes 2 hours, 30 minutes. The patient is otherwise normal and healthy. List the procedure and diagnostic code numbers with appropriate modifiers for each physician.

Professional Service Rendered by Dr. Input

_____   CPT # _____

_____   ICD # _____

Professional Service Rendered by Dr. Scott

_____   CPT # _____

_____   ICD # _____

Professional Service Rendered by Dr. Cutler

_____   CPT # _____

_____   ICD # _____

10. Dr. Rumsey assists Dr. Cutler with a total colectomy (intraperitoneal procedure) with ileostomy. Dr. Scott is the anesthesiologist. Surgery takes 2 hours, 55 minutes. The patient has a secondary malignant neoplasm of the colon (severe systemic disease). List the procedure code numbers with appropriate modifiers and diagnostic code numbers for each physician.

Professional Service Rendered by Dr. Rumsey

_____   CPT # _____

_____   ICD # _____

Professional Service Rendered by Dr. Scott

_____   CPT # _____

_____   ICD # _____

Professional Service Rendered by Dr. Cutler

_____   CPT # _____

_____   ICD # _____

11. Dr. Cutis removes a malignant tumor from a patient's back (1.5 cm) and does the local anesthesia herself.

Description

_____   CPT # _____

_____   ICD# _____

12. Dr. Skeleton sees Mr. Richmond, a new patient worked into the office schedule on an emergency basis after a motor vehicle traffic accident. Mr. Richmond has multiple lacerations of the face, arm, and chest and a fracture of the left tibia. The physician takes a comprehensive history and performs a comprehensive examination. Decision making is moderately complex. Dr. Skeleton orders bilateral radiographs of the tibia

and fibula and two views of the chest and left wrist to be taken in his office. Then he closes the following lacerations: 2.6 cm, simple, face; 2.0 cm, intermediate, face; 7.5 cm, intermediate, right arm; 4.5 cm, intermediate, chest. All radiographs are negative except that of the left tibia. Dr. Skeleton performs a manipulative reduction of the left tibial shaft and applies a cast. Code this case as if you were actually listing the codes on the CMS-1500 (08-05) claim form.

Description

_____   CPT # _____ and _____

_____   CPT # _____

_____   CPT # _____

_____   CPT # _____

_____   CPT # _____

_____   CPT # _____

_____   CPT # _____

_____   CPT # _____

_____   CPT # _____

_____   CPT # _____

_____   CPT # _____

_____   CPT # _____

_____   CPT # _____

_____   CPT # _____

_____   CPT # _____

Six weeks later, Dr. Skeleton sees the same patient for an office visit and obtains radiographs (two views) of the left tibia and fibula. Treatment involves application of a cast below the patient's left knee to the toes, including a walking heel.

Description

_____   CPT # _____

_____   CPT # _____

_____   CPT # _____

_____   ICD # _____

13. Dr. Cutler performs an incisional biopsy of a patient's breast for a breast lump, which requires 40 minutes of anesthesia. Dr. Scott is the anesthesiologist. The patient is otherwise normal and healthy. List the procedure and diagnostic code numbers for each physician.

Professional Service Rendered by Dr. Cutler

_____ CPT # _____

_____ ICD # _____

Professional Service Rendered by Dr. Scott

_____ CPT # _____

_____ ICD # _____

14. Mrs. DeBeau is aware that Dr. Input will be out of town for 6 weeks; however, she decides to have him perform the recommended combined anterior-posterior colporrhaphy with enterocele repair for vaginal enterocele. Dr. Practon agrees to perform the follow-up care and assist. Dr. Scott is the anesthesiologist. The anesthesia time is 2 hours, 15 minutes. The patient is normal and healthy. List the procedure and diagnostic code numbers for each physician. Note: Emphasis for this problem should be placed on the choice of CPT modifiers.

Professional Service Rendered by Dr. Input

_____ CPT # _____

_____ ICD # _____

Professional Service Rendered by Dr. Practon

_____ CPT # _____

_____ CPT modifier _____

_____ CPT modifier _____

_____ ICD # _____

Professional Service Rendered by Dr. Scott

_____ CPT # _____

_____ ICD # _____

15. Mr. Wong, a new patient, is seen in the College Hospital and undergoes a comprehensive history and physical examination (H & P) with moderately complex decision making. Dr. Coccidioides performs a bronchoscopy with biopsy. Results of the biopsy confirm the diagnosis: malignant neoplasm of upper left lobe of lung. The following day the physician performs a total pneumonectomy. Dr. Cutler assists on the total pneumonectomy (pulmonary resection), and Dr. Scott is the anesthesiologist. Surgery takes 3 hours, 45 minutes. The patient has mild systemic disease. List the procedure and diagnostic code numbers for each physician.

Professional Service Rendered by Dr. Coccidioides

_____ CPT # _____

_____ CPT # _____

_____ CPT # _____

_____ ICD # _____

Professional Service Rendered by Dr. Cutler

_____ CPT # _____

_____ ICD # _____

Professional Service Rendered by Dr. Scott

_____ CPT # _____

_____ ICD # _____

When completing the CMS-1500 (08-05) claim form for Dr. Scott, in which block

would you list anesthesia minutes? _____

TEST 3: PROCEDURE (RADIOLOGY AND PATHOLOGY SECTIONS) AND DIAGNOSTIC CODE TEST

Directions. Using a CPT code book or Appendix A in this *Workbook*, insert the correct procedure code numbers and modifiers and diagnostic codes for each service rendered. Give a brief description for each professional service rendered, although this is not needed for completing the CMS-1500 (08-05) claim form.

1. Mrs. Cahn sees Dr. Skeleton because of severe pain in her right shoulder. She is a new patient. Dr. Skeleton takes a detailed history and performs a detailed examination. A complete x-ray study of the right shoulder is done. Decision making is of low complexity. A diagnosis of bursitis is made, and an injection into the bursa is administered.

Description

_____ CPT # _____

_____ CPT # _____

_____ CPT # _____

_____ ICD # _____

2. John Murphy comes into the Broxton Radiologic Group, Inc., for an extended radiation therapy consultation for prostatic cancer. The radiologist takes a detailed history and does a detailed examination. Decision making is of low complexity. The physician determines a simple treatment plan involving simple simulation-aided field settings. Basic dosimetry calculations are done, and the patient returns the following day and receives radiation therapy to a single treatment area (6 to 10 MeV).

Description

_____ CPT # _____

_____ CPT # _____

_____ CPT # _____

_____ CPT # _____

_____ CPT # _____

Diagnosis: _____ ICD # _____

3. Dr. Input refers Mrs. Horner to the Nuclear Medicine department of the Broxton Radiologic Group, Inc., for a bone marrow imaging of the whole body and imaging of the liver and spleen. List the procedure code numbers after each radiologic procedure to show how the radiology group would bill. Also, list the diagnosis of malignant neoplasm of the bone marrow.

Description

Total body bone marrow, imaging   CPT # _____

Radiopharmaceuticals, diagnostic (Iodine I-123)   HCPCS # _____

Liver and spleen imaging   CPT # _____

Radiopharmaceuticals, diagnostic (Iodine I-123)   HCPCS # _____

Diagnosis: _____   ICD # _____

4. Dr. Input also refers Mrs. Horner to XYZ Laboratory for the following tests. List the procedure code numbers to indicate how the laboratory would bill.

Description

CBC, automated and automated differential   CPT # _____

Urinalysis, automated with microscopy   CPT # _____

Urine culture (quantitative, colony count)   CPT # _____

Urine antibiotic sensitivity (microtiter)   CPT # _____

5. The general laboratory at College Hospital receives a surgical tissue specimen (ovarian biopsy) for gross and microscopic examination from a patient with Stein-Leventhal syndrome. List the procedure and diagnostic code numbers to indicate what the hospital pathology department would bill.

Description

_____   CPT # _____

Diagnosis: _____   ICD # _____

6. Dr. Langerhans refers Jerry Cramer to XYZ Laboratory for a lipid panel. He has a family history of cardiovascular disease. List the procedure and diagnostic code number or numbers to indicate how the laboratory would bill.

Description

_____   CPT # _____

Diagnosis: _____   ICD # _____

7. Dr. Caesar is an OB/GYN specialist who has her own ultrasound machine. Carmen Cardoza, age 45, is referred to Dr. Caesar for an obstetric consultation and an amniocentesis with ultrasonic guidance. The diagnosis is Rh incompatibility. The doctor performs a detailed history and physical examination, and decision making is of low complexity.

Description

_____ CPT # _____

_____ CPT # _____

_____ CPT # _____

_____ ICD # _____

8. Mr. Marcos's medical record indicates that a retrograde pyelogram followed by a percutaneous nephrostolithotomy, with basket extraction of a 1-cm stone, was performed by Dr. Ulibarri for nephrolithiasis.

Description

_____ CPT # _____

_____ CPT # _____

Diagnosis: _____ ICD # _____

9. Broxton Radiologic Group, Inc., performs the following procedures on Mrs. Stephens at the request of Dr. Input. List the procedure code numbers after each radiologic procedure. On the laboratory slip, the following congenital diagnoses are listed: Diverticulum of the stomach and colon; cystic lung. Locate the corresponding diagnostic codes.

Barium enema   CPT # _____

Evaluation of upper gastrointestinal tract with small bowel   CPT # _____

Complete chest X-ray   CPT # _____

Diagnosis: _____   ICD # _____

Diagnosis: _____   ICD # _____

Diagnosis: _____   ICD # _____

10. Two weeks later, Mrs. Stephens is referred again for further radiologic studies for flank pain. List the procedure and diagnostic code numbers after each radiologic procedure.

Intravenous pyelogram (IVP) with drip infusion   CPT # _____

Oral cholecystography   CPT # _____

Diagnosis: _____   ICD # _____

TEST 4: COMPLETE A CMS-1500 (08-05) CLAIM FORM

Performance Objective

Task: Complete a CMS-1500 (08-05) claim form for a private case and post transactions to the patient's financial accounting record.

Conditions: Use the patient's record (Figure 1) and financial statement (Figure 2); one health insurance claim form; a typewriter, computer, or pen; procedural and diagnostic code books; and appendices A and B in this *Workbook*.

Standards: Claim Productivity Management

Time: _____ minutes

Accuracy: _____

(Note: The time element and accuracy criteria may be given by your instructor.)

Directions

1. Using OCR guidelines, complete a CMS-1500 (08-05) claim form and direct it to the private carrier. Refer to Jennifer T. Lacey's patient record for information and Appendix A in this *Workbook* to locate the fees to record on the claim, and post them to the financial statement. Date the claim August 15. Dr. Caesar is accepting assignment, and the patient's signatures to release information to the insurance company and to have the payment forwarded directly to the physician are on file.

2. Use your CPT code book or Appendix A in this *Workbook* to determine the correct five-digit code numbers and modifiers for each professional service rendered. Use your HCPCS Level II code book or refer to Appendix B in this *Workbook* for HCPCS procedure codes and modifiers. Use your diagnostic code book to code each active diagnosis.

3. Record the proper information on the financial record and claim form, and note the date when you have billed the insurance company.

4. American Commercial Insurance Company sent a check (voucher number 5586) on November 17 in the amount of $880. The patient's responsibility is $220. Post the payment, write off (adjust) the remaining balance, and circle the amount billed to the patient.

PATIENT RECORD NO. T-4

Lacey	Jennifer	T	11-12-45	F	555-549-0098
LAST NAME	FIRST NAME	MIDDLE NAME	BIRTH DATE	SEX	HOME PHONE

451 Roberts Street	Woodland Hills	XY	12345
ADDRESS	CITY	STATE	ZIP CODE

555-443-9899	555-549-0098		lacey@wb.net
CELL PHONE	PAGER NO.	FAX NO.	E-MAIL ADDRESS

430-XX-7709	Y0053498
PATIENT'S SOC. SEC. NO.	DRIVER'S LICENSE

legal secretary	Higgins and Higgins Attorneys at Law
PATIENT'S OCCUPATION	NAME OF COMPANY

430 Second Avenue, Woodland Hills, XY 12345	555-540-6675
ADDRESS OF EMPLOYER	PHONE

SPOUSE OR PARENT	OCCUPATION

EMPLOYER	ADDRESS	PHONE

American Commercial Insurance Company, 5682 Bendix Blvd., Woodland Hills, XY 12345	
NAME OF INSURANCE	INSURED OR SUB SCRIBER

5789022	444
POLICY/CERTIFICATE NO.	GROUP NO.

REFERRED BY: Clarence Cutler, MD

Figure 1

Continued

DATE	PROGRESS NOTES No. T-4
8-1-xx	New pt referred by Dr. Cutler, came into office for consultation and additional opinion.
	CC: Full feeling in stomach and low abdominal region.
	Irregular menstruation. Ultrasonic report showed
	leiomyomata uteri and rt ovarian mass; however, visualization of mass poor and type
	cannot be identified. Pap smear Class I. No personal or family hx of CA.
	Comprehensive physical examination performed on healthy appearing white female.
	Wt: 136 lbs. BP 128/60. T 98.6 F. Palpated rt adnexal mass and
	enlarged uterus; vulva and cervix appear normal; LMP 7/16/XX.
	Tx plan: Adv hospital admit and additional tests to R/O carcinoma.
	Tentatively scheduled abdominal hysterectomy with bilateral salpingo-oophorectomy.
	(M/MDM).
	BC/llf *Bertha Caesar, MD*
8-2-xx	Adm to College Hosp (C HX/PX M/MDM). Scheduled
	surgery at 7:00 A.M. tomorrow.
	BC/llf *Bertha Caesar, MD*
8-3-xx	Perf abdominal
	hysterectomy with bilateral salpingo-oophorectomy.
	BC/llf *Bertha Caesar, MD*
8-4-xx	HV (EPF HX/PX M/MDM) Path report revealed interstitial leiomyomata uteri and corpus
	luteum cyst of rt ovary. Pt C/O PO pain, otherwise doing well.
	BC/llf *Bertha Caesar, MD*
8-5-xx	HV (EPF HX/PX M/MDM). Pt ambulating well, pain decreased. Dressing changed, wound
	healing well.
	BC/llf *Bertha Caesar, MD*
8-6-xx	HV (PF HX/PX SF/MDM). Pain minimal. Pt ambulating without assistance.
	Removed staples, no redness or swelling. Pln DC tomorrow.
	BC/llf *Bertha Caesar, MD*
8-7-xx	Discharge to home; pt doing well. RTO next wk.
	BC/llf *Bertha Caesar, MD*

Figure 1, cont'd

STATEMENT
COLLEGE CLINIC
4567 Broad Avenue
Woodland Hills, XY 12345-0001
Tel. 555-486-9002
Fax No. 555-487-8976

Acct. No. T-4

Jennifer T. Lacey
451 Roberts Street
Woodland Hills, XY 12345

Phone No. (H) (555) 549-0098   (W) (555) 540-6675   Birthdate 11-12-45

Insurance Co. American Commercial Insurance Company   Policy/Group No. 5789022 / 444

DATE	REFERENCE	DESCRIPTION	CHARGES	CREDITS PYMNTS.	ADJ.	BALANCE	
20XX			BALANCE FORWARD →				
8-1-xx		Consult					
8-2-xx		Admit					
8-3-xx		TAH BSO					
8-4-xx		HV					
8-5-xx		HV					
8-6-xx		HV					
8-7-xx		Discharge					

PLEASE PAY LAST AMOUNT IN BALANCE COLUMN

THIS IS A COPY OF YOUR FINANCIAL ACCOUNT AS IT APPEARS ON OUR RECORDS

Figure 2

TEST 5: COMPLETE A CMS-1500 (08-05) CLAIM FORM

Performance Objective

Task: Complete a CMS-1500 (08-05) claim form for a private case and post transactions to the patient's financial accounting record.

Conditions: Use the patient's record (Figure 3) and financial statement (Figure 4); one health insurance claim form; a typewriter, computer, or pen; procedural and diagnostic code books; and appendices A and B in this *Workbook*.

Standards: Claim Productivity Management

Time: _____ minutes

Accuracy: _____

(Note: The time element and accuracy criteria may be given by your instructor.)

Directions

1. Using OCR guidelines, complete a CMS-1500 (08-05) claim form and direct it to the private carrier. Refer to Hortense N. Hope's patient record for information and Appendix A in this *Workbook* to locate the fees to record on the claim, and post them to the financial statement. Date the claim July 31. Dr. Practon is accepting assignment, and the patient's signatures to release information to the insurance company and to have the payment forwarded directly to the physician are on file.

2. Use your CPT code book or Appendix A in this *Workbook* to determine the correct five-digit code numbers and modifiers for each professional service rendered. Use your HCPCS Level II code book or refer to Appendix B in this *Workbook* for HCPCS procedure codes and modifiers. Use your diagnostic code book to code each active diagnosis.

3. Record the proper information on the financial record and claim form, and note the date you have billed the insurance company.

PATIENT RECORD NO. T-5

Hope	Hortense	N		04-12-46	F	555-666-7821
LAST NAME	FIRST NAME	MIDDLE NAME		BIRTH DATE	SEX	HOME PHONE

247 Lantern Pike	Woodland Hills	XY	12345
ADDRESS	CITY	STATE	ZIP CODE

	555-323-1687	555-666-7821		hope@wb.net
CELL PHONE	PAGER NO.	FAX NO.		E-MAIL ADDRESS

321-XX-8809	N0058921
PATIENT'S SOC. SEC. NO.	DRIVER'S LICENSE

Clerk typist	R and S Manufacturing Company
PATIENT'S OCCUPATION	NAME OF COMPANY

2271 West 74 Street, Torres, XY 12349	555-466-5890
ADDRESS OF EMPLOYER	PHONE

Harry J. Hope	carpenter
SPOUSE OR PARENT	OCCUPATION

Jesse Construction Company, 3861 South Orange Street, Torres, XY 12349	555-765-2318
EMPLOYER ADDRESS	PHONE

Ralston Insurance Company, 2611 Hanley Street, Woodland Hills, XY 12345	
NAME OF INSURANCE	INSURED OR SUBSCRIBER

ATC321458809	T8471811A
POLICY/CERTIFICATE NO.	GROUP NO.

REFERRED BY: Harry J. Hope (husband)

DATE	PROGRESS NOTES
7-1-xx	New F pt comes in complaining of lt great toe pain. Incised, drained, and cleaned area
	around nail on lt great toe. Dx: onychia and paronychia. Started on antibiotic and adv to
	retn in 2 days for permanent excision of nail plate (EPF HX/PX SF/MDM).
	GP/llf *Gerald Practon, MD*
7-3-xx	Pt returns for nail excision. Injected procaine in lt great toe; removed entire toenail.
	Drs applied. PTR in 5 days for PO check.
	GP/llf *Gerald Practon, MD*
7-7-xx	PO check. Dressing changed, nail bed healing well. Pt to continue on AB until gone.
	Retn PRN (PF HX/PX SF/MDM).
	GP/llf *Gerald Practon, MD*

Figure 3

Acct No. T-5

STATEMENT
Financial Account
COLLEGE CLINIC
4567 Broad Avenue
Woodland Hills, XY 12345-0001
Tel. 555-486-9002
Fax No. 555-487-8976

Hortense N. Hope
247 Lantern Pike
Woodland Hills, XY 123345

Phone No. (H) 555-666-7821   (W)   555-466-5890   Birthdate 4/12/46

Primary Insurance Co.   Ralston Insurance Company   Policy/Group No. ATC321458809 / T8471811A

Secondary Insurance Co.   None   Policy/Group No.

DATE	REFERENCE	DESCRIPTION	CHARGES	PYMNTS.	ADJ.	BALANCE
20xx		BALANCE FORWARD ➡				
7-1-xx		NP OV				
7-1-xx		I & D lt great toe				
7-3-xx		Excision lt great toenail				
7-7-xx		PO check				

PLEASE PAY LAST AMOUNT IN BALANCE COLUMN ⬆

THIS IS A COPY OF YOUR FINANCIAL ACCOUNT AS IT APPEARS ON OUR RECORDS

Figure 4

TEST 6: COMPLETE A CLAIM FORM FOR A MEDICARE CASE

Performance Objective

Task: Complete a CMS-1500 (08-05) claim form and post transactions to the patient's financial accounting record.

Conditions: Use the patient's record (Figure 5) and financial statement (Figure 6); one health insurance claim form; a typewriter, computer, or pen; procedural and diagnostic code books; and appendices A and B in this *Workbook*.

Standards: Claim Productivity Management

                 Time: _____ minutes

                 Accuracy: _____

                 (Note: The time element and accuracy criteria may be given by your instructor.)

Directions

1. Using OCR guidelines, complete a CMS-1500 (08-05) claim form and direct it to the Medicare fiscal intermediary. To locate your local fiscal intermediary, go to website http://www.cms.hhs.gov/contacts/incardir.asp. Refer to Frances F. Foote's patient record for information and Appendix A in this *Workbook* to locate the fees to record on the claim, and post them to the financial statement. Date the claim October 31. Dr. Practon is a participating provider, and the patient's signatures to release information to the insurance company and to have the payment forwarded directly to the physician are on file.

2. Use your CPT code book or Appendix A in this *Workbook* to determine the correct five-digit code numbers and modifiers for each professional service rendered. Use your HCPCS Level II code book or refer to Appendix B in this *Workbook* for HCPCS procedure codes and modifiers. Use your diagnostic code book to code each active diagnosis.

3. Record the proper information on the patient's financial accounting record and claim form, and note the date when you have billed the insurance company.

PATIENT RECORD NO. T-6

Foote	Frances	F		08-10-32	F	555-678-0943
LAST NAME	FIRST NAME	MIDDLE NAME		BIRTH DATE	SEX	HOME PHONE

984 North A Street	Woodland Hills	XY	12345
ADDRESS	CITY	STATE	ZIP CODE

555-443-9908	555-320-7789	555-678-0943	foote@wb.net
CELL PHONE	PAGER NO.	FAX NO.	E-MAIL ADDRESS

578-XX-8924	B4309811
PATIENT'S SOC. SEC. NO.	DRIVER'S LICENSE

retired legal secretary	
PATIENT'S OCCUPATION	NAME OF COMPANY

ADDRESS OF EMPLOYER	PHONE

Harry L. Foote	roofer
SPOUSE OR PARENT	OCCUPATION

BDO Construction Company, 340 North 6th Street, Woodland Hills, XY 12345	555-478-9083
EMPLOYER ADDRESS	PHONE

Medicare	self
NAME OF INSURANCE	INSURED OR SUB SCRIBER

578-XX-8924A	
POLICY/CERTIFICATE NO.	GROUP NO.

REFERRED BY: G. U. Curette, MD, 4780 Main Street, Ehrlich, XY 12350 Tel: 555-430-8788   NPI #34216600XX

DATE	PROGRESS NOTES
10-11-xx	NP pt referred by Dr. Curette with a CC of foot pain centering around rt great toe and
	sometimes shooting up her leg. PF history taken. PF exam revealed severe overgrowth
	of nail into surrounding tissues. AP and lat right foot x-rays taken & interpreted which
	indicate no fractures or arthritis. Pt has had a N workup for gout by Dr. Curette.
	DX: Severe onychocryptosis both margins of rt hallux. Adv to sched. OP surgery at
	College Hospital for wedge resection of skin of nail fold to repair ingrown nail.
	No disability from work (SF/MDM).
	NP/llf *Nick Pedro, MD*
10-13-xx	Pt admitted for OP surgery at College Hospital. Complete wedge resection performed for
	repair of rt hallux ingrown nail. Pt will stay off foot over the weekend and retn next wk for
	PO re ch.
	NP/llf *Nick Pedro, MD*
10-20-xx	PO visit (PF HX/PX SF/MDM). Rt hallux healing well. RTC as necessary.
	NP/llf *Nick Pedro, MD*

Figure 5

Acct No. T-6

STATEMENT
Financial Account

COLLEGE CLINIC
4567 Broad Avenue
Woodland Hills, XY 12345-0001
Tel. 555-486-9002
Fax No. 555-487-8976

Frances F. Foote
984 North A Street
Woodland Hills, XY 12345

Phone No. (H)   555-678-0943   (W)   Birthdate   8/10/32

Primary Insurance Co.   Medicare   Policy/Group No.   578-XX-8924A

| DATE | REFERENCE | DESCRIPTION | CHARGES | CREDITS | | BALANCE |
				PYMNTS.	ADJ.	
20xx		BALANCE FORWARD ➡				
10-11-xx		NP OV				
10-11-xx		X-rays				
10-13-xx		Wedge excision/skin of nail fold				
10-20-xx		PO				

PLEASE PAY LAST AMOUNT IN BALANCE COLUMN ⬆

THIS IS A COPY OF YOUR FINANCIAL ACCOUNT AS IT APPEARS ON OUR RECORDS

Figure 6

TEST 7: COMPLETE A CLAIM FORM FOR A MEDICARE/MEDIGAP CASE

Performance Objective

Task: Complete two CMS-1500 (08-05) claim forms for a Medicare/Medigap case and post transactions to the patient's financial accounting record.

Conditions: Use patient's record (Figure 7) and financial statement (Figure 8); two health insurance claim forms; a typewriter, computer, or pen; procedural and diagnostic code books; and appendices A and B in this *Workbook*.

Standards: Claim Productivity Management

Time: _____ minutes

Accuracy: _____

(Note: The time element and accuracy criteria may be given by your instructor.)

Directions

1. Using OCR guidelines, complete two CMS-1500 (08-05) claim forms and direct them to the Medicare fiscal intermediary. To locate your local fiscal intermediary, go to website http://www.cms.hhs.gov/contacts/incardir.asp. Refer to Charles B. Kamb's patient record for information and Appendix A to locate the fees to record on the claim, and post them to the financial statement. Be sure to include the Medigap information on the claim form so that it will be crossed over (sent to the Medigap insurance carrier) automatically. Date the claim June 30. Dr. Practon is a participating provider with both Medicare and the Medigap program, and the patient's signatures to release information to the insurance companies and to have the payment forwarded directly to the physician are on file.

2. Use your CPT code book or Appendix A in this *Workbook* to determine the correct five-digit code numbers and modifiers for each professional service rendered. Use your HCPCS Level II code book or refer to Appendix B in this *Workbook* for HCPCS procedure codes and modifiers. Use your diagnostic code book to code each active diagnosis.

3. Record the proper information on the patient's financial accounting record and claim form, and note the date when you have billed the insurance company.

PATIENT RECORD NO. T-7

Kamb	Charles	B	01-26-27	M	555-467-2601
LAST NAME	FIRST NAME	MIDDLE NAME	BIRTH DATE	SEX	HOME PHONE

2600 West Nautilus Street	Woodland Hills	XY	12345	
ADDRESS	CITY	STATE	ZIP CODE	

CELL PHONE	PAGER NO.	FAX NO.	E-MAIL ADDRESS

454-XX-9569	M3200563	
PATIENT'S SOC. SEC. NO.	DRIVER'S LICENSE	

Retired TV actor	Amer. Federation of TV & Radio Artists (AFTRA)
PATIENT'S OCCUPATION	NAME OF COMPANY

30077 Ventura Boulevard, Woodland Hills, XY 12345	555-466-3331
ADDRESS OF EMPLOYER	PHONE

Jane C. Kamb	homemaker
SPOUSE OR PARENT	OCCUPATION

EMPLOYER	ADDRESS	PHONE

Medicare (Primary)	self	National Insurance Company (Medigap)
NAME OF INSURANCE	INSURED OR SUBSCRIBER	

454-XX-9569A	Medigap Policy No. 5789002	
POLICY/CERTIFICATE NO.	GROUP NO.	

REFERRED BY: Mrs. O. S. Tomy (friend)   National PAYRID NAT234567

DATE	PROGRESS NOTES
6-1-xx	New pt comes into ofc to est new PCP in area; recently moved from Ohio. W obese M c/o
	nasal bleeding for two and a half months c̄ headaches and nasal congestion. Pt states he
	has had HBP for 1 yr. Taking med: Serpasil prescribed by dr in Ohio; does not know dosage.
	Took a C HX and performed a C PX which revealed post nasal hemorrhage. Coagulation
	time (Lee and White) and microhematocrit (spun) done in ofc are WNL. BP 180/100.
	Used nasal cautery and post nasal packs to control hemorrhage. Rx prophylactic antibiotic
	to guard against sinusitis NKA. Adv retn tomorrow, bring hypertensive medication.
	Pt signed authorization to request med records from dr in Ohio. D: Recurrent epistaxis
	due to nonspecific hypertension. No disability from work.
	GP/llf *Gerald Practon, MD*
6-2-xx	Pt retns and nasal hemorrhage is reevaluated (PF HX/PX SF/MDM). Postnasal packs
	removed and replaced. BP 182/98. Pt forgot medication for hypertension but states he is
	taking it 2 X d. Adv retn in 1 day, bring medication.
	GP/llf *Gerald Practon, MD*
6-3-xx	Pt retns and nasal hemorrhage is reevaluated (PF HX/PX SF/MDM). Postnasal packs
	removed. BP 178/100. Verified hypertensive medication. Pt to increase dosage to 4 X d.
	Adv retn in 5 days.
	GP/llf *Gerald Practon, MD*
6-3-xx	Pt retns and nasal hemorrhage is reevaluated (EPF HX/PX L/MDM). Prev medical records
	arrived and reviewed. BP 190/102. Pt referred to Dr. Perry Cardi (int) for future care of
	hypertension.
	GP/llf *Gerald Practon, MD*

Figure 7

Acct No. ___T-7___

STATEMENT
Financial Account
COLLEGE CLINIC
4567 Broad Avenue
Woodland Hills, XY 12345-0001
Tel. 555-486-9002
Fax No. 555-487-8976

Charles B. Kamb
2600 West Nautilus Street
Woodland Hills, XY 12345

Phone No. (H) ___555-467-2601___ (W) ___None/retired___ Birthdate ___1-26-27___

Primary Insurance Co. ___Medicare___ Policy/Group No. ___454-XX-9569A___

Secondary Insurance Co. ___National Insurance Company (Medigap)___ Policy/Group No. ___5789002___

DATE	REFERENCE	DESCRIPTION	CHARGES	CREDITS PYMNTS.	ADJ.	BALANCE	
20xx		BALANCE FORWARD					
6-1-xx		NP OV					
6-1-xx		Coagulation time					
6-1-xx		Microhematocrit					
6-1-xx		Post nasal pack/cautery					
6-2-xx		OV					
6-2-xx		Subsequent nasal pack					
6-3-xx		OV					
6-8-xx		OV					

PLEASE PAY LAST AMOUNT IN BALANCE COLUMN

THIS IS A COPY OF YOUR FINANCIAL ACCOUNT AS IT APPEARS ON OUR RECORDS

Figure 8

TEST 8: COMPLETE A CLAIM FORM FOR A MEDICAID CASE

Performance Objective

Task: Complete a CMS-1500 (08-05) claim form for a Medicaid case and post transactions to the patient's financial accounting record.

Conditions: Use the patient's record (Figure 9) and financial statement (Figure 10); one health insurance claim form; a typewriter, computer, or pen; procedural and diagnostic code books; and appendices A and B in this *Workbook*.

Standards: Claim Productivity Management

Time: _____ minutes

Accuracy: _____

(Note: The time element and accuracy criteria may be given by your instructor.)

Directions

1. Using OCR guidelines, complete a CMS-1500 (08-05) claim form and direct it to the Medicaid fiscal intermediary. Obtain the address of your Medicaid fiscal agent by first going to website http://www.cms.hhs.gov/medicaid/geninfo and then either sending an e-mail message to the Medicaid contact or using the toll-free number to obtain the Medicaid carrier name and address. An option might be to contact your local state medical society. Refer to Louise K. Herman's patient record for information and Appendix A to locate the fees to record on the claim, and post them to the financial statement. Date the claim May 31.

2. Use your CPT code book or Appendix A in this *Workbook* to determine the correct five-digit code numbers and modifiers for each professional service rendered. Use your HCPCS Level II code book or refer to Appendix B in this *Workbook* for HCPCS procedure codes and modifiers. Use your diagnostic code book to code each active diagnosis.

3. Record the proper information on the patient's financial accounting record and claim form and note the date when you have billed the insurance company.

4. Post the payment of $350 (voucher number 4300), received from the Medicaid fiscal intermediary 40 days after claim submission, and write off (adjust) the balance of the account.

PATIENT RECORD NO. T-8

Herman	Louise	K	11-04-50	F	555-266-9085
LAST NAME	FIRST NAME	MIDDLE NAME	BIRTH DATE	SEX	HOME PHONE

13453 Burbank Boulevard	Woodland Hills	XY	12345
ADDRESS	CITY	STATE	ZIP CODE

555-466-7003		555-266-9085	herman@wb.net
CELL PHONE	PAGER NO.	FAX NO.	E-MAIL ADDRESS

519-XX-0018	T0943995
PATIENT'S SOC. SEC. NO.	DRIVER'S LICENSE

unemployed budget analyst	
PATIENT'S OCCUPATION	NAME OF COMPANY

ADDRESS OF EMPLOYER	PHONE

Harold D. Herman	retired salesman
SPOUSE OR PARENT	OCCUPATION

EMPLOYER	ADDRESS	PHONE

Medicaid	self
NAME OF INSURANCE	INSURED OR SUBSCRIBER

0051936001X	
MEDICAID NO.	GROUP NO.

REFERRED BY: Raymond Skeleton, MD

DATE	PROGRESS NOTES
5-6-xx	NP pt referred by Dr. Skeleton. CC: Rectal bleeding. Took a comprehensive history and
	performed a comprehensive physical examination. Diagnostic anoscopy revealed
	bleeding int and ext hemorrhoids and 2 infected rectal polyps. Rx antibiotics. Retn in
	2 days for removal of hemorrhoids and polyps (M/MDM)
	RR/llf *Rex Rumsey, MD*
5-8-xx	Pt returned to office for simple internal/external hemorrhoidectomy. Rigid
	proctosigmoidoscopy also perf for removal of polyps using snare technique. Adv. sitz
	baths daily. Continue on AB until gone. Retn in 1 wk.
	RR/llf *Rex Rumsey, MD*
5-15-xx	DNS Telephoned pt and rescheduled.
	Mary Bright, CMA
5-17-xx	PO OV (EPF HX/PX LC/MDM). Pt progressing well. No pain, discomfort or bleeding.
	Discharged from care, retn PRN.
	RR/llf *Rex Rumsey, MD*

Figure 9

Acct No. __T-8__

STATEMENT
Financial Account
COLLEGE CLINIC
4567 Broad Avenue
Woodland Hills, XY 12345-0001
Tel. 555-486-9002
Fax No. 555-487-8976

Louise K. Herman
13453 Burbank Boulevard
Woodland Hills, XY 12345

Phone No. (H) __555-266-9085__   (W) _____   Birthdate __11/4/50__

Primary Insurance Co. __Medicaid__   Policy/Group No. __0051936001X__

Secondary Insurance Co._____   Policy/Group No._____

DATE	REFERENCE	DESCRIPTION	CHARGES	CREDITS PYMNTS.	ADJ.	BALANCE	
20xx			BALANCE FORWARD				
5-6-xx		NP OV					
5-6-xx		Dx anoscopy					
5-8-xx		Int/Ext Hemorrhoidectomy					
5-8-xx		Proctosigmoidoscopy with removal of polyps					
5-17-xx		PO OV					

PLEASE PAY LAST AMOUNT IN BALANCE COLUMN

THIS IS A COPY OF YOUR FINANCIAL ACCOUNT AS IT APPEARS ON OUR RECORDS

Figure 10

TEST 9: COMPLETE A CLAIM FORM FOR A TRICARE CASE

Performance Objective

Task: Complete a CMS-1500 (08-05) claim form for a TRICARE case and post transactions to the patient's financial accounting record.

Conditions: Use the patient's record (Figure 11) and financial statement (Figure 12); one health insurance claim form; a typewriter, computer, or pen; procedural and diagnostic code books; and appendices A and B in this *Workbook*.

Standards: Claim Productivity Management

Time: _____ minutes

Accuracy: _____

(Note: The time element and accuracy criteria may be given by your instructor.)

Directions

1. Using OCR guidelines, complete a CMS-1500 (08-05) claim form and direct it to the TRICARE carrier. To locate your local fiscal intermediary, go to website http://www.tricare.osd.mil. Click on the area of the map you are residing in and then choose a state to access claims information for that state. Refer to Darlene M. Cash's patient record for information and Appendix A to locate the fees to record on the claim, and post them to the financial statement. Date the claim February 27. Dr. Cutler is accepting assignment, and the patient's signatures to release information to the insurance company and to have the payment forwarded directly to the physician are on file.

2. Use your CPT code book or Appendix A in this *Workbook* to determine the correct five-digit code numbers and fees for each professional service rendered. Use your HCPCS Level II code book or refer to Appendix B in this Workbook for HCPCS procedure codes and modifiers. Use your diagnostic code book to code each active diagnosis.

3. Record the proper information on the patient's financial accounting record and claim form, and note the date when you have billed the insurance company.

PATIENT RECORD NO. T-9

Cash	Darlene	M	3-15-70	F	555-666-8901
LAST NAME	FIRST NAME	MIDDLE NAME	BIRTH DATE SEX		HOME PHONE

5729 Redwood Avenue   Woodland Hills   XY   12344
ADDRESS   CITY   STATE   ZIP CODE

555-290-5400   555-666-8901   cash@wb.net
CELL PHONE   PAGER NO.   FAX NO.   E-MAIL ADDRESS

298-XX-6754   J3457789
PATIENT'S SOC. SEC. NO.   DRIVER'S LICENSE

Teacher   City Unified School District
PATIENT'S OCCUPATION   NAME OF COMPANY

Century High School, 2031 West Olympic Boulevard, Dorland, XY 12345   555-678-1076
ADDRESS OF EMPLOYER   PHONE

David F. Cash   Navy Petty Officer—Grade 8 (active status)
SPOUSE OR PARENT   OCCUPATION

United States Navy   HHC, 2nd Batt, 26th Infantry, APO New York, NY, 10030
EMPLOYER   ADDRESS   PHONE

TRICARE Standard   David Cash (DOB 4-22-70)
NAME OF INSURANCE   INSURED OR SUBSCRIBER

767-XX-9080
POLICY/CERTIFICATE NO.   GROUP NO.

REFERRED BY: Hugh R. Foot, MD, 2010 Main St., Woodland Hills, XY 12345   Fed Tax ID #61 25099XX

DATE	PROGRESS NOTES
1-4-xx	New pt, referred by Dr. Foot comes in complaining of head pain which began yesterday.
	Performed an EPF history and physical exam. Lt parietal area of skull slightly tender,
	some redness of scalp. Pain localized and not consistent with HA syndromes. Rest of
	exam N. Imp: head pain, undetermined nature, possible cyst. Apply hot compresses and
	observe. Take Ibuprofen for pain prn (200 mg up to 2 q. 4 h). Retn in 1 wk, no disability
	from work (SF/MDM).
	CC/llf *Clarence Cutler, MD*
1-11-xx	Pt retns and states that the hot compresses have helped but is concerned with some
	swelling in area. On exam noticed slt elevation of skin in lt parietal area of scalp, no
	warmth over area. Slt pain on palpation. Exam otherwise neg. Imp: Subcutaneous nodule.
	Continue with same tx plan: Hot compresses daily and Ibuprofen prn. Retn in 2 to 3 wks
	if not resolved (PF HX/PX SF/MDM).
	CC/llf *Clarence Cutler, MD*
2-3-xx	Pt retns for reexamination of parietal skull. Elevation of skin still persisting. It has now
	come to a head, is warm to the touch, and consistent with an inflammatory cystic lesion.
	A decision is made to excise the benign lesion. Scalp cyst, 1.5 cm removed under
	procaine block with knife dissection; closed wound with six #000 black silk sutures.
	Adv to retn 1 wk for removal of sutures (EPF HX/PX LC/MDM).
	CC/llf *Clarence Cutler, MD*
2-10-xx	Pt presents for suture removal. Sutures removed and slight oozing occurs in midsection
	of wound. Wound dressed and pt advised to apply antibacterial cream daily. Retn in 4 to
	5 days for final check (PF HX/PX SF/MDM).
	CC/llf *Clarence Cutler, MD*
2-15-xx	Pt presents for PO check of head wound. Parietal area healed well. RTO prn
	(PF HX/PX SF/MDM).
	CC/llf *Clarence Cutler, MD*

Figure 11

STATEMENT
Financial Account
COLLEGE CLINIC
4567 Broad Avenue
Woodland Hills, XY 12345-0001
Fax No. 555-487-8976

Acct No. ___T-9___

Darlene M. Cash
5729 Redwood Avenue
Woodland Hills, XY 12345

Phone No. (H) ___555-666-8901___ (W) ___555-678-1076___   Birthdate ___3/15/70___

Primary Insurance Co. __TRICARE Standard_____   Policy/Group No. ___767-XX-9080___

Secondary Insurance Co._____   Policy/Group No._____

| DATE | REFERENCE | DESCRIPTION | CHARGES | CREDITS | | BALANCE | |
				PYMNTS.	ADJ.		
20xx			BALANCE FORWARD				
1-4-xx		NP OV					
1-11-xx		OV					
2-3-xx		OV					
2-3-xx		Excision inflammatory cystic scalp lesion					
2-10-xx		OV					
2-15-xx		OV					

PLEASE PAY LAST AMOUNT IN BALANCE COLUMN

THIS IS A COPY OF YOUR FINANCIAL ACCOUNT AS IT APPEARS ON OUR RECORDS

Figure 12

TEST 10: COMPLETE TWO CLAIM FORMS FOR A PRIVATE PLAN

Performance Objective

Task: Complete two CMS-1500 (08-05) claim forms for a private case and post transactions to the patient's financial accounting record.

Conditions: Use the patient's record (Figure 13) and financial statement (Figure 14); two health insurance claim forms; a typewriter, computer, or pen; procedural and diagnostic code books; and appendices A and B in this *Workbook*.

Standards: Claim Productivity Management

Time: _____ minutes

Accuracy: _____

(Note: The time element and accuracy criteria may be given by your instructor.)

Directions

1. Using OCR guidelines, complete two CMS-1500 (08-05) claim forms and direct them to the private carrier. Refer to Gertrude C. Hamilton's patient record for information and Appendix A in this *Workbook* to locate the fees to record on the claim, and post them to the financial statement. Date the first claim August 15 and the second one October 15. Dr. Cardi is accepting assignment, and the patient's signatures to release information to the insurance company and to have the payment forwarded directly to the physician are on file.

2. Use your CPT code book or Appendix A in this *Workbook* to determine the correct five-digit code numbers and modifiers for each professional service rendered. Use your HCPCS Level II code book or refer to Appendix B in this *Workbook* for HCPCS procedure codes and modifiers. Use your diagnostic code books to code each active diagnosis. Frequently, surgeons wait to receive the pathology report before entering a final diagnosis on the claim form. In this case, the claim was submitted before the pathology report was received.

3. Record the proper information on the financial record and claim form, and note the date when you have billed the insurance company.

4. Mrs. Hamilton makes a payment of $200, check number 5362, on her account on October 26. Post the proper entry for this transaction.

PATIENT RECORD NO. T-10

Hamilton	Gertrude	C	03-06-47	F	555-798-3321
LAST NAME	FIRST NAME	MIDDLE NAME	BIRTH DATE	SEX	HOME PHONE

5320 Phillips Street	Woodland Hills	XY	12345	
ADDRESS	CITY	STATE	ZIP CODE	

555-399-4990	555-312-6677	555-798-3321	hamilton@wb.net
CELL PHONE	PAGER NO.	FAX NO.	E-MAIL ADDRESS

540-XX-7677	D9043557
PATIENT'S SOC. SEC. NO.	DRIVER'S LICENSE

retired secretary	
PATIENT'S OCCUPATION	NAME OF COMPANY

ADDRESS OF EMPLOYER	PHONE

deceased	
SPOUSE OR PARENT	OCCUPATION

EMPLOYER	ADDRESS	PHONE

Colonial Health Insurance, 1011 Main Street, Woodland Hills, XY 12345	self
NAME OF INSURANCE	INSURED OR SUBSCRIBER

540XX7677	4566 (through previous employment)
POLICY/CERTIFICATE NO.	GROUP NO.

REFERRED BY: Gerald Practon, MD, 4567 Broad Avenue, Woodland Hills, XY 12345

Figure 13

DATE	PROGRESS NOTES No. T-10
7-29-xx	Dr. Practon asked me to consult on this 57-year-old pt adm to College Hosp today.
	Duplex carotid ultrasonography indicates bilateral carotid stenosis. C/HX: Suffered CVA lt
	hemisphere 1 yr prior to adm. Marked rt arm & leg weakness c̄ weakness of rt face and
	slurring of speech. C/PE revealed lt carotid bruit, II/IV, & right carotid bruit, II/IV.
	Performed hand-held Doppler vascular study on bilateral carotids which indicated
	decreased blood flow. Adv brain scan and lt carotid thromboendarterectomy; rt carotid
	thromboendarterectomy at a later date H/MDM.
	PC/llf *Perry Cardi, MD*
7-30-xx	HV (EPF HX/PX MC/MDM). Dr. Practon asked me to take over pt's care. Pt had brain scan
	done today, ECG, and lab work.
	PC/llf *Perry Cardi, MD*
7-31-xx	HV (EPF HX/PX MC/MDM). Brain scan indicates prior CVA; no new findings. ECG, normal
	sinus rhythm with occasional premature ventricular contractions. Lab work WNL.
	Discussed test results with Mrs. Hamilton.
	PC/llf *Perry Cardi, MD*
8-1-xx	HV (PF HX/PX LC/MDM). Decision made for surgery, to be scheduled tomorrow.
	PC/llf *Perry Cardi, MD*
8-2-xx	Pt taken to the operative suite. Performed lt carotid thromboendarterectomy by neck
	incision (see op report). Surgery went as planned, pt in recovery.
	PC/llf *Perry Cardi, MD*
8-3-xx	HV (PF HX/PX SF/MDM). Operative site appears normal. Pt resting comfortably.
	PC/llf *Perry Cardi, MD*
8-4-xx	DC from hosp. Pt to be seen in ofc in 1 week.
	PC/llf *Perry Cardi, MD*
8-12-xx	PO OV (D HX/PX M/MDM). Discussed outcome of surgery. Pt making satisfactory
	progress. Adv rt carotid thromboendarterectomy. Pt would like it done as soon as possible;
	next month if there is an operative time. Scheduled surgery for September 16, 20XX at
	College Hospital.
	PC/llf *Perry Cardi, MD*
9-16-xx	Adm to College Hospital. Performed a D history, D physical examination, and SF medical
	decision making. Rt. carotid thromboendarterectomy performed by neck incision.
	DX: Rt carotid stenosis.
	PC/llf *Perry Cardi, MD*
9-17-xx	HV (PF HX/PX SF/MDM). Pt stable and doing well. Operative site looks good. Plan for
	discharge tomorrow.
	PC/llf *Perry Cardi, MD*
9-18-xx	DC from hosp to home. RTC 1 wk.
	PC/llf *Perry Cardi, MD*
9-25-xx	PO visit (PF HX/PX SF/MDM). Pt making satisfactory recovery. Her neighbor will monitor
	BP daily. Retn 1 month.
	PC/llf *Perry Cardi, MD*

Figure 13, cont'd

STATEMENT

COLLEGE CLINIC
4567 Broad Avenue
Woodland Hills, XY 12345-0001
Tel. 555-486-9002
Fax No. 555-487-8976

Acct. No . T-10

Gertrude C. Hamilton
5320 Phillips Street
Woodland Hills, XY 12345

Phone No. (H) (555) 798-3321 (W) _____ Birthdate 03-06-47

Insurance Co Colonial Health Insurance _____ Policy/Group No. 540Xx7677 / 4566

	REFERENCE	DESCRIPTION	CHARGES	CREDITS PYMNTS.	ADJ.	BALANCE
20xx			BALANCE FORWARD →			
7-29-xx		Inpatient consult				
7-30-xx		HV				
7-31-xx		HV				
8-1-xx		HV				
8-2-xx		L carotid thromboendarterectmy				
8-3-xx		HV				
8-4-xx		Discharge				
8-12-xx		PO OV				
9-16-xx		Admit				
9-16-xx		R Carotid thromboendarterectomy				
9-17-xx		HV				
9-18-xx		Discharge				
9-25-xx		PO OV				

PLEASE PAY LAST AMOUNT IN BALANCE COLUMN ⇧

THIS IS A COPY OF YOUR FINANCIAL ACCOUNT AS IT APPEARS ON OUR RECORDS

Figure 14

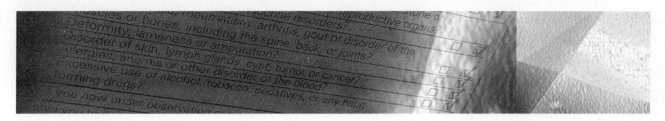

College Clinic Office Policies and Mock Fee Schedule

College Clinic

You are employed as an insurance billing specialist for an incorporated group of medical doctors, other allied health specialists, and podiatrists. These doctors are on the staff of a nearby hospital, College Hospital. Reference information to complete insurance claim forms for each assignment follows.

Office address:
College Clinic
4567 Broad Avenue
Woodland Hills, XY 12345-0001
telephone: 555-486-9002
FAX: 555-487-8976
Group practice national provider identifier: 3664021CC
Medicare Durable Medical Equipment (DME) supplier
  number: 3400760001

Hospital address:
College Hospital
4500 Broad Avenue
Woodland Hills, XY 12345-0001
telephone: 555-487-6789
FAX: 555-486-8900
Hospital national provider identifier: 95-0731067

College Clinic Staff

Patient records in this *Workbook* include the doctors' names, specialties, subspecialties, and physicians' identification numbers of the College Clinic staff.

Table 1. College Clinic Staff

Name	Specialty (abbreviation)	Social Security No.	State License No.	EIN No. or Federal Tax Identification No.	Medicare CMS-Assigned National Provider Identifier (NPI)*
Concha Antrum, MD	Otolaryngologist (OTO) or Ear, Nose, and Throat Specialist (ENT)	082–XX–1707	C 01602X	74–10640XX	12458977XX
Pedro Atrics, MD	Pediatrician (PD)	134–XX–7600	D 06012X	71–32061XX	37640017XX
Bertha Caesar, MD	Obstetrician and Gynecologist (OBG)	230–XX–6700	A 01817X	72–57130XX	43056757XX
Perry Cardi, MD	Internist (I) Subspecialty Cardiovascular Disease (CD)	557–XX–9980	C 02140X	70–64217XX	67805027XX
Brady Coccidioides, MD	Internist (I) Subspecialty Pulmonary Disease (PUD)	670–XX–0874	C 04821X	75–67321XX	64211067XX
Vera Cutis, MD	Dermatologist (D)	409–XX–8620	C 06002X	71–80561XX	70568717XX
Clarence Cutler, MD	General Surgeon (GS)	410–XX–5630	B 07600X	71–57372XX	43050047XX
Dennis Drill, DDS	Dentist	240–XX–8960	70610X	72–46503XX	74301087XX
Max Glutens, RPT	Physical Therapist (PT)	507–XX–4300	87610X	79–36500XX	65132277XX
Cosmo Graff, MD	Plastic Surgeon (PS)	452–XX–9899	C 08104X	74–60789XX	50307117XX
Malvern Grumose, MD	Pathologist (Path)	470–XX–2301	A 01602X	72–73651XX	
Gaston Input, MD	Internist (I) Subspecialty Gastroenterologist: (GE)	211–XX–6734	C 08001X	75–67210XX	32783127XX
Adam Langerhans, MD	Endocrinologist	447–XX–6720	C 06051X	60–57831XX	47680657XX
Cornell Lenser, MD	Ophthalmologist (OPH)	322–XX–8963	C 06046X	61–78941XX	54037217XX
Michael Menter, MD	Psychiatrist (P)	210–XX–5302	C 07140X	73–66577XX	67301237XX
Arthur O. Dont, DDS	Orthodontist	102–XX–4566	80530X	90–51178XX	45378247XX
Astro Parkinson, MD	Neurosurgeon (NS)	210–XX–8533	C 02600X	75–44530XX	46789377XX
Nick Pedro, DPM	Podiatrist	233–XX–4300	E 08340X	62–74109XX	54022287XX
Gerald Practon, MD	General Practitioner (GP) or Family Practitioner (FP)	123–XX–6789	C 01402X	70–34597XX	46278897XX
Walter Radon, MD	Radiologist (R)	344–XX–6540	C 05001X	95–46137XX	40037227XX
Rex Rumsey, MD	Proctologist (Proct)	337–XX–9743	C 03042X	95–32601XX	01999047XX
Sensitive E. Scott, MD	Anesthesiologist (Anes)	220–XX–5655	C 02041X	72–54203XX	99999267XX
Raymond Skeleton, MD	Orthopedist (ORS, Orthop)	432–XX–4589	C 04561X	74–65412XX	12678547XX
Gene Ulibarri, MD	Urologist (U)	990–XX–3245	C 06430X	77–86531XX	25678831XX

*Providers began using the NPI on May 23, 2007, except for small health plans, whose compliance date is May 23, 2008.

Abbreviations and Symbols

Abbreviations and symbols may appear on patient records, prescriptions, hospital charts, and patient ledger cards. Abbreviation styles differ, but the current trend is to omit periods in capital letter abbreviations except for doctors' academic degrees. For information on official American Hospital Association policy, refer to p. 108 in the *Handbook*. Following is a list of abbreviations and symbols used in this *Workbook* and their meanings.

Abbreviations

A	allergy
AB	antibiotics
Abdom	abdomen
abt	about
a.c.	before meals
Adj*	adjustment
adm	admit; admission; admitted
adv	advise(d)
aet	at the age of
agit	shake or stir
AgNO₃	silver nitrate
ALL	allergy
AM, a.m.	ante meridian (time—before noon)
ant	anterior
ante	before
AP	anterior-posterior; anteroposterior
approx	approximate
appt	appointment
apt	apartment
ASA	acetylsalicylic acid (aspirin)
ASAP	as soon as possible
ASCVD	arteriosclerotic cardiovascular disease
ASHD	arteriosclerotic heart disease
asst	assistant
auto	automated, automobile
AV	atrioventricular
Ba	barium (enema)
Bal/fwd*	balance forward
BE	barium enema
B/F*	balance forward; brought forward
b.i.d.	two times daily
BM	bowel movement
BMR	basal metabolic rate
BP	blood pressure
Brev	Brevital sodium
BX, bx	biopsy
C	cervical (vertebrae); comprehensive (history/examination)
Ca, CA	cancer, carcinoma
c/a*	cash on account
CABG	coronary artery bypass graft
CAT	computed axial tomography
cau	Caucasian
CBC	complete blood count
CBS	chronic brain syndrome
cc	cubic centimeter
CC	chief complaint

chr	chronic
ck*	check
cm	centimeter
CO, c/o	complains of; care of
compl, comp	complete; comprehensive
Con, CON, Cons	consultation
Cont	continue
CPX	complete physical examination
C&R	compromise and release
Cr*	credit
C&S	culture and sensitivity
cs, CS*	cash on account
C-section	cesarean section
CT	computed or computerized tomography
CVA	cardiovascular accident; cerebrovascular accident
CXR	chest radiograph
Cysto	cystoscopy
D, d	diagnosis; detailed (history/examination); day(s)
D & C	dilatation and curettage
dc	discontinue
DC	discharge
DDS	Doctor of Dental Surgery
def*	charge deferred
Del	delivery; obstetrics and gynecology
Dg	diagnosis
dia	diameter
diag	diagnosis; diagnostic
dil	dilate (stretch, expand)
Disch	discharge
DM	diabetes mellitus
DNA	does not apply
DNS	did not show
DPM	Doctor of Podiatric Medicine
DPT	diphtheria, pertussis, and tetanus
Dr	Doctor
Dr*	debit
DRG	diagnosis-related group
Drs	dressing
DUB	dysfunctional uterine bleeding
Dx	diagnosis
E	emergency
EC*	error corrected
ECG, EKG	electrocardiogram; electrocardiograph
echo	echocardiogram; echocardiography
ED	emergency department
EDC	estimated date of confinement
EEG	electroencephalograph
EENT	eye, ear, nose, and throat
EGD	esophagogastroduodenoscopy
EKG, ECG	electrocardiogram; electrocardiograph
E/M	Evaluation and Management (Current Procedural Terminology code)
EMG	electromyogram
EPF	expanded problem-focused (history/examination)
epith	epithelial

---

*Bookkeeping abbreviation.

ER	emergency room	IVP	intravenous pyelogram
Er, ER*	error corrected	K 35	Kolman (instrument used in urology)
ESR	erythrocyte sedimentation rate	KUB	kidneys, ureters, and bladder
est	established (patient); estimated	L	left; laboratory
Ex, exam	examination	Lab, LAB	laboratory
exc	excision	lat	lateral; pertaining to the side
Ex MO*	express money order	lbs	pound
ext	external	LC	low complexity (decision making)
24F, 28F	French (size of catheter)	LMP	last menstrual period
F	female	LS	lumbosacral
FBS	fasting blood sugar	lt	left
FH	family history	ltd	limited (office visit)
ft	foot, feet	L & W	living and well
FU	follow-up (examination)	M	medication; married
fwd*	forward	MC	moderate-complexity (decision making)
Fx	fracture	MDM	medical decision making
gb, GB	gallbladder	med	medicine
GGE	generalized glandular enlargement	mg	milligram(s)
GI	gastrointestinal	mg/dL	milligrams per deciliter
Grav, grav	gravida, a pregnant woman; used with Roman numerals (I, II, III) to indicate the number of pregnancies	MI	myocardial infarction
		micro	microscopy
		mL, ml	milliliter
GU	genitourinary	mo	month(s)
H	hospital call	MO*	money order
HA	headache	N	negative
HBP	high blood pressure	NA	not applicable
HC	hospital call or consultation; high-complexity (decision making)	NAD	no appreciable disease
		NC, N/C*	no charge
HCD	house call (day)	NEC	not elsewhere classifiable
HCN	house call (night)	neg	negative
Hct	hematocrit	NKA	no known allergies
HCVD	hypertensive cardiovascular disease	NOS	not otherwise specified
Hgb	hemoglobin	NP	new patient
hist	history	NYD	not yet diagnosed
hosp	hospital	OB, Ob-Gyn	obstetrics and gynecology
H & P	history and physical (examination)	OC	office call
hr, hrs	hour, hours	occ	occasional
h.s.	before bedtime	OD	right eye
HS	hospital surgery	ofc	office
Ht	height	OP	outpatient
HV	hospital visit	Op, op	operation
HX, hx	history	OR	operating room
HX PX	history and physical examination	orig	original
I	injection	OS	office surgery; left eye
IC	initial consultation	OV	office visit
I & D	incision and drainage	oz	ounce
I/f*	in full	PA	posterior-anterior; posteroanterior
IM	intramuscular (injection)	Pap	Papanicolaou (smear, stain, test)
imp, imp.	impression (diagnosis)	Para I	woman having borne one child
incl.	include; including	PC	present complaint
inflam	inflammation	p.c.	after meals
init	initial (office visit)	PCP	primary care physician
inj, INJ	injection	PD	permanent disability
ins, INS*	insurance	Pd, PD*	professional discount
int	internal	PE	physical examination
intermed	intermediate (office visit)	perf	performed
interpret	interpretation	PF	problem-focused (history/examination)
IUD	intrauterine device	PFT	pulmonary function test
IV	intravenous (injection)	PH	past history
		Ph ex	physical examination
		phys	physical

*Bookkeeping abbreviation.

PID	pelvic inflammatory disease	SOB	shortness of breath
PM, p.m.	post meridian (time—after noon)	Sp gr	specific gravity
PND	postnasal drip	SQ	subcutaneous (injection)
PO, P Op	postoperative	STAT	immediately
p.o.	by mouth (per os)	strep	*Streptococcus*
post	posterior	surg	surgery
postop	postoperative	Sx	symptom(s)
PPD	purified protein derivative (such as in tuberculin test)	T	temperature
		T & A	tonsillectomy and adenoidectomy
preop	preoperative	Tb, tb	tuberculosis
prep	prepared	TD	temporary disability
PRN, p.r.n.	as necessary (pro re nata)	tech	technician
Proc	procedure	temp	temperature
Prog	prognosis	tet. tox.	tetanus toxoid
P & S	permanent and stationary	t.i.d.	three times daily
PSA	prostate-specific antigen (blood test to determine cancer in prostate gland)	TPR	temperature, pulse, and respiration
		Tr, trt	treatment
Pt, pt	patient	TURB	transurethral resection of bladder
PT	physical therapy	TURP	transurethral resection of prostate
PTR	patient to return	TX	treatment
PVC	premature ventricular contraction	u	units
PVT ck*	private check received	UA, ua	urinalysis
PX	physical examination	UCHD	usual childhood diseases
q	every	UCR	usual, customary, and reasonable (fees)
qd	one time daily, every day	UGI	upper gastrointestinal
qh	every hour	UPJ	ureteropelvic junction or joint
q.i.d.	four times daily	UR	urinalysis
QNS	insufficient quantity	URI	upper respiratory infection
qod	every other day	Urn	urinalysis
R	right; residence call; report	UTI	urinary tract infection
RBC, rbc	red blood cell (count)	W	work; white
rec	recommend	WBC, wbc	white blood cell (count); well baby care
rec'd	received	WC	workers' compensation
re ch	recheck	wk	week; work
re-exam	reexamination	wks	weeks
Reg	regular	WNL	within normal limits
ret, retn, rtn	return	Wr	Wassermann reaction (test for syphilis)
rev	review	Wt, wt	weight
RHD	rheumatic heart disease	X	xray, x-ray(s); times (e.g., 3X means three times)
RN	registered nurse		
R/O	rule out	XR	xray, x-ray(s)
ROA*	received on account	yr(s)	year(s)
RPT	registered physical therapist		
rt	right	**Symbols**	
RTC	return to clinic		
RTO	return to office	+	positive
RTW	return to work	#	pound(s)
RX, Rx, Rx	prescribe; prescription; any medication or treatment ordered	c̄, /c	with
		s̄, /s	without
S	surgery	c̄c, c̄/c	with correction (eye glasses)
SC	subcutaneous	s̄c, s̄/c	without correction (eye glasses)
sched.	scheduled	~	negative
SD	state disability	ō	negative
SE	special examination	⊕, +	positive
SF	straightforward (decision making)		left
Sig	directions on prescription	(R)	right
SLR	straight leg raising	♂	male
slt	slight	♀	female
Smr	smear	–*	charge already made
		⊖*	no balance due
		√*	posted
		($0.00)*	credit

*Bookkeeping abbreviation.

Laboratory Abbreviations

Abbreviation	*Definition*
ABG	arterial blood gas(es)
AcG	factor V (AcG or proaccelerin); a factor in coagulation that converts prothrombin to thrombin
ACTH	adrenocorticotropic hormone
AFB	acid-fast bacilli
A/C ratio	albumin-coagulin ratio
AHB	alpha-hydroxybutyric (dehydrogenase)
AHG	antihemophilic globulin; antihemolytic globulin (factor)
ALA	aminolevulinic acid
ALT	alanine aminotransferase (see SGPT)
AMP	adenosine monophosphate
APT test	aluminum-precipitated toxoid test
AST	aspartate aminotransferase (see SGOT)
ATP	adenosine triphosphate
BSP	bromsulfophthalein (Bromsulphalein; sodium sulfobromophthalein) (test)
BUN	blood urea nitrogen
CBC	complete blood count
CNS	central nervous system
CO	carbon monoxide
CPB	competitive protein binding: plasma
CPK	creatine phosphokinase
CSF	cerebrospinal fluid
D hemoglobin	hemoglobin fractionation by electrophoresis for hemoglobin D
DAP	direct agglutination pregnancy (Gravindex and DAP)
DEAE	diethylaminoethylcellulose
DHT	dihydrotestosterone
diff	differential
DNA	deoxyribonucleic acid
DRT	test for syphilis
EACA	epsilon-aminocaproic acid (a fibrinolysin)
EMIT	enzyme-multiplied immunoassay technique (for drugs)
ENA	extractable nuclear antigen
esr, ESR	erythrocyte sedimentation (sed) rate
FDP	fibrin degradation products
FIGLU	formiminoglutamic acid
FRAT	free radical assay technique (for drugs)
FSH	follicle-stimulating hormone
FSP	fibrinogen split products
FTA	fluorescent-absorbed treponema antibodies
Gc, Gm, Inv	immunoglobulin typing
GG, gamma G, A, D, G, M	gamma-globulin (immunoglobulin fractionation by electrophoresis)
GG, gamma G E, RIA	immunization E fractionation by radioimmunoassay
GGT	gamma-glutamyl transpeptidase
GLC	gas liquid chromatography
GMP	guanosine monophosphate
GTT	glucose tolerance test
G6PD	glucose-6-phosphate dehydrogenase
HAA	hepatitis-associated agent (antigen)
HBD, HBDH	hydroxybutyrate dehydrogenase
HCT	hematocrit
hemoglobin, electrophoresis	letters of the alphabet used for different types or factors of hemoglobins (e.g., A_2, S, C)
Hgb	hemoglobin, qualitative
HGH	human growth hormone
HI	hemagglutination inhibition
HIA	hemagglutination inhibition antibody
HIAA	hydroxyindoleacetic acid (urine), 24-hour specimen
HIV	human immunodeficiency virus
HLA	human leukocyte antigen (tissue typing)

HPL	human placental lactogen
HTLV-III	antibody detection; confirmatory test
HVA	homovanillic acid
ICSH	interstitial cell–stimulating hormone
IFA	intrinsic factor, antibody (fluorescent screen)
IgA, IgE, IgG, IgM	immunoglobulins: quantitative by gel diffusion
INH	isonicotinic hydrazide, isoniazid
LAP	leucine aminopeptidase
LATS	long-acting thyroid-stimulating (hormone)
LDH	lactic dehydrogenase
LE Prep	lupus erythematosus cell preparation
L.E. factor	antinuclear antibody
LH	luteinizing hormone
LSD	lysergic acid diethylamide
L/S ratio	lecithin-sphingomyelin ratio
MC (Streptococcus)	antibody titer
MIC	minimum inhibitory concentration
NBT	nitro-blue tetrazolium (test)
OCT	ornithine carbamyl transferase
PAH	para-aminohippuric acid
PBI	protein-bound iodine
pCO_2	arterial carbon dioxide pressure (or tension)
PCP	phencyclidine piperidine
pcv	packed cell volume
pH	symbol for expression of concentration of hydrogen ions (degree of acidity)
PHA	phenylalanine
PIT	prothrombin inhibition test
PKU	phenylketonuria—a metabolic disease affecting mental development
PO_2	oxygen pressure
P & P	prothrombin-proconvertin
PSP	phenolsulfonphthalein
PT	prothrombin time
PTA	plasma thromboplastin antecedent
PTC	plasma thromboplastin component; phenylthiocarbamide
PTT	prothrombin time; partial thromboplastin time (plasma or whole blood)
RBC, rbc	red blood cells (count)
RIA	radioimmunoassay
RISA	radioiodinated human serum albumin
RIST	radioimmunosorbent test
RPR	rapid plasma reagin (test)
RT3U	resin triiodothyronine uptake
S-D	strength-duration (curve)
SGOT	serum glutamic oxaloacetic transaminase (see AST)
SGPT	serum glutamic pyruvic transaminase (see ALT)
STS	serologic test for syphilis
T3	triiodothyronine (uptake)
TB	tubercle bacillus, tuberculosis
TBG	thyroxine-binding globulin
T & B differentiation, lymphocytes	thymus-dependent lymphs and bursa-dependent lymphs
THC	tetrahydrocannabinol (marijuana)
TIBC	total iron-binding capacity, chemical
TLC screen	thin-layer chromatography screen
TRP	tubular reabsorption of phosphates
UA	urinalysis
VDRL	Venereal Disease Research Laboratory (agglutination test for syphilis)
VMA	vanillylmandelic acid
WBC, wbc	white blood cells (count)

Mock Fee Schedule

Refer to the mock fee schedule (Table 2) to complete the financial accounting statements (ledgers) and claim forms in this *Workbook*. The fees listed are hypothetical and are intended only for use in completing the questions. For the cases that are private, Medicaid, TRICARE, and workers' compensation, use the amounts in the column labeled Mock Fees. For Medicare cases, refer to the three columns pertaining to Medicare and use the amounts in the column labeled Limiting Charge. Follow these instructions unless your instructor wishes you to round out the amounts on the fee schedule to the next dollar.

In a real medical practice, some offices round out the amounts to the next dollar unless the physician is nonparticipating with Medicare and then by Medicare regulations the provider can only bill the exact limiting amount. Other offices may have two fee schedules. Schedule B is for Medicare participating physicians and amounts are listed in dollars and cents. Schedule A is used for other plans and the amounts are rounded to the next dollar. However, if a fee schedule is sent by the insurance plan, then the medical practice may use the dollars and cents provided.

When completing the insurance claim forms, use the latest edition of *Current Procedural Terminology* (CPT), the professional code book published by the American Medical Association, to find the correct code numbers and modifiers for the services rendered. If you do not have access to the latest edition of CPT, you may use the code numbers provided in the mock fee schedule; however, do so with the understanding that the code numbers and descriptions provided in this schedule are not comprehensive. They are based on the information found in CPT; however, students are cautioned not to use it as a substitute for CPT. Because the code numbers are subject to change, every medical office must have on hand the most recent edition of CPT.

The mock fee schedule (Tables 2 and 3) is arranged in the same sequence as the six CPT code book sections (i.e., Evaluation and Management; Anesthesia; Surgery; Radiology, Nuclear Medicine, and Diagnostic Ultrasound; Pathology and Laboratory; and Medicine), with a comprehensive list of modifiers placed at the beginning. An index at the end of the mock fee schedule can assist you in locating code numbers. Mock fees for the modifiers are not listed, because these can vary from one claim to another, depending on the circumstances.

Remember that fees can vary with the region of the United States (West, Midwest, South, East), the specialty of the practitioner, the type of community (urban, suburban, or rural), the type of practice (incorporated or unincorporated, solo, partners, or shareholders), the overhead, and a number of other factors.

Table 2. College Clinic Mock Fee Schedule

Modifier Code Number	Description	Mock Fee ($)
-21	*Prolonged Evaluation and Management Services:* When the face-to-face or floor/unit service(s) provided is prolonged or otherwise greater than that usually required for the highest level of evaluation and management service within a given category, it may be identified by adding modifier -21 to the evaluation and management code number. A report may also be appropriate.	Increase fee
-22	*Unusual Services:* When the service(s) provided is greater than that usually required for the listed procedure, it may be identified by adding modifier -22 to the usual procedure code number. A report may also be appropriate.	Increase fee
-23	*Unusual Anesthesia:* Occasionally a procedure that usually requires either no anesthesia or local anesthesia must be done under general anesthesia because of unusual circumstances. These circumstances may be reported by adding the modifier -23 to the procedure code number of the basic service.	Increase fee
-24	*Unrelated Evaluation and Management Service by the Same Physician During a Postoperative Period:* The physician may need to indicate that an evaluation and management service was performed during a postoperative period for a reason(s) unrelated to the original procedure. This circumstance may be reported by adding the modifier -24 to the appropriate level of E/M service.	Variable per E/M fee
-25	*Significant, Separately Identifiable Evaluation and Management Service by the Same Physician on the Same Day of a Procedure or Other Service:* The physician may need to indicate that on the day a procedure or service identified by a CPT code was performed, the patient's condition required a significant, separately identifiable E/M service above and beyond the other service provided or beyond the usual preoperative and postoperative care associated with the procedure that was performed. The E/M service may be prompted by the symptom or condition for which the procedure and/or service was provided. As such, different diagnoses are not	Variable per E/M fee

Table 2. College Clinic Mock Fee Schedule—cont'd

Modifier Code Number	Description	Mock Fee ($)
	required for reporting of the E/M services on the same date. This circumstance may be reported by adding the modifier -25 to the appropriate level of E/M service. **NOTE:** This modifier is not used to report an E/M service that resulted in a decision to perform surgery. See modifier -57.	
-26	*Professional Component:* Certain procedures are a combination of a physician component and a technical component. When the physician component is reported separately, the service may be identified by adding the modifier -26 to the usual procedure code number.	Decrease fee
-27	*Multiple Outpatient Hospital E/M Encounters on the Same Date:* For hospital outpatient reporting purposes, utilization of hospital resources related to separate and distinct E/M encounters performed in multiple outpatient hospital settings on the same date may be reported by adding the modifier -27 to each appropriate level outpatient and/or emergency department E/M code(s). This modifier provides a means of reporting circumstances involving E/M services provided by physician(s) in more than one (multiple) outpatient hospital setting(s) (e.g., hospital emergency department, clinic). Do not use this modifier for physician reporting of multiple E/M services performed by the same physician on the same date. See E/M, emergency department, or preventive medicine services codes.	Variable
-32	*Mandated Services:* Services related to mandated consultation and/or related services (e.g., PRO, third party payer) may be identified by adding the modifier -32 to the basic procedure.	Use standard fee
-47	*Anesthesia by Surgeon:* Regional or general anesthesia provided by the surgeon may be reported by adding the modifier -47 to the basic service or by using the separate five-digit modifier code number 09947 (this does not include local anesthesia). **NOTE:** Modifier -47 or code number 09947 would not be used as a modifier for the anesthesia procedures 00100 through 01999.	Increase fee
-50	*Bilateral Procedure:* Unless otherwise identified in the listings, bilateral procedures that are performed at the same operative session should be identified by the appropriate five-digit code number describing the first procedure. The second (bilateral) procedure is identified either by adding modifier -50 to the procedure code number.	Paid at 50% of standard fee
-51	*Multiple Procedures:* When multiple procedures other than E/M services are performed at the same session by the same provider, the primary procedure or service may be reported as listed. The additional procedure(s) may be identified by adding the modifier -51 to the additional procedure or service code(s). **NOTE:** This modifier should not be appended to designated "add-on" codes.	Second procedure usually paid at 50% of fee. Third procedure usually paid at 25% of fee. Fourth and subsequent procedures usually paid at 10% of fee.
-52	*Reduced Services:* Under certain circumstances a service or procedure is partially reduced or eliminated at the physician's discretion. Under these circumstances, the service provided can be identified by its usual procedure number and the addition of the modifier -52, signifying that the service is reduced. This provides a means of reporting reduced services without disturbing the identification of the basic service. Modifier code 09952 may be used as an alternative to modifier -52. **NOTE:** For hospital outpatient reporting of a previously scheduled procedure/service that is partially reduced or canceled as a result of extenuating circumstances or those that threaten the well-being of the patient before or after administration of anesthesia, see modifiers -73 and -74.	Decrease fee
-53	*Discontinued Procedure:* Under certain circumstances, the physician may elect to terminate a surgical or diagnostic procedure. Due to extenuating circumstances or those that threaten the well-being of the patient, it may be necessary to indicate that a surgical or diagnostic procedure was started but discontinued.	Decrease fee

Continued

Table 2. College Clinic Mock Fee Schedule—cont'd

Modifier Code Number	Description	Mock Fee ($)
	This circumstance may be reported by adding modifier -53 to the code reported by the physician for the discontinued procedure. NOTE: This modifier is not used to report the elective cancellation of a procedure before the patient's anesthesia induction and/or surgical preparation in the operating suite. For outpatient hospital/ambulatory surgery center (ASC) reporting of a previously scheduled procedure/service that is partially reduced or canceled as a result of extenuating circumstances or those that threaten the well-being of the patient before or after administration of anesthesia, see modifiers -73 and -74 (see modifiers approved for ASC hospital outpatient use).	
-54	*Surgical Care Only:* When one physician performs a surgical procedure and another provides preoperative and/or postoperative management, surgical services may be identified by adding the modifier -54 to the usual procedure number.	Decrease fee
-55	*Postoperative Management Only:* When one physician performs the postoperative management and another physician performs the surgical procedure, the postoperative component may be identified by adding modifier -55 to the usual procedure number.	Decrease fee
-56	*Preoperative Management Only:* When one physician performs the preoperative care and evaluation and another physician performs the surgical procedure, the preoperative component may be identified by adding the modifier -56 to the usual procedure number.	Decrease fee
-57	*Decision for Surgery:* An evaluation and management service that resulted in the initial decision to perform the surgery may be identified by adding the modifier -57 to the appropriate level of E/M service.	Use standard fee
-58	*Staged or Related Procedure or Service by the Same Physician During the Postoperative Period:* The physician may need to indicate that the performance of a procedure or service during the postoperative period was (a) planned prospectively at the time of the original procedure (staged); (b) more extensive than the original procedure; or (c) for therapy following a diagnostic surgical procedure. This circumstance may be reported by adding the modifier -58 to the staged or related procedure. NOTE: This modifier is not used to report the treatment of a problem that requires a return to the operating room. See modifier -78.	Variable
-59	*Distinct Procedural Service:* Under certain circumstances, the physician may need to indicate that a procedure or service was distinct or independent from other services performed on the same day. Modifier -59 is used to identify procedures/services that are not normally reported together, but are appropriate under the circumstances. This may represent a different session or patient encounter, different procedure or surgery, different site or organ system, separate incision/excision, separate lesion, or separate injury (or area of injury in extensive injuries) not ordinarily encountered or performed on the same day by the same physician. However, when another already established modifier is appropriate it should be used rather than modifier -59. Only if no more descriptive modifier is available, and the use of modifier -59 best explains the circumstances, should modifier -59 be used.	Variable
-62	*Two Surgeons:* Under certain circumstances the skills of two surgeons (usually with different skills) may be required in the management of a specific surgical procedure. Under such circumstances the separate services may be identified by adding the modifier -62 to the procedure number used by each surgeon for reporting his or her services. NOTE: If a co-surgeon acts as an assistant in the performance of additional procedure(s) during the same surgical session, those services may be reported using separate procedure code(s) with the modifier -80 or modifier -81 added, as appropriate.	Use standard fee
-63	*Procedure Performed on Infants less than 4 kg:* Procedures performed on neonates and infants up to a present body weight of 4 kg may involve significantly increased complexity and physician work commonly associated with these patients. This circumstance may be reported by adding the modifier -63 to the procedure number.	Variable
-66	*Surgical Team:* Under some circumstances, highly complex procedures (requiring the concomitant services of several physicians, often of different specialties, plus other highly skilled, specially trained personnel and various types of complex equipment)	Variable

Table 2. College Clinic Mock Fee Schedule—cont'd

Modifier Code Number	Description	Mock Fee ($)
	are carried out under the "surgical team" concept. Such circumstances may be identified by each participating physician with the addition of the modifier -66 to the basic procedure code number used for reporting services.	
-73	Discontinued Outpatient Hospital/Ambulatory Center (ASC) Procedure Prior to the Administration of Anesthesia: Due to extenuating circumstances or those that threaten the well-being of the patient, the physician may cancel a surgical or diagnostic procedure subsequent to the patient's surgical preparation (including sedation when provided, and being taken to the room where the procedure is to be performed), but before the administration of anesthesia (local, regional block[s] or general). Under these circumstances, the intended service that is prepared for but canceled can be reported by its usual procedure number and the addition of the modifier -73. NOTE: The elective cancellation of a service before the administration of anesthesia and/or surgical preparation of the patient should not be reported. For physician reporting of a discontinued procedure, see modifier -53.	Decrease fee
-74	*Discontinued Outpatient Hospital/Ambulatory Surgery Center (ASC) Procedure After Administration of Anesthesia:* Due to extenuating circumstances or those that threaten the well-being of the patient, the physician may terminate a surgical or diagnostic procedure after the administration of anesthesia (local, regional block[s] or general) or after the procedure was started (e.g., incision made, intubation started, scope inserted). Under these circumstances, the procedure started but terminated can be reported by its usual procedure number and the addition of the modifier -74. NOTE: The elective cancellation of a service before the administration of anesthesia and/or surgical preparation of the patient should not be reported. For physician reporting of a discontinued procedure, see modifier -53.	Decrease fee
-76	*Repeat Procedure by Same Physician:* The physician may need to indicate that a procedure or service was repeated subsequent to the original procedure or service. This circumstance may be reported by adding modifier -76 to the repeated service/procedure.	Decrease fee
-77	*Repeat Procedure by Another Physician:* The physician may need to indicate that a basic procedure or service performed by another physician had to be repeated. This situation may be reported by adding modifier -77 to the repeated procedure/service.	Decrease fee
-78	*Return to the Operating Room for a Related Procedure During the Postoperative Period:* The physician may need to indicate that another procedure was performed during the postoperative period of the initial procedure. When this subsequent procedure is related to the first and requires the use of the operating room, it may be reported by adding the modifier -78 to the related procedure. (For repeat procedures on the same day, see -76.)	Decrease fee
-79	*Unrelated Procedure or Service by the Same Physician During the Postoperative Period:* The physician may need to indicate that the performance of a procedure or service during the postoperative period was unrelated to the original procedure. This circumstance may be reported by using the modifier -79. (For repeat procedures on the same day, see -76.)	Use standard fee
-80	*Assistant Surgeon:* Surgical assistant services may be identified by adding the modifier -80 to the usual procedure number(s).	Billed and/or paid at approximately 20% of surgeon's fee
-81	*Minimum Assistant Surgeon:* Minimum surgical assistant services are identified by adding the modifier -81 to the usual procedure number.	Billed and/or paid at approximately 10% of surgeon's fee
-82	*Assistant Surgeon When Qualified Resident Surgeon Not Available:* The unavailability of a qualified resident surgeon is a prerequisite for use of modifier -82 appended to the usual procedure code number(s).	Decrease fee
-90	*Reference (Outside) Laboratory:* When laboratory procedures are performed by a party other than the treating or reporting physician and billed by the treating physician, the procedure may be identified by adding the modifier -90 to the usual procedure number.	Fee according to contract

Continued

Table 2. College Clinic Mock Fee Schedule—cont'd

Modifier Code Number	Description	Mock Fee ($)
-91	*Repeat Clinical Diagnostic Laboratory Test:* In the course of treatment of the patient, it may be necessary to repeat the same laboratory test on the same day to obtain subsequent (multiple) test results. Under these circumstances, the laboratory test performed can be identified by its usual procedure number and the addition of modifier -91. **NOTE:** This modifier may not be used when tests are rerun to confirm initial results; due to testing problems with specimens or equipment; or for any other reason when a normal, one-time, reportable result is all that is required. This modifier may not be used when other code(s) describe a series of test results (e.g., glucose tolerance tests, evocative/suppression testing). This modifier may only be used for laboratory test(s) performed more than once on the same day on the same patient.	Decrease fee
-99	Multiple Modifiers: Under certain circumstances, two or more modifiers may be necessary to completely delineate a service. In such situations, modifier -99 should be added to the basic procedure, and other applicable modifiers may be listed as part of the description of the service.	Variable

Table 3. Mock Fee Schedule

Code Number and Description		Mock Fees	Medicare* Participating	Medicare* Nonparticipating	Medicare* Limiting Charge
EVALUATION AND MANAGEMENT†					
Office					
New Patient					
99201	Level 1	33.25	30.43	28.91	33.25
99202	Level 2	51.91	47.52	45.14	51.91
99203	Level 3	70.92	64.92	61.67	70.92
99204	Level 4	106.11	97.13	92.27	106.11
99205	Level 5	132.28	121.08	115.03	132.38
Established Patient					
99211	Level 1	16.07	14.70	13.97	16.07
99212	Level 2	28.55	26.14	24.83	28.55
99213	Level 3	40.20	36.80	34.96	40.20
99214	Level 4	61.51	56.31	53.79	61.51
99215	Level 5	96.97	88.76	84.32	96.97
Hospital					
Observation Services (new or established patient)					
99217	Discharge	66.88	61.22	58.16	66.88
99218	Dhx/exam SF/LC DM	74.22	67.94	64.54	74.22
99219	Chx/exam MC DM	117.75	107.78	102.39	117.75
99220	Chx/exam HC DM	147.48	134.99	128.24	147.48
Inpatient Services (new or established patient)					
99221	30 min	73.00	66.84	63.48	73.00
99222	50 min	120.80	110.57	105.04	120.80
99223	70 min	152.98	140.03	133.03	152.98
Subsequent Hospital Care					
99231	15 min	37.74	34.55	32.82	37.74
99232	25 min	55.56	50.85	48.31	55.56
99233	35 min	76.97	70.45	66.93	76.97
99238	Discharge	65.26	59.74	56.75	65.26

*Some services and procedures may not be considered a benefit under the Medicare program and when listed on a claim form, no reimbursement may be received. However, it is important to include these codes when billing because Medicare policies may change without an individual knowing of a new benefit. For this reason, some of the services shown in this mock fee schedule do not have any amounts listed under the three Medicare columns.
†See Tables 6–3 and 6-4 in the *Handbook* for more descriptions of E/M codes 99201 through 99275.

Table 3. Mock Fee Schedule—cont'd

Code Number and Description		Mock Fees	Medicare*		
			Participating	Nonparticipating	Limiting Charge
Consultations					
Office (new or established patient)					
99241	Level 1	51.93	47.54	45.16	51.93
99242	Level 2	80.24	73.44	69.77	80.24
99243	Level 3	103.51	94.75	90.01	103.51
99244	Level 4	145.05	132.77	126.13	145.05
99245	Level 5	195.48	178.93	169.98	195.45
Inpatient (new or established patient)					
99251	Level 1	53.29	48.78	46.34	53.29
99252	Level 2	80.56	73.74	70.05	80.56
99253	Level 3	106.10	97.12	92.26	106.10
99254	Level 4	145.26	132.96	126.31	145.26
99255	Level 5	196.55	179.91	170.91	196.55
Follow-up Inpatient (new or established patient)					
99261	Focused	29.66	27.15	25.79	29.66
99262	Expanded	50.57	46.28	43.97	50.57
99263	Detailed	76.36	69.90	66.40	76.36
Confirmatory Second or Third Opinion (new or established patient)					
99271	Focused	45.47	41.62	39.54	45.47
99272	Expanded	67.02	61.35	58.28	67.02
99273	Detailed	95.14	87.08	82.73	95.14
99274	Comprehensive	125.15	114.56	108.83	125.15
99275	Comprehensive	172.73	158.10	150.20	172.73
Emergency Department (new/established patient)					
99281	PF hx/exam SF DM	24.32	22.26	21.15	24.32
99282	EPF hx/exam LC DM	37.02	33.88	32.19	37.02
99283	EPF hx/exam MC DM	66.23	60.62	57.59	66.23
99284	D hx/exam MC DM	100.71	92.18	87.57	100.71
99285	C hx/exam HC DM	158.86	145.41	138.14	158.86
Critical Care Services					
99291	First hour	208.91	191.22	181.66	208.91
99292	Each addl. 30 min	102.02	92.46	87.84	102.02
Neonatal Intensive Care					
99295	Initial	892.74	817.16	776.30	892.74
99296	Subsequent unstable case	418.73	383.27	364.11	418.73
Nursing Facility					
99301	30 min	64.11	58.68	55.75	64.11
99302	40 min	90.55	82.88	78.74	90.55
99303	50 min	136.76	125.18	118.92	136.76
Subsequent (new/established patient)					
99311	15 min	37.95	34.74	33.00	37.95
99312	25 min	55.11	50.44	47.92	55.11
99313	35 min	69.61	63.72	60.53	69.61
Domiciliary, Rest Home, Custodial Care					
New Patient					
99321	PF hx/exam LC DM	46.10	42.20	40.09	46.10
99322	EPF hx/exam MC DM	65.02	59.53	56.54	65.02
99323	D hx/exam HC DM	86.18	78.88	74.94	86.18

*Some services and procedures may not be considered a benefit under the Medicare program and when listed on a claim form, no reimbursement may be received. However, it is important to include these codes when billing because Medicare policies may change without an individual knowing of a new benefit. For this reason, some of the services shown in this mock fee schedule do not have any amounts listed under the three Medicare columns.

Continued

Table 3. Mock Fee Schedule—cont'd

Code Number and Description		Mock Fees	Medicare*		
			Participating	Nonparticipating	Limiting Charge
99331	PF hx/exam LC DM	37.31	34.15	32.44	37.31
99332	EPF hx/exam MC DM	49.22	45.05	42.80	49.22
99333	D hx/exam HC DM	60.61	55.47	52.70	60.61
Home Services					
New Patient					
99341	PF hx/exam SF DM	70.32	64.37	61.15	70.32
99342	EPF hx/exam LC DM	91.85	84.07	79.87	91.85
99343	D hx/exam MC DM	120.24	110.06	104.56	120.24
Established Patient					
99347	PF hx/exam SF DM	54.83	50.19	47.68	54.83
99348	EPF hx/exam LC DM	70.06	64.13	60.92	70.06
99349	D hx/exam MC DM	88.33	80.85	76.81	88.33
Prolonged Services with Contact					
Outpatient					
99354	First hour	96.97	88.76	84.32	96.97
99355	Each addl. 30 min	96.97	88.76	84.32	96.97
Inpatient					
99356	First hour	96.42	88.25	83.84	96.42
99357	Each addl. 30 min	96.42	88.25	83.84	96.42
Prolonged Services Without Direct Contact					
99358	First hour	90.00			
99359	Each addl. 30 min	90.00			
Physician Standby Service					
99360	Each 30 min	95.00			
Case Management Services					
Team Conferences					
99361		85.00			
99362		105.00			
Telephone Calls					
99371	Simple or brief	30.00			
99372	Intermediate	40.00			
99373	Complex	60.00			
Care Plan Oversight Services					
99375	30 min or more	93.40	85.49	81.22	93.40
Preventive Medicine					
New Patient					
99381	Infant younger than 1 year	50.00			
99382	1-4 years	50.00			
99383	5-11 years	45.00			
99384	12-17 years	45.00			
99385	18-39 years	50.00			
99386	40-64 years	50.00			
99387	65 years and older	55.00			
Established Patient					
99391	Infant younger than year	35.00			
99392	1-4 years	35.00			
99393	5-11 years	30.00			
99394	12-17 years	30.00			

*Some services and procedures may not be considered a benefit under the Medicare program and when listed on a claim form, no reimbursement may be received. However, it is important to include these codes when billing because Medicare policies may change without an individual knowing of a new benefit. For this reason, some of the services shown in this mock fee schedule do not have any amounts listed under the three Medicare columns.

Table 3. Mock Fee Schedule—cont'd

Code Number and Description		Mock Fees	Medicare*		
			Participating	Nonparticipating	Limiting Charge
99395	18-39 years	35.00			
99396	40-64 years	35.00			
99397	65 years and older	40.00			
Counseling (new/est pt)					
Individual					
99401	15 min	35.00			
99402	30 min	50.00			
99403	45 min	65.00			
99404	60 min	80.00			
Group					
99411	30 min	30.00			
99412	60 min	50.00			
Other preventive medicine services					
99420	Health hazard appraisal	50.00			
99429	Unlisted preventive med serv	variable			
Newborn Care					
99431	Birthing room delivery	102.50	93.50	88.83	102.15
99432	Other than birthing room	110.16	100.83	95.79	110.16
99433	Subsequent hospital care	54.02	49.44	46.97	54.02
99440	Newborn resuscitation	255.98	234.30	222.59	255.98
99499	Unlisted E/M service	variable			
Anesthesiology					

Anesthesiology fees are presented here for CPT codes. However, each case would require a fee for time, e.g., every 15 minutes would be worth $55. This fee is determined according to the relative value system, calculated, and added into the anesthesia (CPT) fee. Some anesthetists may list a surgical code using an anesthesia modifier on a subsequent line for carriers that do not acknowledge anesthesia codes.

99100	Anes for pt younger than 1 yr or older than 70 years	55.00			
99116	Anes complicated use total hypothermia	275.00			
99135	Anes complicated use hypotension	275.00			
99140	Anes complicated emer cond	110.00			
Physician Status Modifier Codes					
P-1	Normal healthy patient	00.00			
P-2	Patient with mild systemic disease	00.00			
P-3	Patient with severe systemic disease	55.00			
P-4	Patient with severe systemic (disease constant threat to life)	110.00			

*Some services and procedures may not be considered a benefit under the Medicare program and when listed on a claim form, no reimbursement may be received. However, it is important to include these codes when billing because Medicare policies may change without an individual knowing of a new benefit. For this reason, some of the services shown in this mock fee schedule do not have any amounts listed under the three Medicare columns.

Continued

Table 3. Mock Fee Schedule—cont'd

Code Number and Description		Mock Fees	Medicare*		
			Participating	Nonparticipating	Limiting Charge
P-5	Moribund pt not expected to survive for 24 hr with or without operation	165.00			
P-6	Declared brain-dead pt, organs being removed for donor	00.00			
Head					
00160	Anes for proc nose & accessory sinuses: NOS	275.00			
00172	Anes repair cleft palate	165.00			
Thorax					
00400	Anes for procant integumentary system of chest, incl SC tissue	165.00			
00402	Anes breast reconstruction	275.00			
00546	Anes pulmonary resection with thoracoplasty	275.00			
00600	Anes cervical spine and cord	550.00			
Lower Abdomen					
00800	Anes for proc lower ant abdominal wall	165.00			
00840	Anes intraperitoneal proc lower abdomen: NOS	330.00			
00842	Amniocentesis	220.00			
00914	Anes TURP	275.00			
00942	Anes colporrhaphy, colpotomy, colpectomy	220.00			
Upper Leg					
01210	Anes open proc hip joint; NOS	330.00			
01214	Total hip replacement	440.00			
Upper Arm and Elbow					
01740	Anes open proc humerus/ elbow; NOS	220.00			
01758	Exc cyst/tumor humerus	275.00			
Radiologic Procedures					
01922	Anes CAT scan	385.00			
Miscellaneous Procedure(s)					
01999	Unlisted anes proc	variable			
Neurology					
95812	Electroencephalogram	129.32	118.37	112.45	129.32
95819	Electroencephalogram— awake and asleep	126.81	116.07	110.27	126.81
95860	Electromyography, 1 extremity	88.83	81.31	77.24	88.83
95864	Electromyography, 4 extremities	239.99	219.67	208.69	239.99
96100	Psychological testing (per hour)	80.95	74.10	70.39	80.95

*Some services and procedures may not be considered a benefit under the Medicare program and when listed on a claim form, no reimbursement may be received. However, it is important to include these codes when billing because Medicare policies may change without an individual knowing of a new benefit. For this reason, some of the services shown in this mock fee schedule do not have any amounts listed under the three Medicare columns.

Table 3. Mock Fee Schedule—cont'd

Code Number and Description		Mock Fees	Medicare*		
			Participating	Nonparticipating	Limiting Charge
Physical Medicine					
97024	Diathermy	14.27	13.06	12.41	14.27
97036	Hubbard tank, each 15 min	24.77	22.67	21.54	24.77
97110	Physical therapy, initial 30 min	23.89	21.86	20.77	23.89
97140	Manual therapy (manipulation, traction), one or more regions, each 15 min	16.93	15.49	14.72	16.93
Special Services and Reports					
99000	Handling of specimen (transfer from Dr.'s office to lab)	5.00			
99025	Initial surg eval (new pt) with starred procedure	50.00			
99050	Services requested after office hours in addition to basic service	25.00			
99052	Services between 10 p.m. and 8 a.m. in addition to basic service	35.00			
99054	Services on Sundays and holidays in addition to basic service	35.00			
99056	Services normally provided in office requested by pt in location other than office	20.00			
99058	Office services provided on an emergency basis	65.00			
99070	Supplies and materials (itemize drugs and materials provided)	25.00			
99080	Special reports:				
	Insurance forms	10.00			
	Review of data to clarify pt's status	20.00			
	WC reports	50.00			
	WC extensive review report	250.00			

*Some services and procedures may not be considered a benefit under the Medicare program and when listed on a claim form, no reimbursement may be received. However, it is important to include these codes when billing because Medicare policies may change without an individual knowing of a new benefit. For this reason, some of the services shown in this mock fee schedule do not have any amounts listed under the three Medicare columns.

Continued

Table 3. Mock Fee Schedule—cont'd

			Medicare*		
Code Number and Description	Mock Fees	Participating	Non participating	Limiting Charge	Follow-up Days†
10060	I & D furuncle, onychia, paronychia; single	75.92	69.49	66.02	75.92	10
11040	Debridement; skin, partial thickness	79.32	75.60	68.97	79.32	10
11044	Debridement; skin, subcu. muscle, bone	269.28	246.48	234.16	269.28	10
11100	Biopsy of skin, SC tissue &/or mucous membrane; 1 lesion	65.43	59.89	56.90	65.43	10
11200	Exc, skin tags; up to 15	55.68	50.97	45.42	55.68	10
11401	Exc, benign lesion, 0.6–1.0 cm trunk, arms, legs	95.62	87.53	83.15	96.62	10
11402	1.1–2.0 cm	121.52	111.23	105.67	121.52	10
11403	2.1–3.0 cm	151.82	138.97	132.02	151.82	10
11420	Exc, benign lesion, 0.5 cm or less scalp, neck, hands, feet, genitalia	75.44	69.05	65.60	75.44	10
11422	Exc, benign lesion scalp, neck, hands, feet, or genitalia; 1.1–2.0 cm	131.35	120.23	114.22	131.35	10
11441	Exc, benign lesion face, ears, eyelids, nose, lips, or mucous membrane; 0.6–1.0 cm dia or less	119.08	109.00	103.55	119.08	10
11602	Exc, malignant lesion, trunk, arms, or legs; 1.1–2.0 cm dia	195.06	178.55	169.62	195.06	10
11719	Trimming of nondystrophic nails, any number	30.58	27.82	26.33	30.58	0
11720	Debridement of nails, any method, 1–5	32.58	29.82	28.33	32.58	0
11721	6 or more	32.58	29.82	28.33	32.58	0
11730	Avulsion nail plate, partial or complete, simple repair; single	76.91	70.40	66.88	76.91	0
11750	Exc, nail or nail matrix, partial or complete	193.45	177.07	168.22	193.45	10
11765	Wedge excision of nail fold	57.95	53.04	50.39	57.95	10
12001	Simple repair (scalp, neck, axillae, ext genitalia, trunk, or extremities incl hands & feet); 2.5 cm or less	91.17	83.45	79.28	91.17	10
12011	Simple repair (face, ears, eyelids, nose, lips, or mucous membranes); 2.5 cm or less	101.44	92.85	88.21	101.44	10
12013	2.6–5.0 cm	123.98	113.48	107.81	123.98	10
12032	Repair, scalp, axillae, trunk (intermediate)	169.73	155.36	147.59	169.73	10
12034	Repair, intermediate, layer closure of wounds (scalp, axillae, trunk, or extremities) excl hands or feet; 7.6–12.5 cm	214.20	196.06	186.26	214.20	10
12051	Repair, intermediate, layer closure of wounds (face, ears, eyelids, nose, lips, or mucous membranes); 2.5 cm	167.60	153.41	145.74	167.60	10
17000	Cauterization, 1 lesion	52.56	48.11	45.70	52.56	10
17003	Second through 14 lesions, each	15.21	17.77	16.88	15.21	10
17100	Destruction, any method, skin lesion (benign) any area except face—one	44.86	41.06	39.01	44.86	10
17004	Destruction (laser surgery), 15 or more lesions	52.56	48.11	45.70	52.56	10

*Some services and procedures may not be considered a benefit under the Medicare program and when listed on a claim form, no reimbursement may be received. However, it is important to include these codes when billing because Medicare policies may change without an individual knowing of a new benefit. For this reason, some of the services shown in this mock fee schedule do not have any amounts listed under the three Medicare columns.

†Data for the surgical follow-up days from *St. Anthony's CPT '96 Companion: A Guide to Medicare Billing.*

Table 3. Mock Fee Schedule—cont'd

Code Number and Description		Mock Fees	Medicare*			
			Participating	Non participating	Limiting Charge	Follow-up Days
19020	Mastotomy, drainage/exploration deep abscess	237.36	217.26	206.40	237.36	90
19100	Biopsy, breast, needle	96.17	88.03	83.63	96.17	0
19101	Biopsy, breast, incisional	281.51	257.67	244.79	281.51	10
20610	Arthrocentesis, aspiration or injection joint (shoulder, hip, knee) or bursa	52.33	47.89	45.50	52.33	0
21330	Nasal fracture, open treatment complicated	599.46	548.71	521.27	599.46	90
24066	Biopsy, deep, soft tissue, upper arm, elbow	383.34	350.88	333.34	383.34	90
27455	Osteotomy, proximal tibia	1248.03	1142.36	1085.24	1248.03	90
27500	Treatment closed femoral shaft fracture without manipulation	554.90	507.92	482.52	554.90	90
27530	Treatment closed tibial fracture, proximal, without manipulation	344.24	315.09	299.34	344.24	90
27750	Treatment closed tibial shaft fracture without manipulation	400.94	366.99	348.64	400.94	90
27752	With manipulation	531.63	486.62	462.29	531.63	90
29280	Strapping of hand	35.13	31.36	29.79	35.13	0
29345	Appl long leg cast (thigh to toes)	123.23	112.80	107.16	123.23	0
29355	Walker or ambulatory type	133.75	122.42	116.30	133.75	0
29425	Appl short leg walking cast	102.10	93.45	88.78	102.10	0
30110	Excision, simple nasal polyp	145.21	132.92	126.27	145.21	10
30520	Septoplasty	660.88	604.93	574.68	660.88	90
30903	Control nasal hemorrhage; unilateral	118.17	108.17	102.76	118.17	0
30905	Control nasal hemorrhage, posterior with posterior nasal packs; initial	190.57	174.43	165.71	190.57	0
30906	Subsequent	173.01	158.36	150.44	173.01	0
31540	Laryngoscopy with excision of tumor and/or stripping of vocal cords	488.95	447.55	425.17	488.95	0
31541	With operating microscope	428.33	392.06	372.46	428.33	0
31575	Laryngoscopy, flexible fiberoptic; diagnostic	138.48	126.76	120.42	138.48	0
31625	Bronchoscopy with biopsy	312.87	286.38	272.06	312.87	0
32310	Pleurectomy	1234.79	1130.24	1073.73	1234.79	90
32440	Pneumonectomy, total	1972.10	1805.13	1714.87	1972.10	90
33020	Pericardiotomy	1289.25	1180.09	1121.09	1289.25	90
33206	Insertion of pacemaker; atrial	728.42	666.75	633.41	728.42	90
33208	AV sequential	751.57	687.89	653.50	751.57	90
35301	Thromboendarterectomy, with or without patch graft; carotid, vertebral, subclavian, by neck incision	1585.02	1450.82	1378.28	1585.02	90
36005	Intravenous injection for contrast venography	59.18	54.17	51.46	59.18	0
36248	Catheter placement (selective) arterial system, 2nd, 3rd and beyond	68.54	62.74	59.60	68.54	0
36415	Routine venipuncture for collection of specimen(s)	10.00	—	—	—	XXX
38101	Splenectomy, partial	994.44	910.24	864.73	994.44	90
38510	Biopsy/excision deep cervical node/s	327.42	299.69	284.71	327.42	90
39520	Excision tumor, mediastinal	1436.50	1314.87	1249.13	1436.50	90
42820	T & A under age 12 years	341.63	312.71	297.07	341.63	90
42821	T & A over age 12 years	410.73	375.96	357.16	410.73	90

*Some services and procedures may not be considered a benefit under the Medicare program and when listed on a claim form, no reimbursement may be received. However, it is important to include these codes when billing because Medicare policies may change without an individual knowing of a new benefit. For this reason, some of the services shown in this mock fee schedule do not have any amounts listed under the three Medicare columns.

Continued

Table 3. Mock Fee Schedule—cont'd

Code Number and Description		Mock Fees	Medicare*			
			Participating	Non participating	Limiting Charge	Follow-up Days
43234	Upper GI endoscopy, simple primary exam	201.86	184.77	175.53	201.86	0
43235	Upper GI endoscopy incl esophagus, stomach, duodenum, or jejunum; complex	238.92	218.69	207.76	238.92	0
43456	Dilation esophagus	254.52	232.97	221.32	254.52	0
43820	Gastrojejunostomy	971.86	889.58	845.10	971.86	90
44150	Colectomy, total, abdominal	1757.81	108.98	1528.53	1757.81	90
44320	Colostomy or skin level cecostomy	966.25	884.44	840.22	966.25	90
44950	Appendectomy	568.36	520.24	494.23	568.36	90
45308	Proctosigmoidoscopy for removal of polyp	135.34	123.88	117.69	135.34	0
45315	Multiple polyps	185.12	169.44	160.97	185.12	0
45330	Sigmoidoscopy (rigid), diagnostic (for biopsy or collection of specimen by brushing or washing)	95.92	87.80	83.41	95.92	0
45333	Sigmoidoscopy (flexible) with removal of polyps	183.99	168.41	159.99	183.99	0
45380	Colonoscopy with biopsy	382.35	349.98	332.48	382.35	0
46255	Hemorrhoidectomy int & ext, simple	503.57	460.94	437.89	503.57	90
46258	Hemorrhoidectomy with fistulectomy	636.02	582.17	553.06	636.02	90
46600	Anoscopy; diagnostic	32.86	30.07	28.57	32.86	0
46614	With control of hemorrhage	182.10	166.68	158.35	182.10	0
46700	Anoplastic, for stricture, adult	657.39	601.73	571.64	657.39	90
47562	Cholecystectomy; laparoscopic	714.99	654.45	621.73	714.99	90
47600	Cholecystectomy; abdominal excision	937.74	858.35	815.43	937.74	90
49505	Inguinal hernia repair, age 5 or over	551.07	504.41	479.19	551.07	90
49520	Repair, inguinal hernia, any age; recurrent	671.89	615.00	584.25	671.89	90
50080	Nephrostolithotomy, percutaneous	1323.93	1211.83	1151.24	1323.93	90
50780	Ureteroneocystostomy	1561.23	1429.84	1357.59	1561.23	90
51900	Closure of vesicovaginal fistula, abdominal approach	1196.82	1095.48	1040.71	1196.82	90
52000	Cystourethroscopy	167.05	152.90	145.26	167.05	0
52601	Transurethral resection of prostate	1193.53	1092.47	1037.85	1193.53	90
53040	Drainage of deep periurethral abscess	379.48	347.35	329.98	379.48	90
53060	Drainage of Skene's gland	147.45	134.97	128.22	147.45	10
53230	Excision, female diverticulum (urethral)	859.69	786.91	747.56	859.69	90
53240	Marsupialization of urethral diverticulum, M or F	520.11	476.07	452.27	520.11	90
53270	Excision of Skene's gland(s)	184.39	168.78	160.34	184.39	10
53620	Dilation, urethra, male	100.73	92.20	87.59	100.73	0
53660	Dilation urethra, female	48.32	44.23	42.02	48.32	0
54150	Circumcision–newborn	111.78	102.32	97.20	111.78	0
54520	Orchiectomy, simple	523.92	479.56	455.58	523.92	10
55700	Biopsy of prostate, needle or punch	156.22	142.99	135.84	156.22	90
55801	Prostatectomy, perineal subtotal	1466.56	1342.39	1275.27	1466.56	0
57265	Colporrhaphy AP with enterocele repair	902.24	825.85	784.56	902.24	90
57452	Colposcopy	84.18	77.05	73.20	84.18	90
57510	Cauterization of cervix, electro or thermal	115.15	105.40	100.13	115.15	0
57520	Circumferential (cone) of cervix with or without D & C, with or without Sturmdorff-type repair	387.08	354.30	336.59	387.08	10
58100	Endometrial biopsy	71.88	65.79	62.50	71.88	90
						0

*Some services and procedures may not be considered a benefit under the Medicare program and when listed on a claim form, no reimbursement may be received. However, it is important to include these codes when billing because Medicare policies may change without an individual knowing of a new benefit. For this reason, some of the services shown in this mock fee schedule do not have any amounts listed under the three Medicare columns.

Table 3. Mock Fee Schedule—cont'd

| | | | Medicare* | | |
Code Number and Description		Mock Fees	Participating	Non participating	Limiting Charge	Follow-up Days
58120	D & C, diagnostic and/or therapeutic (nonOB)	272.83	249.73	237.24	272.83	10
58150	TAH w/without salpingo-oophorectomy	1167.72	1068.85	1015.41	1167.72	90
58200	Total hysterectomy, extended, corpus cancer, including partial vaginectomy	1707.24	1562.69	1484.56	1707.24	90
58210	With bilateral radical pelvic lymphadenectomy	2160.78	1977.83	1878.94	2160.78	90
58300	Insertion of intrauterine device	100.00				0
58340	Hysterosalpingography, inj proc for	73.06	66.87	63.53	73.06	0
58720	Salpingo-oophorectomy, complete or partial, unilateral or bilateral surgical treatment of ectopic pregnancy	732.40	670.39	636.87	732.40	90
59120	Salpingectomy and/or oophorectomy	789.26	722.43	686.31	789.26	90
59121	Without salpingectomy and/or oophorectomy	638.84	584.75	555.51	638.84	90
59130	Abdominal pregnancy	699.12	639.93	607.93	699.12	90
59135	Total hysterectomy, interstitial, uterine pregnancy	1154.16	1056.44	1003.62	1154.16	90
59136	Partial uterine resection, interstitial uterine pregnancy	772.69	707.26	671.90	772.69	90
59140	Cervical, with evacuation	489.68	448.22	425.81	489.68	90
59160	D & C postpartum hemorrhage (separate proc)	293.46	268.61	255.18	293.46	10
59400	OB Care—routine, inc. antepartum/ postpartum care	1864.30	1706.45	1621.13	1864.30	N/A
59515	C-section, low cervical, incl in-hosp postpartum care (separate proc)	1469.80	1345.36	1278.09	1469.80	N/A
59510	Including antepartum and postpartum care	2102.33	1924.33	1828.11	2102.33	N/A
59812	Treatment of incomplete abortion, any trimester; completed surgically	357.39	327.13	310.77	357.39	90
61314	Craniotomy infratentorial	2548.09	2332.35	2215.73	2548.09	90
62270	Spinal puncture, lumbar; diagnostic	77.52	70.96	67.41	77.52	0
65091	Excision of eye, without implant	708.22	648.25	615.84	708.22	90
65205	Removal of foreign body, ext eye	56.02	51.27	48.71	56.02	0
65222	Corneal, with slit lamp	73.81	67.56	64.18	73.81	0
69420	Myringotomy	97.76	89.48	85.01	97.76	10

*Some services and procedures may not be considered a benefit under the Medicare program and when listed on a claim form, no reimbursement may be received. However, it is important to include these codes when billing because Medicare policies may change without an individual knowing of a new benefit. For this reason, some of the services shown in this mock fee schedule do not have any amounts listed under the three Medicare columns.

Continued

Table 3. Mock Fee Schedule—cont'd

Code Number and Description		Mock Fees	Medicare*		
			Participating	Nonparticipating	Limiting Charge
RADIOLOGY, NUCLEAR MEDICINE, AND DIAGNOSTIC ULTRASOUND					
70120	X-ray mastoids, 2 less than 3 views per side	38.96	35.66	33.88	38.96
70130	Complete, min., 3 views per side	56.07	51.33	48.76	56.07
71010	X-ray chest, 1 view	31.95	29.24	27.78	31.95
71020	Chest x-ray, 2 views	40.97	37.50	35.63	40.97
71030	Chest x-ray, compl. 4 views	54.02	49.44	46.97	54.02
71060	Bronchogram, bilateral	143.75	131.58	125.00	143.75
72100	X-ray spine, LS; AP & lat views	43.23	39.57	37.59	43.23
72114	Complete, incl bending views	74.97	68.62	65.19	74.97
73100	X-ray wrist, 2 views	31.61	28.94	27.49	31.61
73500	X-ray hip, 1 view	31.56	28.88	27.44	31.56
73540	X-ray pelvis & hips, infant or child, 2 views	37.94	34.73	32.99	37.94
73590	X-ray tibia & fibula, 2 views	33.35	30.53	29.00	33.35
73620	Radiologic exam, foot; AP & lat views	31.61	28.94	27.49	31.61
73650	X-ray calcaneus, 2 views	30.71	28.11	26.70	30.71
74241	Radiologic exam, upper gastrointestinal tract, with/without delayed films with KUB	108.93	99.71	94.72	108.93
74245	Upper GI tract with small bowel	161.70	148.01	140.61	161.70
74270	Barium enema	118.47	108.44	103.02	118.47
74290	Oral cholecystography	52.59	48.14	45.73	52.59
74400	Urography (pyelography), intravenous, with or without KUB	104.78	95.90	91.11	104.78
74410	Urography, infusion	116.76	106.87	101.53	116.76
74420	Urography, retrograde	138.89	127.13	120.77	138.89
75982	Percutaneous placement of drainage catheter	359.08	328.67	312.24	359.08
76090	Mammography, unilateral	62.57	57.27	54.41	62.57
76091	Mammography, bilateral	82.83	75.82	72.03	82.83
76805	Echography, pregnant uterus, B-scan or real time; complete	154.18	141.13	134.07	154.18
76810	Echography, pregnant uterus, complete: multiple gestation, after first trimester	306.54	280.59	266.56	306.54
76946	Ultrasonic guidance for amniocentesis	91.22	83.49	79.32	91.22
77300	Radiation dosimetry	97.58	89.32	84.85	97.58
77315	Teletherapy, isodose plan, complex	213.59	195.51	185.73	213.59
78104	Bone marrow imaging, whole body	230.56	211.04	200.49	230.56
78215	Liver and spleen imaging	160.44	146.85	139.51	160.44
78800	Tumor localization, limited area	191.53	175.32	166.55	191.53

*Some services and procedures may not be considered a benefit under the Medicare program and when listed on a claim form, no reimbursement may be received. However, it is important to include these codes when billing because Medicare policies may change without an individual knowing of a new benefit. For this reason, some of the services shown in this mock fee schedule do not have any amounts listed under the three Medicare columns.

PATHOLOGY AND LABORATORY[1]

Laboratory tests done as groups or combination "profiles" performed on multichannel equipment should be billed using the appropriate code number (80048 through 80076). Following is a list of the tests. The subsequent listing illustrates how to find the correct code.

Alanine aminotransferase (ALT, SGPT)
Albumin
Aspartate aminotransferase (AST, SGOT)
Bilirubin, direct
Bilirubin, total
Calcium
Carbon dioxide content

Chloride
Cholesterol
Creatinine
Glucose (sugar)
Lactate dehydrogenase (LD)
Phosphatase, alkaline

Phosphorus (inorganic phosphate)
Potassium
Protein, total
Sodium
Urea nitrogen (BUN)
Uric acid

[1]Mock fees for laboratory tests presented in this schedule may not be representative of fees in your region because of the variety of capitation and managed care contracts, as well as discount policies made by laboratories. At the time of this edition, Medicare guidelines may or may not pay for automatic multichannel tests where a large number of tests are performed per panel. Some cases require documentation and a related diagnostic code for each test performed. Provider must have the CLIA level of licensure to bill for tests, and test results must be documented.

Table 3. Mock Fee Schedule—cont'd

Code Number and Description		Mock Fees	Medicare*		
			Participating	Nonparticipating	Limiting Charge
ORGAN OR DISEASE-ORIENTED PANELS					
80048	Basic metabolic panel	15.00	14.60	13.87	16.64
80050	General health panel	20.00	19.20	15.99	21.87
80051	Electrolyte panel	20.00	19.20	15.99	21.87
80053	Comprehensive metabolic panel	25.00	20.99	19.94	23.93
80055	Obstetric panel	25.00	20.99	19.94	23.93
80076	Hepatic function panel	27.00	25.00	20.88	24.98
80074	Acute hepatitis panel	27.00	25.00	20.88	24.88
80061	Lipid panel	30.00	28.60	25.97	32.16
81000	Urinalysis, non-automated, with microscopy	8.00	7.44	5.98	8.84
81001	Urinalysis, automated, with microscopy	8.00	7.44	5.98	8.84
81002	Urinalysis, non-automated without microscopy	8.00	7.44	5.98	8.84
81015	Urinalysis, microscopy only	8.00	7.44	5.98	8.84
82270	Blood, occult; feces screening 1–3	4.05	3.56	3.31	4.05
82565	Creatinine; blood	10.00	9.80	8.88	12.03
82947	Glucose; quantitative	15.00			
82951	Glucose tol test, 3 spec	40.00	41.00	36.80	45.16
82952	Each add spec beyond 3	30.00	28.60	25.97	32.16
83020	Hemoglobin, electrophoresis	25.00	20.00	19.94	23.93
83715	Lipoprotein, blood; electrophoretic separation	25.00	20.00	19.94	23.93
84478	Triglycerides, blood	20.00	19.20	15.999	21.87
84479	Triiodothyronine (T–3)	20.00	19.20	15.99	21.87
84520	Urea nitrogen, blood (BUN); quantitative	25.00	20.99	19.94	23.93
84550	Uric acid, blood chemical	20.00	19.20	15.99	21.87
84702	Gonadotropin, chorionic; quantitative	20.00	19.20	15.99	21.87
84703	Qualitative	20.00	19.20	15.99	21.87
85013	Microhematocrit (spun)	20.00	19.20	15.99	21.87
85025	Complete blood count (hemogram), platelet count, automated, differential WBC count	25.00	20.00	19.94	23.93
38220	Bone marrow, aspiration only	73.52	67.29	63.93	73.52
38221	Bone marrow aspiration (biopsy)	90.65	82.98	78.83	90.65
85345	Coagulation time; Lee & White	20.00	19.20	15.99	21.87
85032	Platelet count (manual)	20.00	19.20	15.99	21.87
86038	Antinuclear antibodies	25.00	20.00	19.94	23.93
86580	Skin test; TB, intradermal	11.34	10.38	9.86	11.34
87081	Culture, bacterial, screening for single organisms	25.00	20.00	19.94	23.93
87181	Sensitivity studies, antibiotic; per antibiotic	20.00	19.20	15.99	21.87
87184	Disk method, per plate (12 disks or less)	20.00	19.20	15.99	21.87
87210	Smear, primary source, wet mount with simple stain, for bacteria, fungi, ova, and/or parasites	35.00	48.35	45.93	55.12
88150	Papanicolaou, cytopath	35.00	48.35	45.93	55.12
88302	Surgical pathology, gross & micro exam (skin, fingers, nerve, testis)	24.14	22.09	20.99	24.14
88305	Bone marrow, interpret	77.69	71.12	67.56	77.69

*Some services and procedures may not be considered a benefit under the Medicare program and when listed on a claim form, no reimbursement may be received. However, it is important to include these codes when billing because Medicare policies may change without an individual knowing of a new benefit. For this reason, some of the services shown in this mock fee schedule do not have any amounts listed under the three Medicare columns.

Continued

Table 3. Mock Fee Schedule—cont'd

Code Number and Description		Mock Fees	Medicare*		
			Participating	Nonparticipating	Limiting Charge
MEDICINE PROCEDURES					
Immunization Injections					
90701	Diphtheria, tetanus, pertussis	34.00			
90703	Tetanus toxoid	28.00			
90712	Poliovirus vaccine, oral	28.00			
Therapeutic Injections					
90782	IM or SC medication	4.77	4.37	4.15	4.77
90784	IV	21.33	19.53	18.55	21.33
90788	IM antibiotic	5.22	4.78	4.54	5.22
Psychiatry					
90816	Individual psychotherapy 20–30 min	60.25	55.15	52.39	60.25
90853	Group therapy	29.22	26.75	25.41	29.22
Hemodialysis					
90935	Single phys evaluation	117.23	107.31	101.94	117.23
90937	Repeat evaluation	206.24	188.78	179.34	206.24
Gastroenterology					
91000	Esophageal incubation	69.82	63.91	60.71	69.82
91055	Gastric incubation	87.41	80.01	76.01	87.41
Ophthalmologic Services					
92004	Comprehensive eye exam	90.86	83.17	79.01	90.86
92100	Tonometry	47.31	43.31	41.14	47.31
92230	Fluorescein angioscopy	55.49	50.79	48.25	55.49
92275	Electroretinography	81.17	74.29	70.58	81.17
92531	Spontaneous nystagmus	26.00			
Audiologic Function Tests					
92557	Comprehensive audiometry	54.33	49.73	47.24	54.33
92596	Ear measurements	26.81	24.54	23.31	26.81
Cardiovascular Therapeutic Services					
93000	Electrocardiogram (ECG)	34.26	31.36	29.79	34.26
93015	Treadmill ECG	140.71	128.80	122.36	140.71
93040	Rhythm ECG, 1–3 leads	18.47	16.90	16.06	18.47
93307	Echocardiography	250.73	229.50	218.03	250.73
93320	Doppler echocardiography	114.60	104.90	99.65	114.60
Pulmonary					
94010	Spirometry	38.57	35.31	33.54	38.57
94060	Spirometry before and after bronchodilator	71.67	65.60	62.32	71.67
94150	Vital capacity, total	13.82	12.65	12.02	13.82
Allergy and Clinical Immunology					
95024	Intradermal tests; immediate reaction	6.58	6.02	5.72	6.85
95028	Intradermal tests; delayed reaction	9.32	8.85	10.18	9.32
93320	Doppler echocardiography	114.60	104.90	99.65	114.60
95044	Patch tests	8.83	8.08	7.68	8.83
95115	Treatment for allergy, single inj.	17.20	15.75	14.96	17.20
95117	2 or more inj.	22.17	20.29	19.28	22.17
95165	Allergen immunotherapy, single or multiple antigens, multiple-dose vials		6.50	6.18	7.11

*Some services and procedures may not be considered a benefit under the Medicare program and when listed on a claim form, no reimbursement may be received. However, it is important to include these codes when billing because Medicare policies may change without an individual knowing of a new benefit. For this reason, some of the services shown in this mock fee schedule do not have any amounts listed under the three Medicare columns.

Table 3. Mock Fee Schedule—cont'd

Code Number and Description		Mock Fees	Medicare*		
			Participating	Nonparticipating	Limiting Charge
Neurology					
95812	Electroencephalogram, up to 1 hr.	129.32	118.37	112.45	129.32
95819	Electroencephalogram—awake and asleep	126.81	116.07	110.27	126.81
95860	Electromyography, 1 extremity	88.83	81.31	77.24	88.83
95864	Electromyography, 4 extremities	239.99	219.67	208.69	239.99
96100	Psychological testing (per hour)	80.95	74.10	70.39	80.95
Physical Medicine					
97024	Diathermy	14.27	13.06	12.41	14.27
97036	Hubbard tank, each 15 min	24.77	22.67	21.54	24.77
97110	Physical therapy, initial 30 min	23.89	21.86	20.77	23.89
97140	Manual therapy (manipulation, traction), one or more regions, each 15 min	16.93	15.49	14.72	16.93
Special Services and Reports					
99000	Handling of specimen (transfer from Dr.'s office to lab)	5.00			
99025	Initial surg eval (new pt) with starred procedure	50.00			
99050	Services requested after office hours in addition to basic service	25.00			
99052	Services between 10 p.m. and 8 a.m. in addition to basic service	35.00			
99054	Services on Sundays and holidays in addition to basic service	35.00			
99056	Services normally provided in office requested by pt in location other than office	20.00			
99058	Office services provided on an emergency basis	65.00			
99070	Supplies and materials (itemize drugs and materials provided)	25.00			
99080	Special reports:				
	Insurance forms	10.00			
	Review of data to clarify pt's status	20.00			
	WC reports	50.00			
	WC extensive review report	250.00			

*Some services and procedures may not be considered a benefit under the Medicare program and when listed on a claim form, no reimbursement may be received. However, it is important to include these codes when billing because Medicare policies may change without an individual knowing of a new benefit. For this reason, some of the services shown in this mock fee schedule do not have any amounts listed under the three Medicare columns.

INDEX

A

B

C

Colectomy	44140-44160
Colonoscopy, fiberoptic	45355-45385
Colostomy, separate procedure	44320
Colporrhaphy	57240-57265, 57289
Colposcopy	57452-57460
Complete blood count	85022-85031
Conization, cervix	57520-57522
Consultation	
confirmatory	99271-99275
during surgery (pathology)	88329-88332
initial	99251-99255
inpatient follow-up	99261-99263
office	99241-99245
telephone calls	99371-99373
telephone, psychiatric patient	99371-99373
with examination and evaluation	99241-99255
Counseling	
group	99411, 99412
individual	99401-99404
Craniotomy	61314
Creatinine	82540, 82565-82570
Critical care	
initial	99291
follow-up visit	99292
neonatal	99295-99297
Culture, bacterial	87040-87088
Custodial care medical services	
established patient	99331-99333
new patient	99321-99323
Cystourethroscopy	52000-52340

D

Debridement	
nails	11720-11721
skin	11040-11044
Destruction benign lesion, any method	
face	17000-17010
other than face	17100-17105
Dentition, prolonged physician attendance	99354-99360
Dilation	
dilatation and curettage	57820, 58120, 59160, 59840, 59851
esophagus	43450-43460
urethra, female	53660-53661
urethra, male	53620-53621
Diathermy	97024
Domiciliary visits	
established patient	99331-99333
new patient	99321-99323
Dosimetry	77300, 77331

E

Ear	
excision, benign lesion, external	11440-11446
layer closure, wounds	12051-12057
simple repair, wounds	12011-12018
Echocardiography	93307
Echography, pregnant uterus	76805-76816
Electrocardiogram	93000-93042

Electroencephalogram	95819-95827
Electromyography	95858, 95860-95869
Electroretinography	92275
Emergency department services	99281-99288
Endoscopy, gastrointestinal, upper	43234-43264
Esophageal intubation	91000
Excision—see organ, region, or structure involved	
Eye	
excision	65091
removal foreign body	65205-65222
Eyelid	
excision, benign lesion	11440-11446
layer closure, wounds	12051-12057
repair, simple	12011-12018

F

Face	
excision, benign lesion	11440-11446
layer closure, wounds (intermediate)	12051-12057
simple repair, wounds	12011-12018
Feces screening; blood occult	82270
Feet—see foot	
Fluorescein angioscopy, ophthalmoscopy	92230
Foot	
excision, benign lesion, skin	11420-11426
radiologic exam	73620-73630
simple repair, wounds	12001-12007
Fracture	
femur shaft	27500-27508
nasal	21300-21339
tibia proximal, plateau	27530-27537
tibia shaft	27750-27758

G

Gastric intubation	91055
Gastrointestinal tract, radiologic examination	74210-74340
Gastrojejunostomy	43632, 43820-43825, 43860-43865
Genitalia	
excision, benign lesion	11420-11426
repair, simple	12001-12007
Glucose, quantitative	82947
Glucose tolerance test	82951, 82952
Gonadotropin, chorionic	84702, 84703

H

Handling or specimen	99000
Hands	
excision, benign lesion	11420-11426
simple repair, wounds	12001-12007
Hemodialysis	90935-90937
insertion of cannula	36800-36815
placement, venous catheter	36245-36248
Hemoglobin electrophoresis	83020
Hemorrhage, nasal	30901-30906
Hemorrhoidectomy	46221-46262
Hernia, inguinal	49495-49525
Hip, radiologic examination	73500-73540

Home visits
 established patient 99351-99353
 new patient 99341-99343
Hospital visits
 discharge day 99238
 first day 99221-99223
 newborn, initial care 99431
 prolonged service 99356, 99357
 subsequent care 99231-99233
 subsequent day 99433
Hubbard tank 97036, 97113
Hysterectomy 58150-58285
 ectopic pregnancy 59135-59140
 supracervical 58180
 total 58150-58152, 58200-58240
 vaginal 58260-58285
Hysterosalpingography 74740
 injection procedure for 58340

I

Imaging
 bone marrow 78102-78104
 liver 78201-78220
Immunotherapy 95120-95199
Incision and drainage, furuncle 10060
Incision, breast 19000-19030
Injection
 allergies, steroids 95115-95117
 antibiotic 90788
 arthrocentesis, small joint or bursa 20600-20610
 catheter placement 36245-36248
 immunization 90700-90749
 intravenous 90784
 IV for contrast venography 36005
 medication, intravenous 90784
 medication, subcutaneous or intramuscular 90782
 therapeutic 90782-90784
Intrauterine device (IUD)
 insertion 58300
 removal 58301

J

Joint fluid, cell count 89050, 89051

K

KUB 74400-74405, 74420

L

Laryngoscopy 31540-31575
Leg, excision, malignant lesion 11600-11606
Lip
 excision, benign lesion 11440-11446
 layer closure, wounds 12051-12057
 repair, superficial wound 12011-12018
Lipoprotein 83715, 83717

M

Mammography	76090, 76091
Manipulation, spine	22505, 97260
Manipulation (physical therapy)	97260, 97261
Marsupialization, urethral diverticulum	53240
Mastoids, radiologic exam	70120, 70130
Mucous membrane, cutaneous	
excision, benign lesion	11440-11446
layer closure, wounds	12051-12057
simple repair, wounds	12011-12018
Myringotomy	69420

N

Nail	
excision	11750
trim	11719
wedge excision	11765
Nasal polyp, excision	30110
Neck	
excision, benign lesion	11420-11426
simple repair, wounds	12001-12007
Neonatal critical care	99295-99297
Nephrostolithotomy	50080
Newborn care	99431-99440
Nose	
excision, benign lesion	11440-11446
layer closure	12051-12057
simple repair	12011-12018
Nursing facility care	
assessment	99301-99303
subsequent care	99311-99313
Nystagmus	
optokinetic	92534
optokinetic test	92544
positional	92532
spontaneous	92531
spontaneous test	92541

O

Obstetric care	59400-59410
Office medical service	
after hours	99050-99054
emergency care	99058
Office visit	
established patient	99211-99215
new patient	99201-99205
service at another location	99056
with surgical procedure	99025
Ophthalmologic examination	92002-92019
Orchiectomy	54520-54535
Organ- or disease-oriented laboratory panels	80049-80091
Osteotomy, tibia	27455, 27457, 27705, 27709
Outpatient visit	
established patient	99211-99215
new patient	99201-99205

P

Pacemaker, insertion	33200-33217, 71090
Papanicolaou cytopathology	88150-88155
Patch skin test	95044-95052
Pathology, surgical gross and microscopic	88302-88309
Pericardiotomy	33020
Physical medicine services	97010-97150
Platelet count	85590
Pleurectomy	32310
Pneumonectomy	32440-32450
Preventive medicine	
established patient	99391-99397
health hazard appraisal	99420
new patient	99381-99387
unlisted	99429
Proctosigmoidoscopy	45300-45321
Prolonged services	
hospital inpatient	99356-99359
office/outpatient	99354, 99355, 99358, 99359
Prostatectomy, perineal, subtotal	55801
Psychiatric evaluation of records, reports, and/or tests	90825
Psychological testing	96100
Psychotherapy	
pharmacologic management	90862
family (conjoint)	90847
group medical	90853
individual	90816
multiple-family	90849
Puncture, lumbar spine	62270, 62272

Q

Quadriceps repair	27430

R

Radiology	
dosimetry	77300, 77331
teletherapy	77305-77315, 77321
therapeutic	77261-77799
treatment delivery	77401-77417
Repair—see procedure, organ, structure, or region involved	
Reports, special	99080
Resection, prostate, transurethral	52601-54640

S

Salpingo-oophorectomy	58720
Salpingectomy and/or oophorectomy	59120-59140
excision, benign lesion	11420-11422
layer closure, wounds	12031-12037
simple repair, wounds	12001-12007
Sensitivity studies, antibiotic	87181-87192
Septum, nasal septoplasty	30520
Sigmoidoscopy	45330-45333
Skene's gland	53060-53270
Skin excision, skin tags	11200, 11201
Splenectomy	38100-38115
Smear, primary source	87205-87211
Spine, radiologic exam	72010-72120

Spirometry	94010-94070
Standby services	99360
Supplies and materials	99070, 99071

T

TB skin test	86580
Teletherapy	77305-77321
Thromboendarterectomy	35301-35381
Tibia, radiologic exam	73590
Tonometry	92100
Tonsillectomy	42820-42826
TURP	52601-52648
Treadmill exercise	93015-93018
Triglycerides	84478
Triiodothyronine	84479-84482
Trunk	
excision, malignant lesion	11600-11606
layer closure—intermediate	12031-12037
simple repair	12001-12007
Tumor localization	78800-78803

U

Ureteroneocystostomy	50780-50800
Urethral diverticulum, excision	53230-53235
Uric acid	84550-84560
Urinalysis	81000-81099
Urography	74400-74425

V

Venipuncture	36400-36425
Vesicovaginal fistula, closure	51900, 57320, 57330
Vital capacity	94010, 94150, 94160

W

Wrist, radiologic examination	73100, 73110

X

Xenograft	15400

Y

Y-plasty, bladder	51800

Z

Z-plasty	14000, 26121, 41520

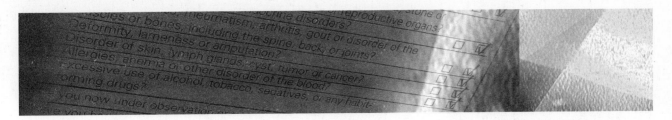

Medicare Level II HCPCS Codes

The following pages provide a partial alphanumeric list of the Centers for Medicare and Medicaid Services, referred to as Healthcare Common Procedure Coding System (HCPCS) (pronounced "hick-picks"). These Level II codes and modifiers were adopted by the Medicare program in 1984; additional codes and modifiers are added and deleted every year. This system was developed to code procedures not listed in the American Medical Association's *Current Procedural Terminology* (CPT) code book. This second level is a national standard used by all regional Medicare carriers.

Partial List of the Medicare Healthcare Common Procedure Coding System (HCPCS)

In certain circumstances, a code may need a modifier to show that the procedure has been changed by a specific situation. Remember that CPT and national modifiers apply to both CPT and HCPCS code systems. When applicable, indicate the appropriate modifier on the insurance claim form (Tables 1 and 2). Sometimes a special report may be needed to clarify the use of the modifier to the insurance company.

Table 1. Medicare HCPCS Modifiers

Modifier	Short Description	Modifier	Short Description
A1	Dressing for one wound	AK	Nonparticipating physician
A2	Dressing for two wounds	AM	Physician, team member service
A3	Dressing for three wounds	AP	No determination of refractive state
A4	Dressing for four wounds	AR	Physician scarcity area
A5	Dressing for five wounds	AS	Assistant-at-surgery service
A6	Dressing for six wounds	AT	Acute treatment
A7	Dressing for seven wounds	AU	Uro, ostomy, or trach item
A8	Dressing for eight wounds	AV	Item with prosthetic/orthotic
A9	Dressing for nine or more wounds	AW	Item with a surgical dressing.
AA	Anesthesia performed by anesthetist	AX	Item with dialysis services
AD	MD supervision; more than four anesthesia procedures	BA	Item with pen services
		BO	Nutrition oral admin no tube
AE	Registered dietitian	BP	Beneficiary elected to purchase item
AF	Specialty physician	BR	Beneficiary elected to rent item
AG	Primary physician	BU	Beneficiary undecided on purch/rent
AH	Clinical psychologist	CA	Procedure payable inpatient
AJ	Clinical social worker	CB	ESRD beneficiary Part A SNF-sep pay

Continued

Table 1. Medicare HCPCS Modifiers—cont'd

Modifier	Short Description	Modifier	Short Description
CC	Procedure code change	HB	Adult program nongeriatric
CD	AMCC test for ESRD or MCP MD	HC	Adult program geriatric
CE	Med necessity AMCC test sep reimbursement	HD	Pregnant/parenting program
CF	AMCC test not composite rate	HE	Mental health program
CG	Innovator drug dispensed	HF	Substance abuse program
E1	Upper left eyelid	HG	Opioid addiction tx program
E2	Lower left eyelid	HH	Mental hlth/substance abs pr
E3	Upper right eyelid	HI	M health/m retrdtn/dev dis pro
E4	Lower right eyelid	HJ	Employee assistance program
EJ	Subsequent claim	HK	spec high risk mntl hlth pop p
EM	Emergency reserve supply (ESRD)	HL	Intern
EP	Medicaid EPSDT program SVC	HM	Less than bachelor degree LV
ET	Emergency treatment	HN	Bachelors degree level
EY	No MD order for item/service	HO	Masters degree level
FA	Left hand, thumb	HP	Doctoral level
FP	Service part of family planning program	HQ	Group setting
F1	Left hand, second digit	HR	Family/couple W client presnt
F2	Left hand, third digit	HS	Family/couple W/O client prs
F3	Left hand, fourth digit	HT	Multi-disciplinary team
F4	Left hand, fifth digit	HU	Child welfare agency funded
F5	Right hand, thumb	HV	Funded state addiction agency
F6	Right hand, second digit	HW	State mntl hlth agency funded
F7	Right hand, third digit	HX	County/local agency funded
F8	Right hand, fourth digit	HY	Funded by juvenile justice
F9	Right hand, fifth digit	HZ	Criminal justice agency fund
G1	URR reading of less than 60	JW	Discarded drug not administered
G2	URR reading of 60 to 64.9	K0	LWR EXT PROST FUNCTNL LVL 0
G3	Urr reading of 65 to 69.9	K1	LWR EXT PROST FUNCTNL LVL 1
G4	URR reading of 70 to 74.9	K2	LWR EXT PROST FUNCTNL LVL 2
G5	URR reading of 75 or greater	K3	LWR EXT PROST FUNCTNL LVL 3
G6	ERSD patient <6 dialysis/mth	K4	LWR EXT PROST FUNCTNL LVL 4
G7	Payment limits do not apply	KA	Wheelchair add-on option/acc
G8	Monitored anesthesia care	KB	>4 modifiers on claim
G9	MAC for at risk patient	KC	Repl special pwr wc intrface
GA	Waiver of liability on file	KD	Drug/biological dme infused
GB	Claim resubmitted	KF	FDA class III device
GC	Resident/teaching phys serv	KH	DME POS INI CLM, PUR/1 MO RNT
GE	Resident primary care exception	KI	DME POS 2nd or 3rd mo rental
GF	Nonphysician serv C A hosp	KJ	DME POS PEN PMP or 4-15 mo rent
GG	Payment screen mam + diag mam	KM	RPLC facial prosth new imp
GH	Diag mammo to screening mamo	KN	RPLC facial prosth old mod
GJ	Opt out provider of ER serv	K0	Single drug unit dose form
GK	Actual item/service ordered	KP	First drug of multidrug UD
GL	Upgraded item, no charge	KQ	2nd/subsqnt drg multi DRG UD
GM	Multiple transports	KR	Rental item partial month
GN	OP speech language service	KS	Glucose monitor supply
GO	OP occupational therapy serv	KX	Documentation on file
GP	OP PT services	KZ	New cov not implement by MC
GQ	Telehealth store and forward	LC	Left circumflex coronary artery.
GT	Interactive telecommunication	LD	Left anterior descending coronary artery.
GV	Attending phys not hospice	LL	Lease/rental (Appld to pur)
GW	Service unrelated to term CO	LR	Laboratory round trip
GY	Statutorily excluded	LS	FDA-monitored intraocular lens implant
GZ	Not reasonable and necessary	LT	Left side
H9	Court ordered	MS	6 mo maint/svc fee parts/lbr
HA	Child/adolescent program	NR	New when rented

Table 1. Medicare HCPCS Modifiers—cont'd

Modifier	Short Description	Modifier	Short Description
NU	New equipment	SW	Serv by cert diab educator
PL	Progressive addition lenses	SY	Contact w/high-risk pop
Q2	HCFA/ord demo procedure/svc	T1	Left foot, second digit
Q3	Live donor surgery/services	T2	Left foot, third digit
Q4	Service exempt ordering/referring MD	T3	Left foot, fourth digit
Q5	Substitute MD service, recip bill arrangement	T4	Left foot, fifth digit
Q6	Locum tenens MD service	T5	Right foot, great toe
Q7	One Class A finding	T6	Right foot, second digit
Q8	Two Class B findings	T7	Right foot, third digit
Q9	One Class B and two Class C findings	T8	Right foot, fourth digit
QA	FDA investigational device	T9	Right foot, fifth digit
QB	MD providing SVC in rural HPSA	TA	Left foot, great toe
QC	Single-channel monitoring	TC	Technical component
QD	Recording/storage in solid-state memory	TD	RN
QE	Prescribed oxygen <1 LPM	TE	LPN/LVN
QF	Prescribed oxygen >4 LPM & port	TF	Intermediate level of care
QG	Prescribed oxygen >4 LPM	TG	Complex/high tech level care
QH	Oxygen-conserving device with delivery system	TH	OB tx/servcs prenatl/postpart
QJ	Patient in state/local custody	TJ	Child/adolescent program GP
QK	Med dir 2-4 concurrent anes proc	TK	Extra patient or passenger
QL	Patient died after Amb call	TL	Early intervention IFSP
QM	Ambulance arrangement by hospital	TM	Individualized ED prrm (EP)
QN	Ambulance furnished by provider	TN	Rural/out or service area
QP	Individually ordered lab test	TP	Med transprt unloaded vehicle
QQ	SOI submitted	TQ	Bls by volunteer amb provider
QS	Monitored anesthesia care	TR	School-based IEP out of district
QT	Recording/storage tape analog recorder	TS	Follow-up service
QU	MD providing service urban HPSA	TT	Additional patient
QV	Item or service provided	TU	Overtime payment rate
QW	CLIA waived test	TV	Holiday/weekend payment rate
QX	CRNA service with MD med direction	TW	Back-up equipment
QY	Medically directed CRNA	U1	Medicaid care Level 1 state def
QZ	CRNA service: without medical direction by MD	U2	Medicaid care Level 2 state def
RC	Right coronary artery	U3	Medicaid care Level 3 state def
RD	Drug admin not incident-to	U4	Medicaid care Level 4 state def
RP	Replacement and repair (DMEPOS)	U5	Medicaid care Level 5 state def
RR	Rental (DME)	U6	Medicaid care Level 6 state def
RT	Right side	U7	Medicaid care Level 7 state def
SA	Nurse practitioner with physician	U8	Medicaid care Level 8 state def
SB	Nurse midwife	U9	Medicaid care Level 9 state def
SC	Medically necessary serv/sup	UA	Medicaid care Level 10 state def
SD	Service by home infusion RN	UB	Medicaid care Level 11 state def
SE	State/Fed funded program/ser	UC	Medicaid care Level 12 state def
SF	2nd opinion ordered by PRO	UD	Medicaid care Level 13 state def
SG	Ambulatory surgical center facility service	UE	Used durable medical equipment
SH	2nd concurrent infusion therapy	UF	Services provided, morning
SJ	3rd concurrent infusion therapy	UG	Services provided afternoon
SK	High risk population	UH	Services provided, evening
SL	State supplied vaccine	UJ	Services provided, night
SM	Second opinion	UK	Service on behalf client-collateral
SN	Third opinion	UN	Two patients served
SQ	Item ordered by home health	UP	Three patients served
ST	Related to trauma or injury	UQ	Four patients served
SU	Performed in phys office	UR	Five patients served
SV	Drugs delivered not used	US	Six or more patients served
		VP	Aphakic patient

Continued

Table 2. HCPCS Alphanumeric Index

Description	Code
A	
above-elbow endoskeletal prostheses	L6500
above-elbow prostheses	L6250
above-knee endoskeletal prostheses	L5320
acetazolamide sodium (Diamox), injection	J1120
actinomycin D, injection	J9120
adjustable arms, wheelchair	E0973
adjustable chair, dialysis	E1570
adrenaline, injection	J0170
air ambulance	A0030
air bubble detector, dialysis	E1530
air travel and nonemergency transport	A0140
alarm, pressure dialysis	E1540
alcohol	A4244
alcohol wipes	A4245
alternating pressure pad	E0180
aminophylline, injection	J0280
amitriptyline HCl (Elavil), injection	J1320
ammonia test paper	A4774
amobarbital sodium (Amytal sodium), injection	J0300
ampicillin, injection	J0290
ampicillin sodium (Omnipen-N), injection	J2430
amputee adapter, wheelchair	E0959
amputee wheelchair, detachable elevating leg rests	E1170
amputee wheelchair, detachable foot rests	E1200
amygdalin, injection	J3570
anesthetics for dialysis	A4735
ankle prostheses, Symes, metal frame	L5060
ankle prostheses, Symes, molded socket	L5050
antineoplastic drugs, not otherwise classified (NOC)	J9999
antitipping device, wheelchair	E0971
apnea monitor	E0608
appliance, pneumatic	E0655
arm rest, wheelchair	E0994
arms, adjustable, wheelchair	E0973
asparaginase (Elspar), injection	J9020
atropine sulfate, injection	J0460
aurothioglucose (Solganal), injection	J2910
axillary crutch extension	L0978
B	
back, upholstery, wheelchair	E0993
bacterial sensitivity study	P7001
bandage, elastic	A4460
bandages, gauze	A4202
bath conductivity meter, dialysis	E1550
bathroom equipment, miscellaneous	E0179
battery charger, wheelchair	E1066
BCNU (carmustine, bis-chloroethyl-nitrosourea), injection	J9050
bed accessories: boards, tables	E0315
bed pan	E0276
below-elbow endoskeletal prostheses	L6400
below-knee endoskeletal prostheses	L5300
belt, extremity	E0945

Table 2. HCPCS Alphanumeric Index—cont'd

Description	Code
belt, ostomy	A4367
belt, pelvic	E0944
bench, bathtub	E0245
benzquinamide HCl (Emete-Con), injection	J0510
benztropine, injection	J0515
bethanechol chloride, injection	J0520
bethanechol chloride (Myotonachol), injection	J0520
bethanechol chloride (Urecholine), injection	J0520
bicarbonate dialysate	A4705
bilirubin (phototherapy) light	E0202
biperiden HCl (Akineton), injection	J0190
bis-chloroethyl-nitrosourea, injection	J9050
bleomycin sulfate, injection	J9040
blood, mucoprotein	P2038
blood (split unit), specify amount	P9011
blood (whole), for transfusion, per unit	P9010
blood leak detector, dialysis	E1560
blood pressure monitor	A4670
blood pump, dialysis	E1620
blood strips	A4253
blood testing supplies	A4770
bond or cement, ostomy skin	A4364
brompheniramine maleate (Dehist), injection	J0945

C

Description	Code
calcitonin (salmon) (Calcimar), injection	J0630
calcium disodium edetate (Versenate), injection	J0600
calcium gluconate, injection	J0610
calcium glycerophosphate and calcium lactate (Calphosan), injection	J0620
calcium leucovorin, injection	J0640
calf rest, wheelchair	E0995
calibrator solution	A4256
canes	E0100
carbon filters	A4680
carmustine, injection	J9050
cast supplies	
long leg, adult (11 years +), cylinder, fiberglass	Q4034
long leg, adult (11 years +), cylinder, plaster	Q4033
long leg, adult (11 years +), fiberglass	Q4030
catheter caps, disposable (dialysis)	A4860
catheter insertion tray	A4354
catheter irrigation set	A4355
cefazolin sodium, injection	J0690
ceftriaxone sodium (Rocepin), 250-mg injection	J0696
cellular therapy	M0075
cement, ostomy	A4364
centrifuge	A4650
cephalin flocculation, blood	P2028
cephalothin sodium (Keflin), injection	J1890
cephapirin sodium, injection	J0710
cervical head harness/halter	E0942
cervical pillow	E0943
chair, adjustable, dialysis	E1570
chelation therapy, intravenous (chemical endarterectomy)	M0300
chin cup, cervical	L0150

Continued

Table 2. HCPCS Alphanumeric Index—cont'd

Description	Code
chiropractor, manipulation of spine	A2000
chloramphenicol (Chloromycetin Sodium Succinate), injection	J0720
chlordiazepoxide HCl (Librium), injection	J1990
chloroprocaine HCl (Nesacaine), injection	J2400
chloroquine HCl (Aralen HCl), injection	J0390
chlorothiazide sodium (Diuril), injection	J1205
chlorpheniramine maleate (Chlor-Trimeton), injection	J0730
chlorpromazine (Thorazine), injection	J3230
chlorprothixene (Taractan), injection	J3080
chorionic gonadotropin, injection	J0725
clamps, dialysis, venous pressure	A4918
clamps, Harvard pressure	A4920
cleansing agent, dialysis equipment	A4790
clotting time tube	A4771
codeine phosphate, injection	J0745
colchicine, injection	J0760
colistimethate sodium (Coly-Mycin M), injection	J0770
commode seat, wheelchair	E0968
compressor	E0565
compressor, pneumatic	E0650
conductive paste or gel	A4558
Congo red blood	P2029
continuous cycling peritoneal dialysis (CCPD) supply kit	A4901
contracts, repair and maintenance, ESRD	A4890
corticotropin, injection	J0800
cortisone, injection	J0810
crutches	E0110
cryoprecipitate, each unit	P9012
culture sensitivity study	P7001
cushion, one-inch, for wheelchair	E0962
Cycler, hemodialysis	E1590
Cycler dialysis machine	E1594
cyclophosphamide, injection	J9070

D

Description	Code
dactinomycin (Cosmegen) or actinomycin, injection	J9120
daunorubicin HCl, injection	J9150
decubitus care pad	E0185
deionizer, water purification system	E1615
detector, blood leak, dialysis	E1560
dexamethasone sodium phosphate, injection	J1100
dextrose/normal saline, solution	J7042
Dextrostix	A4772
dialysate concentrate additives	A4765
dialysate testing solution	A4760
dialysis, bath conductivity, meter	E1550
dialysis supplies, miscellaneous	A4913
dialyzer holder	A4919
dialyzers	A4690
diazepam (Valium), injection	J3360
diazoxide (Hyperstat), injection	J1730
dicyclomine HCl (Bentyl), injection	J0500
digoxin, injection	J1160
dihydroergotamine mesylate (D.H.E. 45), injection	J1110
dimenhydrinate (Dramamine), injection	J1240

Table 2. HCPCS Alphanumeric Index—cont'd

Description	Code
dimercaprol in peanut oil (BAL in Oil), injection	J0470
dimethyl imidazole carboxamide (DIC) (dacarbazine, DTIC-DOME), 100-mg vial	J9130
dimethyl sulfoxide, injection	J1212
dimethyl sulfoxide (DMSO) (Rimso-50), injection	J1212
diphenhydramine HCl (Benadryl), injection	J1200
disarticulation, elbow, prostheses	L6200
doxorubicin (Adriamycin), injection	J9000
drainage bag	A4358
drainage board	E0606
droperidol (Inapsine), injection	J1790
droperidol and fentanyl citrate (Innovar), injection	J1810
drugs, nonprescription	A9150
drugs, prescription, oral chemotherapy	J7150
durable medical equipment (DME) medical supplies	A4610
dyphylline (Dilor), injection	J1180

E

Description	Code
edetate sodium (ethylenediaminetetraacetic acid [EDTA], Endrate), injection	J3520
elbow protector	E0191
electrical work or plumbing, home, dialysis equipment	A4870
electrodes	A4556
elevating leg rest, wheelchair	E0990
endarterectomy, chemical	M0300
epinephrine, injection	J0170
ergonovine maleate (Ergotrate Maleate), injection	J1330
estradiol cypionate (Depo-Estradiol Cypionate), injection	J1000
estradiol valerate (Delestrogen), injection	J0970
estradiol valerate, up to 20 mg (Estraval-2X), injection	J1390
estradiol valerate, up to 10 mg (Estraval P.A.), injection	J1380
estrone, injection	J1435
ethylnorepinephrine HCl (Bronkephrine HCl), injection	J0590
etoposide, 50 mg, injection	J9181
external ambulatory infusion pump with administration equipment	E0781
extremity belt-harness	E0945

F

Description	Code
faceplate, ostomy	A4361
fentanyl citrate (Sublimaze), injection	J3010
fibrinogen unit	P9013
fistula cannulation set	A4730
flotation mattress	E0184
flotation pad gel pressure	E0185
floxuridine, 500 mg, injection	J9200
fluid barriers, dialysis	E1575
fluorouracil, injection	J9190
fluphenazine decanoate (Prolixin Decanoate), injection	J2680
foot rest, for use with commode chair	E0175
footplates, wheelchair	E0970
forearm crutches	E0110
furosemide (Lasix), injection	J1940

G

Description	Code
gamma globulin, 1 ml, injection	J1460
gauze bandages (gauze elastic)	A4202
gauze, non-impregnated, sterile, 16 sq-in pad	A4200

Continued

Table 2. HCPCS Alphanumeric Index—cont'd

Description	Code
gel, conductive	A4558
gel flotation pad	E0185
gentamicin, injection	J1580
gentamicin sulfate (Garamycin), injection	J1580
globulin, gamma, 1 ml, injection	P9014
globulin, Rh immune, 1 ml, injection	P9015
gloves, dialysis	A4927
glucose test strips	A4772
gold sodium thiosulfate, injection	J1600
Gomco drain bottle	A4912
Grade-Aid, wheelchair	E0974
gravity traction device	E0941
Gravlee Jet Washer	A4470

H

Description	Code
hair analysis	P2031
hallux-valgus dynamic splint	L3100
haloperidol (Haldol), injection	J1630
halter, cervical head	E0942
hand rims, wheelchair	E0967
harness, extremity	E0945
harness, pelvic	E0944
harness/halter, cervical head	E0942
Harvard pressure clamp, dialysis	A4920
head rest extension, wheelchair	E0966
heater for nebulizer	E1372
heel or elbow protector	E0191
heel stabilizer	L3170
helicopter ambulance	A0040
hemipelvectomy, endoskeletal prostheses	L5340
hemipelvectomy prostheses	L5280
hemodialysis, monthly capitation	E0945
hemodialysis kit	A4820
hemodialysis unit	E1590
hemostats	A4850
Hemostix	A4773
heparin	A4800
heparin infusion pump, dialysis	E1520
hexachlorophene (pHisoHex) solution	A4246
Hexcelite, cast material—see Q codes under "cast supplies" for specific casts	A4590
HN2 (nitrogen mustard)	J9230
hot water bottle	E0220
hyaluronidase (Wydase), injection	J3470
hydralazine HCl (Apresoline), injection	J0360
hydrochlorides of opium alkaloids (Pantopon), injection	J2480
hydrocortisone, injection	J1720
hydrocortisone acetate, up to 25 mg, injection	J1700
hydrocortisone phosphate, injection	J1710
hydrocortisone sodium succinate (Solu-Cortef), injection	J1720
hydromorphone (Dilaudid), injection	J1170
hydroxyzine HCl (Vistaril), injection	J3410
hyoscyamine sulfate (Levsin), injection	J1980
hypertonic saline solution	J7130

Table 2. HCPCS Alphanumeric Index—cont'd

Description	Code
I	
ice cap or collar	E0230
imipramine HCl (Tofranil), injection	J3270
incontinence clamp	A4356
infusion pump, external ambulatory with administration equipment	E0781
infusion pump, heparin, dialysis	E1520
infusion pump, implantable	E0782
installation and/or delivery charges for ESRD equipment	E1600
insulin, injection	J1815
intercapsular thoracic endoskeletal prostheses	L6570
interferon, injection	J9213
intermittent peritoneal dialysis (IPD) supply kit	A4905
intermittent peritoneal dialysis (IPD) system, automatic	E1592
intermittent positive-pressure breathing (IPPB) machine	E0500
intraocular lenses, anterior chamber	V2630
intraocular lenses, iris supported	V2631
intraocular lenses, posterior chamber	V2632
iodine I-123 sod. iodide capsule(s) diag.	A9516
iodine swabs/wipes	A4247
iron dextran (Imferon), injection	J1760
irrigation kits, ostomy	A4400
irrigation set, catheter	A4355
IV pole	E0776
J	
jacket, Risser	A4581
K	
kanamycin sulfate, injection	J1840
kanamycin sulfate (Kantrex), up to 75 mg, pediatric, injection	J1850
Kartop patient lift, toilet or bathroom	E0625
kit, chronic ambulatory peritoneal dialysis (CAPD) supply	A4900
kit, CCPD supply	A4901
kit, hemodialysis	A4820
L	
laetrile, amygdalin (vitamin B17), injection	J3570
lancets	A4259
lead wires	A4557
leg extension, walker	E1058
leg rest, wheelchair, elevating	E0990
leukocyte-poor blood, each unit	P9016
levorphanol tartrate (Levo-Dromoran), injection	J1960
lidocaine (Xylocaine), injection	J2001
lightweight wheelchair	E1087
lincomycin, injection	J2010
liquid barrier, ostomy	A4363
liver derivative complex (Kutapressin), injection	J1910
liver injection	J2050
lubricant, ostomy	A4402
M	
manipulation, of spine, by chiropractor	A2000
mannitol, injection	J2150
measuring cylinder, dialysis	A4921

Continued

Table 2. HCPCS Alphanumeric Index—cont'd

Description	Code
mechlorethamine, injection	J9230
mechlorethamine HCl (Mustargen), injection	J9230
medical supplies used in DME	A4610
medroxyprogesterone acetate (Depo-Provera), injection	J1050
meperidine, injection	J2175
meperidine HCl and promethazine HCl (Mepergan), injection	J2180
mephentermine sulfate (Wyamine Sulfate), injection	J3450
mepivacaine HCl (Carbocaine), injection	J0670
metaraminol bitartrate (Aramine), injection	J0380
meter, bath conductivity, dialysis	E1550
methadone HCl, injection	J1230
methicillin sodium (Staphcillin), injection	J2970
methocarbamol (Robaxin), injection	J2800
methotrimeprazine (Levoprome), injection	J1970
methoxamine HCl (Vasoxyl), injection	J3390
methyldopate HCl (Aldomet Ester HCl)	J0210
methylergonovine maleate (Methergine), injection	J2210
methylprednisolone acetate (Depo-Medrol), injection	J1020
methylprednisolone sodium succinate (Solu Medrol), injection	
up to 40 mg	J2920
up to 125 mg	J2930
metoclopramide HCl (Reglan)	J2765
metocurine iodide (Metubine Iodide), injection	J2240
microbiology tests	P7001
mini-bus, nonemergency transportation	A0120
miscellaneous dialysis supplies	A4913
mithramycin, injection	J9270
mitomycin (Mutamycin), injection	J9280
monitor, apnea	E0608
monitor, blood pressure	A4670
morphine, injection	J2270
mucoprotein, blood	P2038

N

Description	Code
nandrolone decanoate, up to 50 mg, injection	J2320
nandrolone decanoate, up to 200 mg, injection	J2322
nandrolone phenpropionate (Anabolin), injection	J0340
narrowing device, wheelchair	E0969
nasal vaccine inhalation	J3530
nebulizer, portable	E1375
nebulizer, with compressor	E0570
nebulizer heater	E1372
needle with syringe	A4206
needles	A4215
needles, dialysis	A4655
neonatal transport, ambulance, base rate	A0225
neostigmine methylsulfate (Prostigmin), injection	J2710
neuromuscular stimulator	E0745
niacin, injection	J2350
nikethamide (Coramine), injection	J3490
nitrogen mustard, injection	J9230
noncovered procedure	A9270
nonmedical supplies for dialysis (e.g., scale, scissors, stopwatch)	A4910
nonprescription drugs	A9150
nonprofit transport, nonemergency	A0120

Table 2. HCPCS Alphanumeric Index—cont'd

Description	Code
O	
occipital/mandibular support, cervical	L0160
occupational therapy	H5300
opium, injection	J2480
orphenadrine citrate (Norflex), injection	L2360
orthoses, thoracic-lumbar-sacral (scoliosis)	L1200
orthotic, knee	L1830
ostomy supplies	A4421
oxacillin sodium (Bactocill), injection	J2410
oxymorphone HCl (Numorphan), injection	J2700
oxytetracycline, injection	J2460
oxytocin (Pitocin), injection	J2590
P	
pacemaker monitor, includes audible/visible check systems	E0610
pacemaker monitor, includes digital/visible check systems	E0615
pad for water circulating heat unit	E0249
pads, flotation, electric, standard	E0192
pail or pan for use with commode chair	E0167
papaverine HCl, injection	J2440
paraffin	A4265
paraffin bath unit	E0235
paste, conductive	A4558
pelvic belt/harness/boot	E0944
penicillin G benzathine (Bicillin L-A), injection	J0560
penicillin G potassium (Pfizerpen), injection	J2540
penicillin procaine, aqueous, injection	J2510
pentazocine HCl (Talwin), injection	J3070
percussor	E0480
peritoneal straps	L0980
peroxide	A4244
perphenazine (Trilafon), injection	J3310
personal items	A9190
pessary	A4560
phenobarbital, injection	J2560
phenobarbital sodium, injection	J2515
phentolamine mesylate (Regitine), injection	J2760
phenylephrine HCl (Neo-Synephrine), injection	J2370
phenytoin sodium (Dilantin), injection	J1165
phototherapy, light	E0202
phytonadione (AquaMEPHYTON), injection, vitamin K	J3430
pillow, cervical	E0943
plasma, protein fraction, each unit	P9018
plasma, single donor, fresh frozen, each unit	P9017
platelet concentrate, each unit	P9019
platelet-rich plasma, each unit	P9020
podiatric services, noncovered	A9160
portable hemodialyzer system	E1635
portable nebulizer	E1375
postural drainage board	E0606
pralidoxime chloride (Protopam Chloride), injection	J2730
prednisolone acetate, injection	J2650
preparation kits, dialysis	A4914
prescription drug, oral	J7140
prescription drug, oral chemotherapy	J7150

Continued

Table 2. HCPCS Alphanumeric Index—cont'd

Description	Code
pressure alarm, dialysis	E1540
procainamide HCl (Pronestyl), injection	J2690
prochlorperazine (Compazine), injection	J0780
progesterone, injection	J2675
prolotherapy	M0076
promazine HCl (Sparine), injection	J2950
promethazine HCl (Phenergan), injection	J2550
propiomazine (Largon), injection	J1930
propranolol HCl (Inderal), injection	J1800
prostheses, above elbow, endoskeletal	L6500
prostheses, below elbow, endoskeletal	L6400
prostheses, hemipelvectomy	L5280
prostheses, intercapsular thoracic, endoskeletal	L6570
prostheses, knee, endoskeletal	L5300
prostheses, lower extremity, NOC	L5999
prosthetic services, NOC	L8499
protamine sulfate, injection	J2720
protector, heel or elbow	E0191

Q
Quad cane	E0105

R
rack/stand, oxygen	E1355
reciprocating peritoneal dialysis system	E1630
red blood cells, each unit	P9021
regulator, oxygen	E1353
replacement components, ESRD machines	E1640
replacement tanks, dialysis	A4880
reserpine (Sandril), injection	J2820
restraints, any type	E0710
reverse osmosis water purification, ESRD	E1610
Rh$_O$(D) immune globulin, injection	J2790
rib belt	A4572
rims, hand (wheelchair)	E0967
Ringer's injection	J7120
rings, ostomy	A4404
Risser jacket	A4581

S
safety equipment	E0700
safety visit, wheelchair	E0980
sales tax, orthotic/prosthetic/other	L9999
scale or scissors, dialysis	A4910
seat attachment, walker	E0156
seat insert, wheelchair	E0992
secobarbital sodium (seconal sodium), injection	J2860
sensitivity study	P7001
serum clotting time tube	A4771
shunt accessories, for dialysis	A4740
sitz bath, portable	E0160
skin barrier, ostomy	A4362
skin bond or cement, ostomy	A4364
sling, patient lift	E0621
slings	A4565

Table 2. HCPCS Alphanumeric Index—cont'd

Description	Code
social worker, nonemergency transport	A0160
sodium chloride, injection	J2912
sodium succinate, injection	J1720
sorbent cartridges, ESRD	E1636
spectinomycin dihydrochloride (Trobicin), injection	J3320
sphygmomanometer with cuff and stethoscope	A4660
spinal orthosis, NOC	L1499
splint	A4570
splint, hallux-valgus, night, dynamic	L3100
stand/rack, oxygen	E1355
sterilizing agent, dialysis	A4780
streptokinase-streptodornase, injection	J2995
streptomycin, injection	J3000
streptozocin, injection	J9320
succinylcholine chloride (Anectine), injection	J0330
suction pump, portable	E0600
supplies for self-administered injections	A4211
surgical brush, dialysis	A4910
surgical stockings, above-knee length	A4490
surgical supplies, miscellaneous	A4649
surgical trays	A4550
swabs, povidone-iodine (Betadine) or iodine	A4247
syringe	A4213
syringes, dialysis	A4655

T

Description	Code
tape, all types, all sizes	A4454
taxes, orthotic/prosthetic/other	L9999
taxi, nonemergency transportation	A0100
tent, oxygen	E0455
terbutaline sulfate, 0.5 mg, injection	J3105
terminal devices	L6700
testosterone cypionate (Depo-Testosterone), injection	J1070
testosterone cypionate and estradiol cypionate (Depo-Testadiol), injection	J1060
testosterone enanthate and estradiol valerate (Deladumone), injection	L0900
testosterone propionate, injection	J3150
testosterone suspension, injection	J3140
tetanus immune human globulin (Homo-Tet), injection	J1670
tetracycline, injection	J0120
tetracycline HCl (Achromycin), injection	J0120
theophylline and mersalyl (Salyrgan), injection	J2810
thermometer, dialysis	A4910
thiethylperazine maleate (Torecan), injection	J3280
thiotepa (triethylenethiophosphoramide), injection	J9340
thiothixene HCl (Navane IM), injection	J2330
thymol turbidity, blood	P2033
thyrotropin (TSH), exogenous, up to 10 IU, injection	J3240
tobramycin sulfate (Nebcin), injection	J3260
toilet rail	E0243
toilet seat, raised	E0244
tolazoline HCl (Priscoline), injection	J2670
tolls, nonemergency transport	A0170
tool kit, dialysis	A4910
tourniquet, dialysis	A4910

Continued

Table 2. HCPCS Alphanumeric Index—cont'd

Description	Code
tracheotomy collar or mask	A4621
traction device, gravity-assisted	E0941
traction equipment, overdoor	E0860
travel hemodialyzer system	E1635
trays, surgical	A4550
triflupromazine HCl (Vesprin), injection	J3400
trimethaphan camsylate (Arfonad)	J0400
trimethobenzamide HCl (Tigan), injection	J3250
tube-occluding forceps/clamps, dialysis	A4910

U

Description	Code
ultraviolet cabinet	E0690
unclassified drugs (contraceptives)	J3490
underarm crutches, wood	E0112
unipuncture control system, dialysis	E1580
upholstery, reinforced seat, wheelchair	E0975
upholstery seat, wheelchair	E0991
urea (Ureaphil), injection	J3350
urinary drainage bag	A4357
urinary leg bag	A4358
urinary suspensory	A4359
urine control strips or tablets	A4250
urine sensitivity study	P7001

V

Description	Code
vancomycin HCl (Vancocin), injection	J3370
vaporizer	E0605
vascular catheters	A4300
venous pressure clamps, dialysis	A4918
ventilator, volume	E0450
vest, safety, wheelchair	E0980
vinblastine sulfate, injection	J9360
vinblastine sulfate (Velban), injection	J9360
vitamin B12, injection	J3420
vitamin K, injection	J3430
volume ventilator, stationary or portable	E0450

W

Description	Code
walker, wheeled, without seat	E0141
walker attachments, platform	E0154
warfarin sodium (Coumadin), injection—unclassified	J3490
washed red blood cells, each unit	P9022
water, ambulance	A0050
water softening system, ESRD	E1625
water tanks, dialysis	A4880
wearable artificial kidney	E1632
wearable artificial kidney (WAK)	E1632
wheel attachment, walker	E0977
wheelchair, one-inch cushion for	E0962
wheelchair, heavy duty, with detachable arms	E1280
wheelchair, wide, heavy duty with detachable arms and leg rests	E1092
wrist disarticulation prosthesis	L6060

Y

Description	Code
youth wheelchair	E1091

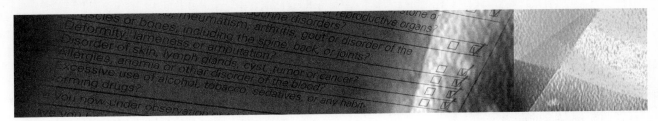
Finding Your Way Around the Practice Management Software

Important Message to New Users

If you are no stranger to using the computer, then you know how important it is to protect your data files. It cannot be said enough, "Back up your data!" It is strongly recommended that you back up data files every time you use this program.

Cycle the media you use for your backups. In other words, use more than one CD/disk and rotate them throughout the week. For example, if you use the program three times in a week, each day you access it and back up the files, there should be a separate CD/disk. In this case, there should be three separate CDs/disks, perhaps labeled "Monday," "Wednesday," and "Friday." This way, you will be assured that a damaged data set can be replaced with a current backup and if one backup CD/disk becomes lost or damaged, there will be a complete set of data files available to recover. Instructions for Backup Data Files appear near the end of this section.

Initial Installation and Log On to the AltaPoint Software

NOTE: During the installation you may see a message that the practice "demo" does not exist. Choose "yes" to create it.

After installing the software onto your computer, double click on the AltaPoint program icon on the desktop.

At the first screen, you will be asked to enter an "EmployeeCode," "Location," and "Password." Select an EmployeeCode by clicking on the magnifying glass (look up) icon. You may choose either Jeffery Lyndon, MD (JHL) or Mitchell Adams (MA). Leave the Password and Location fields blank. Click OK to log in.

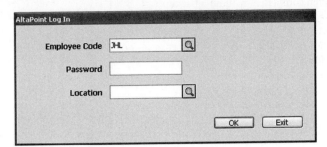

Portions of these general program tips and instruction reprinted with permission from AltaPoint Data Systems, LLC, Midvale, Utah.

Helpful Features and Notes

Toolbar Icons

All toolbar icons are labeled for quick and easy launch of software functions. Each of the functions associated with an icon can be accessed through the menu options as well.

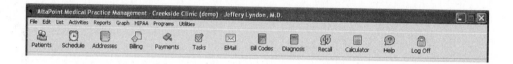

Getting Help

The "Help" feature in AltaPoint answers a wide range of questions. To access assistance, just click on the Question Mark "?" icon on the main toolbar.

Using Shortcut and Alt Keys

In addition to the icon bar, there are several shortcut keys in the program for the user's convenience. These shortcut keys take you directly to certain functions in the software. The shortcuts are generally a series of keystrokes. (They are also listed throughout the program next to their respective menu items.)

For example, you can access a patient file in one of three ways:
1. Click on LIST and then click on "Patients".
2. Click on the "Patients" icon on the toolbar.
3. Press the "Ctrl" key and then the letter "P" on the keyboard. The Patient List pops open.

The following are examples of shortcut keys. The entire list can be found in the Help file.

Keystrokes	Feature
Ctrl + A	Appointments
Ctrl + B	Billing Code File
Ctrl + C	Copy
Ctrl + D	Diagnosis Code File

Temporary Log Off

A user has the ability to log off of the program without exiting the program. This feature is helpful in controlling who has access to the data in your program. Additionally, HIPAA guidelines require that a health care provider control who sees the patient information in the practice. This feature helps a physician's office comply with this HIPAA requirement.

There are two ways to temporarily log off from the program:
1. Click on FILE and then "Log off." This means that another user can log on without having to launch the program again.
2. Press the security lock icon on the toolbar.

Exiting the Program

To exit AltaPoint, click on FILE and then "Exit."

A screen prompts the user to "Backup Data Files," "Cancel," or "Exit AltaPoint." Click the desired action. Selecting "Exit AltaPoint" shuts down the program completely without a backup.

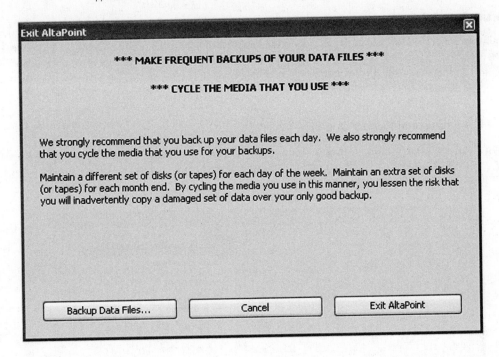

Enter or Tab: Moving from Field to Field

Using the "Tab" key is the Windows standard. However, you can use the "Enter" key to move from field to field. It is simply a matter of user preference. To choose between the "Enter" and "Tab" keys, click on FILE and then select "Practice Information" from the drop-down menu.

In the "Options" tab from the Practice Information screen, place a checkmark in the "Use Enter Key for Next Field" box to use the Enter key. (If this box is checked, you may use both keys.)

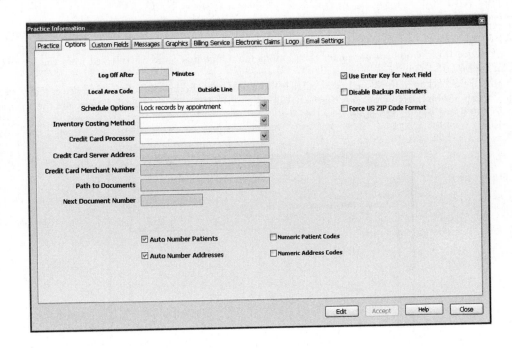

System Date and Date Spin

When performing exercises, you will key in dates. In most date fields throughout the program you have the ability to advance the date forward or backward by pressing the "+" or "–" keys on the number pad on the right side of your keyboard. By default, the current system date will be displayed. Also, if a date field is blank, pressing the "+" or "–" key will input the current system date. Remember to hold down the "Shift" key while depressing the "+"; otherwise, you are pressing the "=" symbol!

Utilities—Data File Backup and Restore Options

Use the "Backup Data Files" and "Restore Data Files" options from the Utilities menu to perform routine backups (as an alternative to running a backup from the Exit AltaPoint option) and restore data when necessary. Before backing up or restoring, read through this entire section to avoid any issues with the system.

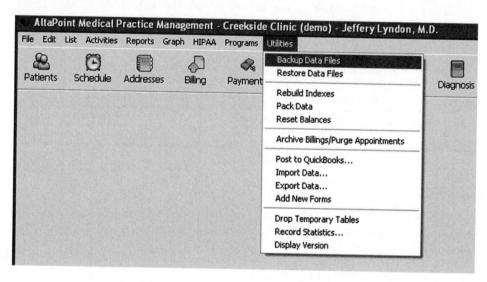

Backup Data Files

From the main menu, click on UTILITIES and select "Backup Data Files" from the drop-down menu. This feature allows the user to specify a location for the data file backup. A backup reminder pops up or appears when exiting the system if this option is selected in the Practice Information feature under the Options tab. Once this option is selected from the Utilities menu, the following screen appears.

Enter the path for the backup in the "File Location" field. The user may also browse to a specific drive, folder, or access point by pressing the lookup button (magnifying glass button to the right of the field). Press the OK button and the system compresses and backs up the files to the specified location.

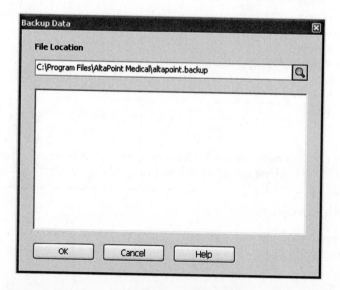

Restore Data Files

Contact your instructor if you have issues with damaged data and only perform "Restore Data" when absolutely necessary. This option allows flexibility in deciding which files to restore to your current data set or system. It may have several purposes, including the following:

Simple example
- Restoring over existing data that may have problems

Advanced examples
- Restoring specific insurance, procedure, or diagnosis files when duplicating a data set for another doctor or for billing services that have a need to duplicate information in other sets of data
- Restoring an old set of data from an old backup to a separately created set of data if archived or deleted data need to be recalled and evaluated

1. From the main menu, click on UTILITIES and select "Restore Data Files" from the drop-down menu.
2. Enter the path for the data files you wish to restore in the "File Location" field. The user may also browse to a specific drive, folder, or access point by pressing the lookup button (magnifying glass to the right of the field). Click OK.

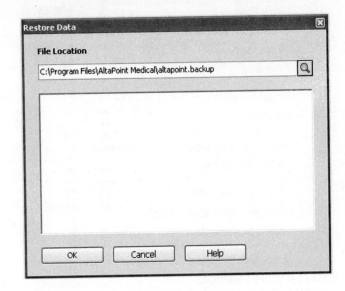

3. A window will open warning you to make sure no other work stations (programs) are running. Click OK and files will be restored.

(**NOTE:** AltaPoint pulls the data to be restored from the most current backup—remember how important it was to back up data daily!)

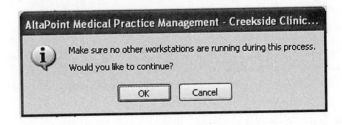

Hands-On Exercises

The student will use the practice management software for "electronic exercises" throughout Chapters 3 through 12. The directions for these assignments are in the *Workbook* and allow for both paper and electronic-based exercises.

More Technical Help and Information

Access the Help functionality in AltaPoint for more detailed information and troubleshooting. Or, contact Elsevier via e-mail at technical.support@elsevier.com.

Practice Management and Billing Software Assignments

NOTE: For assignment purposes, the Social Security, state license, federal tax ID, UPIN, PIN, and NPI numbers associated with the patients and providers have been entered with a mix of zeros and x's so that they are not realistic.

1. The Transaction Entry Screen

Click on ACTIVITIES and choose "Transaction Entry" from the drop-down menu. This can also be done by clicking on the "Billing" icon.

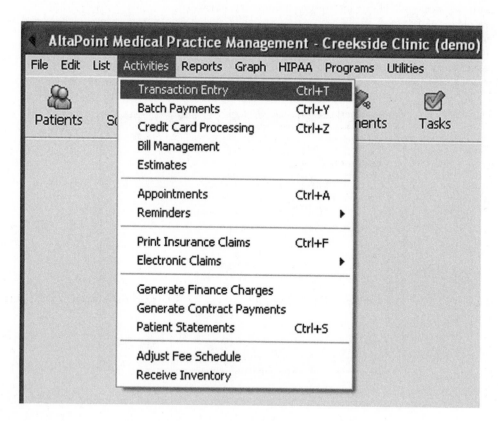

This screen is used for the posting of charges, payments and adjustments to a patient's account.

Helpful Hints When Entering a Transaction

For the system to record and save the entry, there must be a valid SERVICE DATE, PROVIDER, and BILLING CODES!

If there is more than one transaction to post while the "Transaction Entry" screen is open for the same patient, Enter/Tab at the end of the first line entry. This saves the information and compiles it with subsequent lines of entry.

2. The Patient List Screen

Click on LIST and choose "Patients" from the drop-down menu. This can also be done by clicking the "Patients" icon.

This screen shows an alphabetic list of registered patients and basic demographic information on each one. This screen allows you to begin the process of adding, deleting, or editing patients.

How to View a Patient Ledger

1. Click on LIST and choose "Patients" from the drop-down menu, or you can click on the "Patients" icon.
2. On the "Patient" screen, highlight a patient by clicking on that patient's line.
3. Click on "View" or double click the patient's name.
4. Click on the "Ledger" tab. This shows you all of the activity on that patient's account.

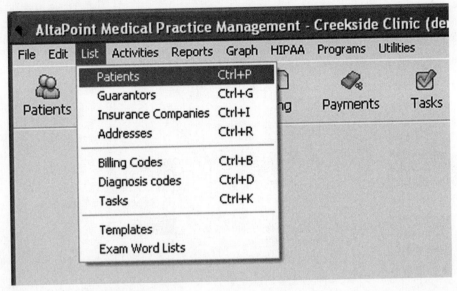

How to Enter a New Patient into the System

1. Click on LIST and choose "Patients" from the drop-down menu, or you can click on the "Patients" icon.
2. Click on "New".
3. Click on the "Page 1", "Page 2", and "Billing" tabs and enter available information on each screen.
(**NOTE:** On the Billing page, be sure, to check the following boxes: Bill Patient, Signature on File, Always Bill, and Accept Assignment.)

3. Insurance Companies

Click on LIST and choose "Insurance Companies" from the drop-down menu. This screen allows you to add, delete, edit, or view insurance company information.

4. CPT Codes

How to Enter New Codes

1. Click on LIST and choose "Billing Codes" from the drop-down menu, or you can click on the "Bill Codes" icon.
2. Click "New".

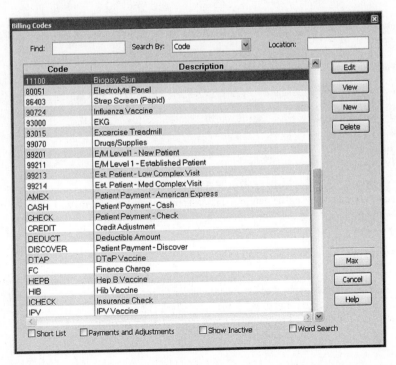

3. Enter the code number in the "Billing Code" box.
4. Enter the code description in the "Name" box.
5. Re-enter the code in the "CPT code" box.

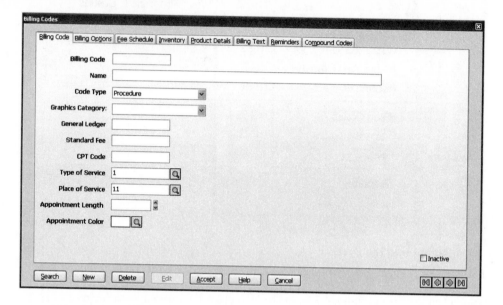

6. Click the magnifying glass in the "Type of Service" box.
7. Click OK to select "Medical (1)" as the type of service.
8. Click the magnifying glass in the "Place of Service" box.
9. Click OK to select "Office (11)" as the "Place of Service" code.
10. Enter the fee for the new code in the "Standard Fee" box.
11. Click "Accept".

How to Change the Fee for an Existing Code

1. Click on LIST and choose "Billing Codes" from the drop-down menu, or click on the "Bill Codes" icon.
2. Select the code you want to change and click "Edit".
3. Change the fee in the "Standard Fee" box to the desired amount.

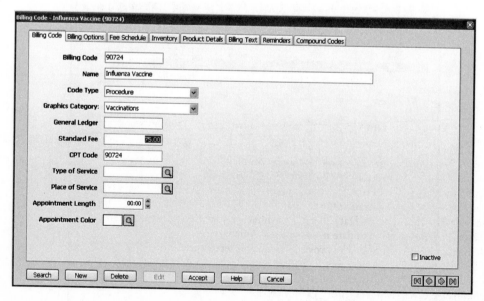

4. Click "Accept".

How to Enter ICD-9-CM Codes into the Practice Management System

1. Click on LIST and choose "Diagnosis Codes" from the drop-down menu, or click on the "Diagnosis" icon.
2. Click "New".

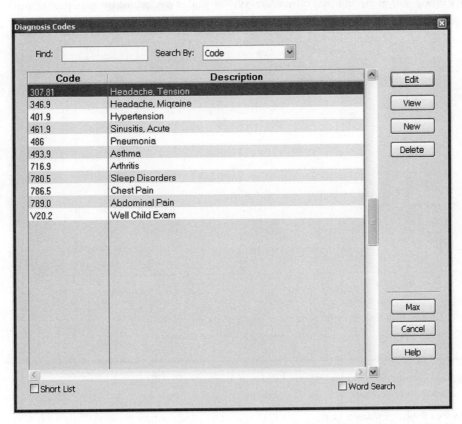

3. Enter the new code in the "Code" box.
4. Enter the code description in the "Description" box. Click OK.

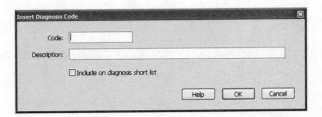

5. The CMS-1500 Form

How to Work from an Encounter Form/Superbill to Complete a CMS-1500 Form

1. Click on ACTIVITIES and choose "Transaction Entry" from the drop-down menu, or click on the "Billing" icon.
2. Click on the magnifying glass in the "Patient" box to select an established patient from the patient list. If this is a new patient, follow the instructions to enter a new patient. Click OK.
3. Click the magnifying glass in the "Provider" box to choose the correct provider. Click OK.
4. Press the tab key to begin entering transactions.
5. Enter the date of service in the "Start Date" box if it is different from the date that appears.
6. Tab to "End Date" and enter the same date if this is a one-time service.
7. Tab to the "Billing Code" box. **NOTE:** The provider name is entered automatically.
8. Enter the CPT codes by typing the numbers in the box or clicking on the "…" button to select the codes from the list of codes already in the system.
9. Tab over to POS (place of service) and enter "11" for office.
10. Tab to the "Diagnosis" box. Type in the diagnosis code or click on the "…" button to choose the code from the list of codes in the system. **NOTE:** Notice that the fee for the procedure is put in automatically.
11. Click "Close"

How to Print a Paper CMS-1500 Claim Form

1. Click ACTIVITIES and choose "Transaction Entry" from the drop-down menu, or click on the "Billing" icon.
2. Click on the magnifying glass in the "Patient" box and select a patient from the list. Click OK.
3. Click on the magnifying glass in the "Bill No." box and choose the date of service for the claim you want to print. Click OK.

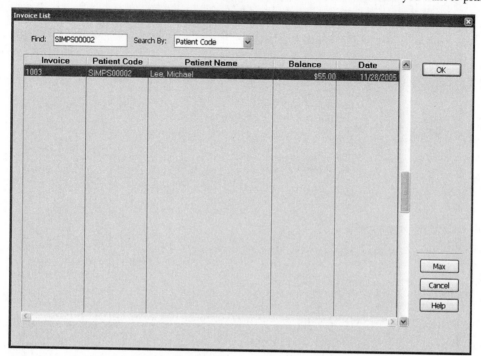

4. Tab down to the transactions and click the "Print" button on the bottom of the screen.
(**NOTE:** Before attempting to print, make sure the "Bill Insurance" box is checked.)

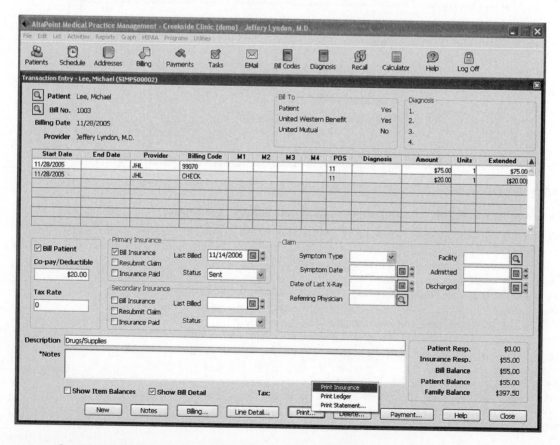

5. Choose "Print insurance" from the drop-down menu.
6. In the "Claim Format" field, choose "CMS1500". (**NOTE:** If CMS1500 does not appear on the list, enter CMS1500 into the Find box and search for it.) Be sure the "Claim Type" field is "Medical Paper."
7. You may preview the claim before or instead of printing it by clicking on the preview button at the bottom of the window.
8. Click "Print" to print the claim on paper.

Helpful Hints When Printing a Paper CMS-1500 Claim Form

You can reprint claims once they have been generated.

In the "Print Insurance Claims" screen, go to [Print Options] and click on the down arrow. From there, choose "Reprint All Claims."

6. The Electronic Claim

An electronic claim is essentially a text file (filename.txt) that is sent to the clearinghouse. So, when an electronic claim is generated, the file must be saved in a directory that will subsequently be sent to the clearinghouse. Think of writing a document in Microsoft Word. The document is then saved to a specific directory in order to be easily accessed later.

How to Transmit a Claim Electronically

1. Click ACTIVITIES and choose "Electronic Claims" from the drop-down menu and select "Create Electronic Claims".
2. ETT should appear in the "Claim Format" box. "Medical Electronic" should appear in the "Claim Type" box. "All Insurance" should appear in the "Insurance to print" box. "Print Pending Only" should appear in the "Print Options" box.
3. Enter the beginning and ending dates for the claims you want to send.

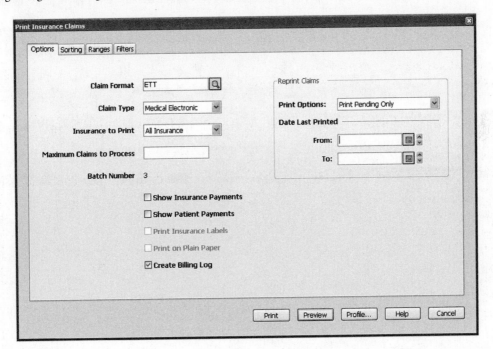

4. Click "Print".
5. In the "Print to File" window, change the file name to "New Folder". Click OK.

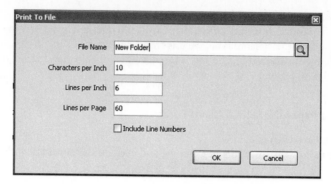

6. If you are trying to send claims more than once, a window will open that says "New Folder already exits" Click on "Replace File".
7. A window will open that says "Report successfully printed to file". Click OK.
8. A window will open that says "Update processed claims as having been sent?" Click yes.

Posting Payments

How to Post Payments from an EOB or Other Source to a Patient's Account

1. Click ACTIVITIES and choose "Transaction Entry" from the drop-down menu, or click on the "Billing" icon.
2. Click the magnifying glass in the "Patient" box and select a patient from the list. Click OK.
3. Click on the magnifying glass in the "Bill No." box and choose the date of service for the payment you are applying.
4. Tab down to the transactions and click the "Payment" button at the bottom of the screen.
5. Click "Apply to item" if the payment is for a specific procedure or click "Apply to bill" of the payment is on the balance.

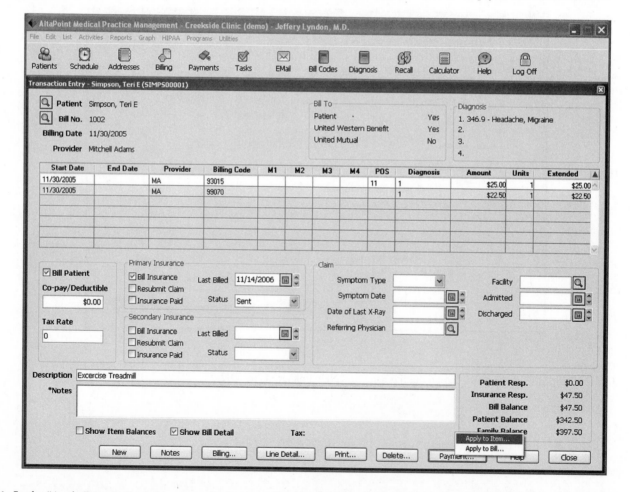

6. In the "Apply Payment" window, enter the amount of the payment in the "Payment Amount" box.
7. Click the magnifying glass in the "Payment Code" box and select the appropriate form of payment from the list. Click OK.